C000173994

SAFETY AS WE WATCH:
Anaesthesia in Ireland 1847–1998

Declan Warde
Joseph Tracey
John Cahill

Eastwood—Dublin

First published by Eastwood Books, 2022
Dublin, Ireland

www.eastwoodbooks.com
www.wordwellbooks.com
@eastwoodbooks

First Edition

Eastwood Books is an imprint of the Wordwell Group

Eastwood Books
The Wordwell Group
Unit 9, 78 Furze Road
Sandyford
Dublin, Ireland

© College of Anaesthesiologists of Ireland

ISBN: 978-1-913934-23-1

Back cover illustration: Facade of 22 Merrion Square, Dublin. Watercolour by Eugene Ward.

British Library Cataloguing in Publication Data.
A catalogue record for this book is available from the British Library.

Typeset in Sabon by Wordwell Ltd.

Copy-editor: Heidi Houlihan

Cover design and artwork: Ronan Colgan

Printed by: Gráficas Castuera, Spain

Contents

Appendices

Foreword

The holy grail of anaesthesia is painless surgery and the consequent reduction in human suffering. Prior to the introduction of anaesthesia in the 1840s, surgery was accompanied by great suffering and distress. This is exemplified by the first-hand account of the English novelist Frances (Fanny) Burney who underwent a mastectomy in France in 1811 under the experienced hands of no less than two senior surgeons, Dominique Jean Larrey, surgeon-in-chief to the Imperial Army, and Antoine Dubois, surgeon to Napoleon himself. She wrote:

> Yet – when the dreadful steel was plunged into the breast – cutting through veins, arteries – flesh – nerves – I needed no injunctions not to restrain my cries. I began a scream that lasted unremittingly during the whole time of the incision – and I almost marvel that it rings not in my Ears still! so excruciating was the agony.

Prior to the 1840s, the surgeon had been reliant on alcohol, opiates, mesmerism and restraint to facilitate surgical interventions. Given the unbearable pain suffered by the patient, speed was of the essence. During the Napoleonic period, time to complete surgical amputation (the most common battlefield surgical intervention) was measured in minutes. Dominique Jean Larrey himself was a believer in early and fast amputation. We are told that, on one occasion, he performed 200 amputations in a 24 hour period during the Battle of Borodino.

William Morton is widely credited with the first successful public demonstration of the use of ether anaesthesia some 30 years later on 16 October 1846 at the Massachusetts General Hospital in Boston. In our world of instant connectivity, it is difficult to conceive nineteenth-century timescales for the dissemination of new knowledge but Ireland's first successful administration of ether was by John MacDonnell, surgeon to the Richmond Hospital, Dublin, on 1 January 1847, around three months after Morton's successful demonstration. MacDonnell anaesthetised an 18 year-old girl named Mary Kane from Drogheda who had developed unresolving suppurative arthritis. Her upper limb amputation was undoubtedly life-saving. She woke up at the end of surgery and recorded feeling no pain. Today, we are the direct professional descendants of both Morton and MacDonnell.

As a former president of the College of Anaesthesiologists of Ireland, it is both a pleasure and honour to be asked to write the foreword of this book. Whilst the conception of this history of our college and of our specialty predated my presidency, its gestation was a constant theme throughout my term of office. Drs Declan Warde, Joseph Tracey and John Cahill of the College of Anaesthesiologists of Ireland Heritage Group were tasked with its writing.

The book details the early years of our specialty including the formation of the Association of Anaesthetists of Great Britain and Ireland in 1932, the establishment of the conjoint Diploma in Anaesthetics (RCPI and RCSI) in 1942, the founding of the Faculty of Anaesthetists, RCSI in 1960 and ultimately the foundation of the College of Anaesthetists of Ireland in 1998. Perhaps more importantly, it brings to life the voices, personalities and stories of those who went before us and in whose footsteps we follow. The title references our college motto and underlines our commitment, as a specialty and a postgraduate training body, to patient safety.

The authors have worked tirelessly over many years in the pursuit of truth and authenticity. We are indebted to them for their tireless commitment, scientific rigor and their passion to record the history of those who have gone before us. While there are three authors, what emerges from the pages before you is one common voice, and I have no doubt it will prove to be the reference source for future generations of anaesthesiologists and researchers.

We owe a debt of gratitude to those who have gone before and this book is a visible link to that past; it not only informs our present but also shapes our future. We write not only for today but for our tomorrows. Enjoy the book.

Dr Brian Kinirons
President,
College of Anaesthesiologists of Ireland 2018–2021

Preface

The year 2022 marks the 175th anniversary of the first use of anaesthesia for painless surgery in Ireland and seems an appropriate one for the publication of a book on the history of the specialty in this country. The project was initiated in December 2016 when Dr Kevin Carson, the president of the College of Anaesthetists of Ireland (CAI), asked us to collaborate in writing the 'story' of Irish anaesthesia. While each of us has had a longstanding interest in medical history, we had never previously considered embarking upon such an ambitious undertaking. However, we soon agreed to accept Kevin's 'invitation' and, in spring 2017, began the work which has culminated five years later in the publication of this book.

We were given complete discretion about how to approach our subject and decided to focus almost entirely on the period of a little over 150 years between 1 January 1847, the date on which the first general anaesthetic was administered in Ireland, and 23 September 1998, the foundation date of the college. Our aim was to produce an all-Ireland history of the specialty and its institutions. We utilised many different resources: books, medical journals and newspapers from the nineteenth and early twentieth century, proceedings and minute books of the various organisations related/linked to the specialty and, invaluably, the personal recollections of a number of our anaesthetic colleagues. The Covid-19 pandemic had a significant effect on our activities as all of the archives and academic libraries that we used were closed for long periods from 2020–22 and this inevitably led to some delay in the book's publication.

Much of the subject matter uncovered during our research fell naturally into two parts. The first section of our book tells the story of the development of the specialty in this country from the first use of ether and chloroform in 1847, through the early anaesthetic appointments towards the end of the nineteenth century, and ends in the early 1940s, by which time the use of both intravenous and regional anaesthetic techniques was well-established. The second part describes the foundation and development of professional bodies such as the Faculty of Anaesthetists of the Royal College of Surgeons in Ireland, the introduction of specialty examinations and the initiation of formal training programmes. This section also covers related groups such as the South of Ireland Society (later Association) of Anaesthetists as well as the development of academic departments and intensive care. We considered it appropriate to include a chapter on the history of 22 Merrion Square, Dublin – the current home of the College of Anaesthesiologists of Ireland.

We had not initially intended to focus on individuals but, during our research, we came to more fully appreciate the significant contribution made by a number of Irish men and women to the development and practice of anaesthesia, both at home and abroad. We considered it appropriate therefore to include a third section consisting of brief biographical sketches in order to bring to life the people behind the names and to highlight their achievements. These included historical figures, the faculty deans, academic figures and others who made noteworthy contributions to anaesthesia. Our 'cut-off' year was 1998; we did not include those who were elected to high office, such as the presidency of CAI, or were appointed to professorial posts after that time.

Working together to write this book has been an exciting and rewarding experience for us. While we have attempted to do so, we are conscious of the fact that we have probably not included every topic that might be considered by some to be worthy of our attention or each individual who contributed to the development of anaesthesia in Ireland over its first 150 years or so. We regret any such 'sins of omission' and hope that the end-result of our efforts will nonetheless be of interest to our readers.

Declan Warde
Joseph Tracey
John Cahill
May 2022

Acknowledgements

We are deeply indebted to the many people who have assisted us in bringing this publication to fruition.

We would especially like to thank Kevin Carson, past-president of the College of Anaesthesiologists of Ireland (CAI), whose idea it was to commission a book of this nature. His successor as president, Brian Kinirons, enthusiastically supported and encouraged us at all times and kindly offered to write the foreword. The current holder of the office, George Shorten, deftly guided the authors through the final stages to publication. We have been ably supported at all times by CAI staff Martin McCormack, Margaret Jenkinson, Rebecca Cornally, Laura Beston and Rebecca Williams, and we thank Denise Johnston in particular for organising and chairing most of the meetings that took place from the time the book was first proposed. It was also Denise who suggested the book title 'Safety as We Watch' to us; it is an English translation of the Latin motto 'Salus dum Vigilamus' on the college coat of arms.

No words can adequately express the debt of gratitude that we owe Harriet Wheelock, Keeper of Collections at the Royal College of Physicians of Ireland. We relied to a great extent, both prior to and during the Covid-19 pandemic, on her assistance in accessing archival material held in the college; she was unfailingly courteous and efficient in responding to our hundreds of requests. Harriet was also involved in and contributed positively to our early discussions on the writing and publication process. We are very grateful to a number of staff members at the Royal College of Surgeons in Ireland (RCSI) including Susan Leyden (Archivist), Ronan Kelly, Carol Creavin, Sarah Timmins, Leanne Harrington and especially Mary O'Doherty, Emeritus Heritage Librarian, who did her utmost to provide documents during the restrictions imposed as a result of the pandemic.

Colum O'Riordan, Chief Executive Officer, and Simon Lincoln of the Irish Architectural Archive supplied much information on 22 Merrion Square, Dublin, the college's home. We appreciate the help provided by Helen Madden (Archivist, Mater Misericordiae University Hospital, Dublin); Clare Foley (Archivist, Blackrock College, Dublin); Mark Gormley (Honorary Archivist, Mater Infirmorum Hospital, Belfast); Timmy O'Connor (University Archivist), Emer Twomey (Archivist, Special Collections and Archives) and Elaine Harrington (Special Collections Librarian) at University College Cork; Caroline Hamson

(Heritage Manager) and Felicia El Kholi (Heritage Assistant) at the Anaesthesia Heritage Centre of the Association of Anaesthetists, London; Holly Peel (Image Services Manager, Wellcome Collection, London); Francesca Charlton-Jones (Sotheby's, London); Helen Theresa Moore (Office Manager, Royal Academy of Medicine in Ireland); Jennifer Warren (Assistant to the Editor, *Irish Medical Journal*); and Barbara Walsh (Secretary, Department of Anaesthesia, University Hospital Galway). In addition, we were assisted by the staff of the National Library of Ireland, the National Archives of Ireland, Dublin City Library and Archive, the Manuscripts and Archives Research Library in Trinity College Dublin, the Public Record Office of Northern Ireland and the General Register Office (Northern Ireland).

Our medical colleagues Pradipta Bhakta, William Blunnie, P.J. Breen, John Cooper, Bob Darling, Howard Fee, Gerry Fitzpatrick, Noel Flynn, Jim Gardiner, Dominic Harmon, Mary Horgan, Brendan Kelly, Peter Kenefick, Andrew Kennedy, Leo Kevin, Ron Kirkham, John Loughrey, Róisín MacSullivan, John McAdoo, Carlos McDowell, Frances Maguire, Rodney Meeke, Denis Moriarty, Patrick Mullin, Brian O'Brien, Rory O'Brien, John O'Dea, Dermot Phelan, Michael Power and Ken Walsh either supplied information which would not otherwise have become known to us or helped in other ways. We were fortunate to have enthusiastic assistance from relatives, friends and indeed 'friends of family' of a number of anaesthetists whose names appear in the following pages – we would particularly like to thank Rosemary Black, Kyleen Clarke, Veronique Coleman, Maurice Delaney, Richard Delaney, Jody Fanagan, Una Flanagan, Sarah Kelly, Nora Lehane, Lynette McCullough, Helen Moore, Oliver O'Brien, Tracey Farrell and Maev-Ann Wren for their support.

David Coleman of Bobby Studio, who foraged for many hours in his attic to find photographic negatives from the early years of the Faculty of Anaesthetists, RCSI and provided high quality digital images from textbooks and journals, was ever-patient with our demands. We also received photographs from other sources and these are acknowledged in the accompanying captions. We thank Ronan Colgan and his colleague Nick Maxwell of the Wordwell Group for their expertise, ongoing reassurance and forbearance as the occasion demanded while the cogent guidance of our copy editor Heidi Houlihan has contributed in no small measure to the final version of the text.

It is quite possible that we have failed to mention some who fully deserve acknowledgement. Should this have happened, we offer our sincere apologies to them.

Abbreviations

AAGBI	Asssociation of Anaesthetists of Great Britain and Ireland
ABA	American Board of Anesthesiology
A.C.E.	Alcohol-chloroform-ether
ACGME	Accreditation Council for Graduate Medical Education
AGM	Annual General Meeting
APAGBI	Association of Paediatric Anaesthetists of Great Britain and Ireland
ASM	Annual Scientific Meeting
ASSERT	Application of Science to Simulation in Education, Research and Technology
ATI	Anaesthetists in Training in Ireland
BA	Bachelor of Arts
BAO	Bachelor of the Art of Obstetrics
Barts	St Bartholomew's Hospital, London
BCh	Bachelor of Surgery
BMA	British Medical Association
BMJ	*British Medical Journal*
BNP	Banque National de Paris
BS	Bachelor of Surgery
BSc	Bachelor of Science
BUPA	British United Provident Association
CAI	College of Anaesthetists of Ireland, later College of Anaesthesiologists of Ireland
CAT	Committee of Anaesthetists in Training of the College of Anaesthesiologists of Ireland
CICM-ANZ	College of Intensive Care Medicine of Australia and New Zealand
CBE	Commander of the Most Excellent Order of the British Empire
CUH	Cork University Hospital
CUS	Catholic University School
DA	Diploma in Anaesthetics
DA (DA, RCP and SEng))	Conjoint Diploma in Anaesthetics of the Royal College of Physicians of London and the Royal College of Surgeons in England
DA (RCP&SI)	Diploma in Anaesthetics of the Conjoint Board of the Royal Colleges of Physicians and Surgeons in Ireland
DABA	Diplomate of the American Board of Anesthesiologists
DIBICM	Diploma of the Irish Board of Intensive Care Medicine
DHSS	Department of Health and Social Security
Dip Med	Diploma in Medical Management
DNA	Deoxyribonucleic acid
DOH	Department of Health
DPH	Diploma in Public Health
DRCOG	Diploma of the Royal College of Obstetricians and Gynaecologists
DSc	Doctor of Science
EBA	European Board of Anaesthesiology
ECG	Electrocardiogram

EMHG	European Malignant Hyperthermia Group
ESICM	European Society of Intensive Care Medicine
FANZCA	Fellow of the Australian and New Zealand College of Anaesthetists
FARACS	Faculty of Anaesthetists of the Royal Australasian College of Surgeons
FCICICM (ANZ)	Fellow of the College of Intensive Care Medicine of Australia and New Zealand
FCMSA	Fellow of the Colleges of Medicine of South Africa
FCPS (Malaysia)	Fellow of the College of Physicians and Surgeons (Malaysia)
FFARCS	Fellow of the Faculty of Anaesthetists of the Royal College of Anaesthetists
FFARCSI	Fellow of the Faculty of Anaesthetists of the Royal College of Surgeons in Ireland
FRCA	Fellow of the Royal College of Anaesthetists
FRCOG	Fellow of the Royal College of Obstetricians and Gynaecologists
FRCP	Fellow of the Royal College of Physicians (London)
FRCP(C)	Fellow of the Royal College of Physicians of Canada
FRCPI	Fellow of the Royal College of Physicians of Ireland
FRCSI	Fellow of the Royal College of Surgeons in Ireland
FFPMCAI	Fellow of the Faculty of Pain Medicine of the College of Anaesthetists of Ireland
GAA	Gaelic Athletic Association
GAT	Group of Anaesthetists in Training of the Association of Anaesthetists of Great Britain and Ireland
GPI	Glucose phosphate isomerase
Hon	Honorary
IACCN	Irish Association of Critical Care Nurses
ICCTG	Irish Critical Care Trials Group
IBICM	Irish Board of Intensive Care Medicine
ICPSA	Irish Clay Pidgeon Shooting Association
ICS	Intensive Care Society
ICSI	Intensive Care Society of Ireland
ICU	Intensive Care Unit
IDEALS	International Disaster & Emergency Aid with Long Term Support
IHCA	Irish Hospital Consultants Association
IJMS	*Irish Journal of Medical Science*
IMA	Irish Medical Association
IMC	Irish Medical Council
IMO	Irish Medical Organisation
IRFU	Irish Rugby Football Union
JAG	Junior Anaesthetists Group of the Association of Anaesthetists of Great Britain and Ireland
JFICMI	Joint Faculty of Intensive Care Medicine of Ireland
JICPS	*Journal of the Irish Colleges of Physicians and Surgeons*
JP	Justice of the Peace
KQCPI	King and Queen's College of Physicians of Ireland
LAH	Licentiate of the Apothecaries Hall, Dublin

LDS	Licentiate in Dental Surgery
LLD	Doctor of Laws
LRCPI	Licentiate of the Royal College of Physicians of Ireland
LRCP & SI	Licentiate of the Royal College of Physicians of Ireland and the Royal College of Surgeons in Ireland
LRCSI	Licentiate of the Royal College of Surgeons in Ireland
MA	Master of Arts, also Massachusetts
MAC	Medical Advisory Committee of the Faculty of Anaesthetists, Royal College of Surgeons in Ireland
MB	Bachelor of Medicine
MBE	Member of the Order of the British Empire
MCQs	Multiple Choice Questions
MD	Doctor of Medicine
MH	Malignant Hyperthermia
MHS	Malignant Hyperthermia Susceptibility
MICAS	Mobile Intensive Care Ambulance Service
MKQCPI	Member of the King and Queen's College of Physicians of Ireland
MMed (Anaesth)	Master of Medicine in Anaesthesiology
MP	Member of Parliament
MRCPI	Member of the Royal College of Physicians of Ireland
MRCS	Member of the Royal College of Surgeons
MSc	Master of Science
NCBI	National Council of the Blind of Ireland
NCHD	Non-Consultant Hospital Doctor
NISA	Northern Ireland Society of Anaesthetists
NUI	National University of Ireland
NUIG	National University of Ireland, Galway (**provisional**)
OAA	Obstetric Anaesthetists Association
OBE	Officer of the Order of the British Empire
OSCE	Objective Structured Clinical Examination
PACT	Patient-centred Acute Care Training
PAYE	Pay As You Earn
PBC	Presentation Brothers College, Cork
PhD	Doctor of Philosophy
PRSI	Pay Related Social Insurance
QUB	Queen's University Belfast
RAMI	Royal Academy of Medicine in Ireland
RCoA	Royal College of Anaesthetists
RCP&SI	Royal College of Physicians of Ireland and Royal College of Surgeons in Ireland
RCPI	Royal College of Physicians of Ireland
RCS	Royal College of Surgeons of England
RCSI	Royal College of Surgeons in Ireland
RDS	Royal Dublin Society
RSM	Royal Society of Medicine
RVH	Royal Victoria Hospital, Belfast

SASWR	Society of Anaesthetists of the South West Region
SAW	Society of Anaesthetists of Wales
SFAR	Societé Française d'Anesthésie et de Réanimation
SFAAR	La Société Française d'Anesthésie et d'Analgésie et d'Réanimation
SHO	Senior House Officer
SIAA	South of Ireland Association of Anaesthetists
SMHS	Shri Maharaja Hari Singh
SpR	Specialist Registrar
SR	Senior Registrar
TCD	Trinity College Dublin
TD	Teachta Dála
UCC	University College Cork
UCD	University College Dublin
UCG	University College Galway
UCH	University College Hospital
UEMS	European Union of Medical Specialists
UWI	University of the West Indies
VAD	Voluntary Aid Detachment
VHI	Voluntary Health Insurance Board
WFSA	World Federation of Societies of Anaesthesiologists
WFSICCM	World Federation of Societies of Intensive and Critical Care Medicine

The authors

Declan Warde is a 1973 medical graduate of University College Dublin (UCD). After postgraduate training in Ireland and Canada, he was appointed Consultant Paediatric Anaesthetist at the Children's University Hospital, Temple Street, Dublin in 1986 and later represented Ireland for many years on the Executive Committee of the Association of Paediatric Anaesthetists of Great Britain and Ireland. His interest in anaesthesia history began during his training; he speaks and writes regularly on the subject and is an active member of both the History of Anaesthesia Society (UK) and the Anesthesia History Association (USA). In retirement he enjoys time with his grandchildren, playing bad golf and supporting the Republic of Ireland and Wolverhampton Wanderers football teams.

Joseph Tracey qualified in medicine from UCD in 1974 and did his postgraduate training in anaesthesia in Dublin, Montreal and Boston before returning to Ireland as consultant anaesthetist in 1985 at Jervis Street/Beaumont Hospital. He was director of the National Poisons Information Centre at that hospital for twenty five years. He was actively involved with the Faculty/College of Anaesthetists throughout his career as an examiner, council member and vice-president and was honoured to receive the Gilmartin Medal in 2015. He retired from clinical practice in 2010. He enjoys swimming, fly-fishing, rugby and French and having time with his grandchildren.

John Cahill graduated MB BCh BAO from UCD in 1975. Following anaesthesia training in Bradford and Leeds, West Yorkshire and in Dublin on the National Senor Registrar Rotation, he was appointed consultant anaesthetist at the Mercy Hospital Cork in 1984. He was elected to council of the College of Anaesthetists of Ireland and acted as chairman of the National Training Committee. He also served as vice president of the Association of Anaesthetists of Great Britain and Ireland and as chairman of its International Relations Committee. Retired from clinical practice since 2012, he is a keen (but not very successful) gardener and enjoys spending time with family and friends.

This book is dedicated to Joyce, Marie and Anne.

PART I

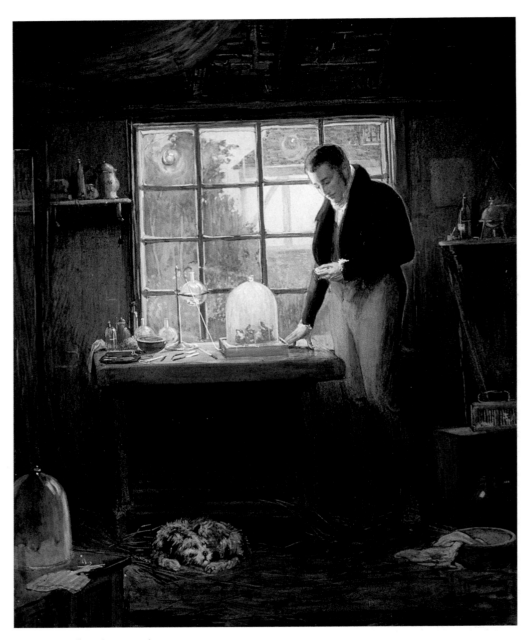

Dr Henry Hill Hickman performing
experiments on suspended animation.
Watercolour by Richard Tennant Cooper.
Wellcome Collection.

Chapter 1

Setting the Stage
Declan Warde

Attempts over the centuries to alleviate the pain of surgical operations often involved the use of alcohol, herbal mixtures containing opium alkaloids or hypnotism.[1] The discovery of the gases oxygen, carbon dioxide and nitrous oxide during the second half of the eighteenth century led to exploration of their therapeutic possibilities and ultimately, a more scientific approach to the quest for painless surgery.

Sir Humphry Davy (1778–1829), born in Penzance, Cornwall was one of the early investigators of nitrous oxide. At the age of just 21 years, while working in Thomas Beddoes' Pneumatic Institution in Bristol, he published his 580-page treatise *Researches Chemical and Philosophical, Chiefly Concerning Nitrous Oxide or Dephlogisticated Nitrous air, and its Respiration*, which contained the following sentence: 'As nitrous oxide in its extensive operation appears capable of destroying physical pain, it may probably be used with advantage during surgical operations in which no great effusion of blood takes place'.[2] This appears to have been the first suggestion that any inhaled agent might successfully relieve the pain of surgery. The young man's proposition received scant attention at the time.

In 1823, **Henry Hill Hickman (1800–1830)**, a physician in Ludlow, Shropshire, used partial asphyxiation by carbon dioxide in a number of small animals to induce what he termed suspended animation and found that he

RESEARCHES,

CHEMICAL AND PHILOSOPHICAL;

CHIEFLY CONCERNING

NITROUS OXIDE,

OR

DEPHLOGISTICATED NITROUS AIR,

AND ITS

RESPIRATION.

By HUMPHRY DAVY,
SUPERINTENDENT OF THE MEDICAL PNEUMATIC INSTITUTION.

LONDON:
PRINTED FOR J. JOHNSON, ST. PAUL'S CHURCH-YARD.
BY BIGGS AND COTTLE, BRISTOL.
1800.

Title page of Humphry Davy's treatise, 1800.

could operate on them without there being any evidence that they were experiencing pain.[3] Despite considerable effort on his part, which included bringing his research to the attention of both Humphry Davy and King Charles X of France, his work was also ignored. It was to be over 100 years before carbon dioxide was proven to have anaesthetic properties.[4]

The first use of inhalational anaesthesia on record took place in Rochester, New York in January 1842 when **William Clarke (1819–1898)**, medical student, administered ether from a towel to a Miss Hobbie, following which a dentist, Elijah Pope, painlessly extracted one of her teeth.[5] Clarke's tutor told him that the entire incident could be explained as the hysterical reaction of women to pain. At his suggestion, the young student refrained from carrying out any further experiments with ether.

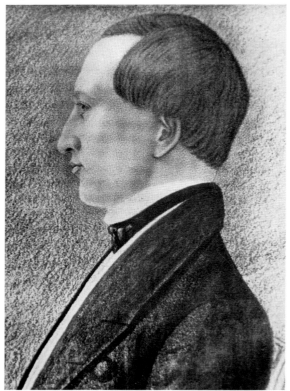

Dr Crawford Williamson Long, aged 26 years. Crayon portrait, drawn by an unknown artist some weeks after Long had administered ether to James Venable.

Crawford Williamson Long (1815–1878), a rural physician working in Jefferson, Georgia, USA, whose paternal grandparents Samuel Long and Ann Williamson had emigrated from Counties Donegal and Tyrone to North America in the mid-eighteenth century, is believed to have been the first to use general anaesthesia in a patient undergoing surgery.[6] On 30 March 1842, Long administered sulphuric ether by inhalation to a friend of his, James Venable, to relieve the pain of excision of a neck tumour and between that date and January 1845, he carried out surgery on at least five further occasions on patients who had inhaled ether beforehand.[7] Long did not publish his work until December 1849, with the result that his efforts went largely unnoticed at the time.[8]

Gardner Quincy Colton (1814–1898), a former medical student, was one of a number of itinerant lecturers who exhibited the effects of nitrous oxide or 'laughing gas' as public entertainment in the early 1840s. One such display, held in Hartford, Connecticut on 10 December 1844, was attended by a local dentist, **Horace Wells (1815–1848)**.[9] During the show, Wells noticed that one of the participants appeared to feel no pain when he gashed his leg while under the influence of nitrous oxide. He spoke with Colton regarding the possibility that the gas might be usefully employed to prevent pain during dental extraction. The following day, Wells had one of his own teeth painlessly removed by his associate John Riggs after inhaling nitrous oxide administered by Colton. Having used the gas successfully

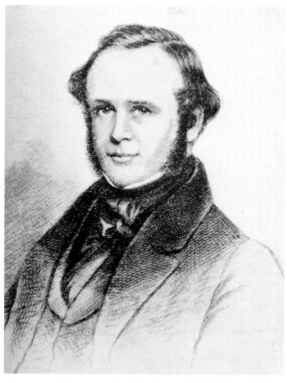

Horace Wells. Engraving by H.B. Hall, from a portrait by James McManus.

on a number of his patients over the next few weeks, he travelled to Boston, Massachusetts in mid-January 1845 in order to demonstrate its efficacy. He sought out **William Thomas Green Morton (1819–1868)**, a fellow dentist and his former student and business partner, who introduced him to a number of Boston doctors. Towards the end of the month, probably in a public hall in the city, Wells administered nitrous oxide to a volunteer medical student about to undergo a dental extraction. The student cried out during the procedure and appeared to be in pain. Most of the observers present considered the demonstration to have been a failure; dejected and disheartened, Wells returned to Hartford the following day.[10] The further development of nitrous oxide anaesthesia was delayed until Colton reintroduced the agent into dentistry in the early 1860s.[9]

Morton was among those who witnessed Wells' failed effort. He tried intoxicants, opium and mesmerism in his own dental practice when endeavouring to alleviate pain. He then attempted to safely induce unconsciousness in goldfish, his pet spaniel, worms, two dental assistants (Thomas Spear and William Leavitt) and himself using ether; the results were inconclusive. He next conferred with **Charles T. Jackson (1805–1880)**, a physician, chemist and geologist. Jackson

5

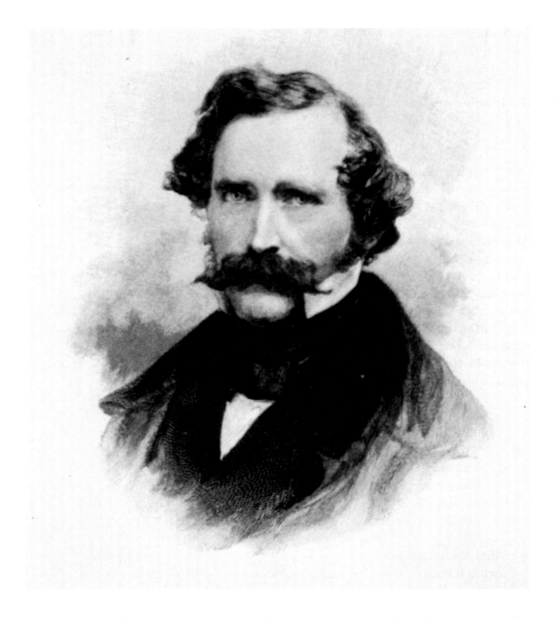

recommended that Morton try pure sulphuric ether rather than the commercially available product. The dentist first used the refined version for dental extraction on Ebenezer Frost on 30 September 1846. On 16 October of the same year, he conducted the first successful *public* demonstration of the agent's ability to prevent surgical pain in what later became known as the Ether Dome at the

Massachusetts General Hospital in Boston.[11-14] News of this momentous event was soon to spread throughout the world and such was its significance that 16 October is, to this day, known as Ether Day or World Anaesthesia Day.

The earliest reference to Morton's demonstration to appear in any Irish publication, lay or medical, was contained in the 22 December edition of *The Belfast News-Letter*:

> An American physician states that he has discovered a mode of producing insensibility to pain, during surgical and dental operations. He affects this by causing his patients to inhale a prepared ether, of which he has not yet revealed the ingredients.

The two sentences appeared in the 'Miscellaneous' column; there was no accompanying attribution as regards the source of this information.

Less than a week later, on 28 December 1846, readers of the Dublin newspaper *Saunders' News-Letter* were made aware of the possibility of painless surgery by a partial reprint of an article titled 'Operations Without Pain', originally published in *The Medical Times*, a London publication, two days earlier.[15] It referred to two operations carried out on 21 December by the surgeon **Robert Liston (1794–1847)** in University College Hospital, London on patients who were under the influence of inhaled ether:

> We have been informed that two operations were performed by Mr Liston at the University College Hospital ... while the patients were under the stupefying influence of vapour of ether. The one was amputation of the leg, the other avulsion of the nail of the great toe ... Neither of the patients knew, when they had recovered from their stupor, that the operation had been performed.

The first such 'operation without pain' in Ireland would take place within the following few days.

References

1   Wildsmith J.A.W., *The History of Anaesthesia*, available at rcoa.ac.uk/about-college/heritage/history-anaesthesia (accessed 5 October 2020).

2   Davy H., *Researches Chemical and Philosophical, Chiefly Concerning Nitrous Oxide, or Dephlogisticated Nitrous Air, and its Respiration*, London: Johnson, 1800, p. 556.

3   Duncum B.M., *The Development of Inhalation Anaesthesia*, London: Oxford University Press, 1947, pp. 77–89.

4 Leake C.D. and Waters R.M., 'The anesthetic value of carbon dioxide', *Journal of Pharmacology and Experimental Therapeutics*, 1928, 33, pp. 280–1.

5 Lyman H.M., *Artificial Anæsthesia and Anæsthetics*, New York: Wood, 1881, p. 6.

6 *Ibid.*, p. 5.

7 Sims J.M., 'The discovery of anæsthesia', *Virginia Medical Monthly*, 1877, 4, pp. 81–99.

8 Long C.W., 'An account of the first use of sulphuric ether by inhalation as an anæsthetic in surgical operations', *Southern Medical and Surgical Journal*, 1849, 5, pp. 705–13.

9 Smith G.B. and Hirsch N.P., 'Gardner Quincy Colton: Pioneer of nitrous oxide anesthesia', *Anesthesia and Analgesia*, 1991, 72, pp. 382–91.

10 Haridas R.P., 'Horace Wells' demonstration of nitrous oxide in Boston', *Anesthesiology*, 2013, 19, pp. 1014–22.

11 Maltby J.R., 'The Ether Dome: William Thomas Green Morton (1819–1868)' in J.R. Maltby (ed.), *Notable Names in Anaesthesia*, London: Royal Society of Medicine Press, 2002, pp. 147–50.

12 Keys T.E., *The History of Surgical Anesthesia*, New York: Schuman's, 1945, pp. 26–7.

13 LeVasseur R. and Desai S.P., 'Ebenezer Hopkins Frost (1824–1866): William T.G. Morton's first identified patient and why he was invited to the ether demonstration of October 16 1846', *Anesthesiology*, 2012, 117, pp. 238–42.

14 Bigelow H.J., 'Insensibility during surgical operations produced by inhalation', *Boston Medical and Surgical Journal*, 1846, 35, pp. 309–17.

15 'Operations without pain', *Medical Times*, 1846, 15, p. 251.

Chapter 2

The First Use of Ether for Surgery in Ireland

Joseph Tracey

I regard this discovery as one of the most important of the century. It will rank with vaccination and other of the greatest benefits that medical science has bestowed upon man

> *John MacDonnell, 1 January 1847,*
> *on the first anaesthetic in Ireland*

On 16 October 1846 at the Massachusetts General Hospital in Boston, William Thomas Green Morton, a dentist, gave the first public demonstration of the successful use of inhaled ether to relieve the pain of surgery. The patient being operated on was Edward Gilbert Abbott and the surgeon was Prof. John Collins Warren. The operation involved an incision near the lower jaw and although the patient muttered a bit during the procedure, he said afterwards that he had 'felt considerable pain but it was mitigated'.[1]

The author of a case report nowadays would usually be one of the people involved, for example Morton or Warren, but on this occasion, it was one of the observers in the operating theatre that day, Dr Henry Bigelow (1818–1890) who would write the first article on the new discovery. He decided that he would observe the use of ether in other cases over the following few weeks before writing an account. He was reluctant to publish a report on the case (of Gilbert Abbott) until he had seen major surgery performed under ether, in particular, amputation of the leg. He was anxious to see how safe it was and also reluctant to endorse the anaesthetic* agent, as he did not yet know its composition. Morton had not revealed what the chemical was that he had used.[1,2] Because of his concerns, Bigelow waited a few weeks before presenting an abstract of his paper[2,3] to the American Academy of Arts and Science on 3 November. He read the full paper titled 'Insensibility during Surgical Operations produced by Inhalation' a few days later[1], on 9 November 1846, to the Boston Society of Medical Improvement. This was published in *The Boston Medical and Surgical Journal* on 18 November, a full month after the Morton demonstration.[1] The report was reprinted the following day in the newspaper *The Boston Daily Advertiser*. Bigelow began by stating:

> It has long been an important problem in medical science, to devise some method of mitigating the pain of surgical operations. An efficient agent for this purpose has at length been discovered. A patient has been rendered completely insensible during an amputation of the thigh, regaining consciousness after a short interval. Other severe operations have been performed without the knowledge of the patients. So remarkable an occurrence will, it is believed, render the following details relating to the history and character of the process not uninteresting. On the 16th of October 1846, an operation was performed at the hospital, upon a patient who had inhaled a preparation administered by Dr Morton, a dentist of this city, with the alleged intention of producing insensibility to pain. Dr Morton was understood to have extracted teeth under similar circumstances, without the knowledge of the patients. The present operation was performed by Dr. Warren, and though comparatively slight, involved an incision near the lower jaw, of some inches in extent. During the operation the patient muttered, as in a semi-conscious state, and afterwards stated that the pain was considerable, though mitigated; in his own words, as though the skin had been scratched with a hoe.[1]

In the rest of his account, Bigelow mentions failures or partial failures but finishes by making it clear that even at this stage, the anaesthetic was efficient.[3] (The term 'anaesthesia' was first suggested by Oliver Wendell Holmes in a letter to Morton on 21 November 1846.[4])

He then described the apparatus needed:

> It remains briefly to describe the process of inhalation by the new method, and to state some of its effects. A small, two-necked glass globe contains the prepared vapour, together with sponges, to

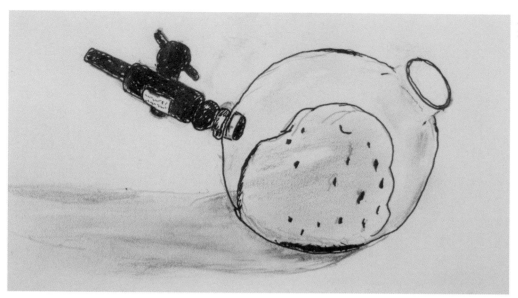

Morton's inhaler.
Sketch by author.

enlarge the evaporating surface. One aperture admits the air to the interior of the globe, whence, charged with vapour, it is drawn through the second into the lungs. The inspired air thus passes through the bottle, but the expiration is diverted by a valve in the mouthpiece, and escaping into the apartment is thus prevented from vitiating the medicated vapour[1]

In 1846, the people of Ireland were experiencing the worst year of the Great Famine which resulted in a million deaths and caused a further million to emigrate. As the famine ships were sailing west to Grosse Isle in Quebec and to Boston, the steamship *Acadia* was travelling east carrying the news of this great new discovery of painless surgery. This was one of the four wooden paddle steamers with which Samuel Cunard had inaugurated his transatlantic steamship service between Britain and North America but it was only available once a month in the wintertime. The steamships were faster and more reliable than sailing ships which could take up to five weeks to make the crossing. The S.S. *Acadia* was a paddle steamer with three masts built by John Wood and Co. of Port Glasgow in 1840; she had an engine capable of doing nine knots and, at one point, held the Blue Riband for the Atlantic having made the crossing from Liverpool to Halifax in 11 days on her maiden voyage.[2]

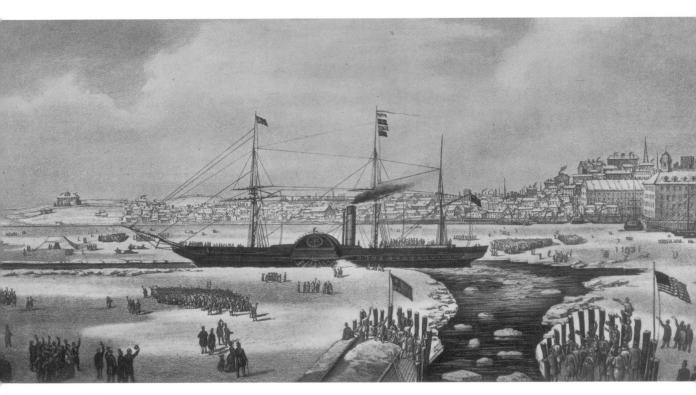

The Cunard steamer Britannia, *sister ship of the SS* Acadia, *leaving Boston bound for Liverpool, February 1844. Reproduced from* Cassier's *Magazine 1893.*

She cleared Boston on Tuesday 1 December and reached Halifax, Nova Scotia on Thursday 3 December, where she refuelled. She finally arrived in Liverpool on 16 December, a full two months after the initial demonstration in Boston.[2] In the mail onboard was a letter from Prof. Jacob Bigelow (the father of Henry Bigelow), dated Boston, 28 November, to his friend and colleague Francis Boott of London telling him the news of ether.[2] Bigelow had waited until the end of November before sending his letter, as he knew that the steamship service was reliable. He also enclosed a copy of *The Boston Daily Advertiser* (dated Thursday 19 November 1846) in which was reprinted Henry Bigelow's paper[2]. He wrote:

> A new anodyne process lately introduced here, which promises to be one of the most important discoveries of the present age. It has rendered many patients insensible to pain during surgical operations and other causes of suffering. Limbs and breasts have been amputated, arteries tied, tumours extirpated, and many

hundreds of teeth extracted, without any consciousness of the least pain on the part of the patient. The inventor is Dr Morton, a dentist of this city, and the process consists of the inhalation of the vapour of ether to the point of intoxication. I send you the *Boston Daily Advertiser*, which contains an article written by my son Henry, and which is extracted from a medical journal, relating to the discovery.[2]

Boott received the letter on 17 December and sent copies of the letter and the article to *The Lancet*. Two days later, on Saturday 19 December, his colleague, the dentist James Robinson, administered ether to a patient for a dental extraction of an infected molar – the first ether anaesthetic given in England. Two days later, on Monday 21 December, the surgeon, Mr Robert Liston, successfully performed a lower limb amputation under ether given by a Mr William Squire at University College Hospital (UCH), London.[5]

John Forbes, the editor of *The British and Foreign Medical Review*, witnessed the operation at UCH. He wrote an editorial in the January edition of the journal, in the final section 'Original reports and memoirs', titled 'On a new means of rendering Surgical operations painless'.[5]

We know nothing more of this new method of eschewing pain than what is contained in the following extracts from two private letters, kindly written to us by our excellent friends, Dr Ware and Dr Warren of Boston. It is impossible however, not to regard the discovery as one of the highest importance. The authors of the discovery are Dr CT Jackson and Dr Morton.

He then reproduced the contents of these two other letters which may also have been brought over to England on the *Acadia*.

Boston November 29th 1846.
It is a mode of rendering patients insensible of the pain of surgical operation by the inhalation of the vapour of the strongest sulphuric ether. They are thrown into a state nearly resembling that of complete intoxication from ardent spirits or of narcotism from opium. The state continues but a few minutes – five to ten – but during it, the patient is insensible to pain. Objections may

13

arise of which we do not dream and evils may be found to follow, which we do not now perceive. It was brought into use by a dentist and is now chiefly employed by that class of practitioner John Ware.

Boston, November 24th 1846.
You may have heard of the respiration of ether to prevent pain in surgical cases. In six cases I have had it applied with satisfactory success and no unpleasant sequela.
I remain yours,
John C Warren.

Forbes then said that he had seen the article published by Dr Bigelow in *The Boston Medical and Surgical Journal* and wrote a detailed account of the cases described including the observed changes in pulse rate as well as changes in pupillary diameter. He continued with an addendum:

Yesterday [i.e. 21 December] we had ourselves the satisfaction of seeing this new mode of cheating pain put into production by a master of chirurgery on our own side of the Atlantic. In the theatre of University College Hospital Mr. Liston amputated the thigh of a man previously narcotised by the inhalation of the ether vapour. He also did a partial removal of an onychia. In these cases the vapour was administered by means of an ingenious apparatus extemporaneously contrived by Mr Squire of Oxford Street. It consisted of the bottom part of a Nooth's apparatus, having a glass funnel filled with a sponge soaked in pure unwashed ether, in the upper orifice and one of Reeds flexible inhaling tubes in the lower. As the ether fell through the neck of the funnel, it became vaporised and the vapour being heavy, descended to the bottom of the vase and was thence inspired through the flexible tube. No heat was applied to the apparatus.[5]

This journal, *The British and Foreign Medical Review*, was usually available to its readers during the last few days of the month before its issue date and thus Mr Edward Hutton, a surgeon at the Richmond Surgical Hospital in Dublin, saw it. He, in turn, showed it to Mr John MacDonnell, one of his colleagues, who read

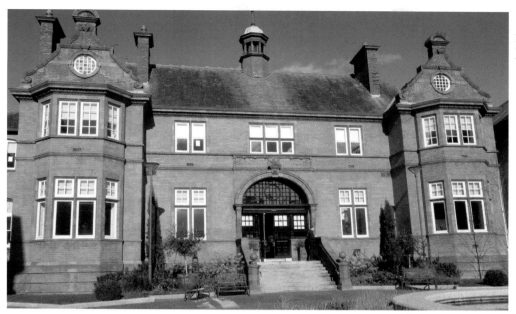

The Richmond Hospital, Dublin. Photograph by the author.

the editorial on Wednesday 30 December.[6] He decided to try it but first wanted to experiment on himself before giving it to a patient, as he wanted to see its effects:

> I procured a bottle with two necks, into one of which I introduced the tube of a funnel, made airtight in the neck of the bottle by adhesive plaster rolled around it – and to the other I adapted a double tube furnished with a Read's ball valve. A sponge being placed in the funnel and saturated with pure sulphuric ether, the apparatus was now fit for use, the only precaution necessary being to maintain the valve-tube perpendicular. – The mouth being applied to the tube, and the nostrils closed, the play of the valves on inspiration opened the communication between the tube and the bottle, and closed that between the tube and the athmosphere, while on expiration, their play closed the communication with the bottle and opened that with the atmosphere. Thus the inspired air necessarily passed through the sponge and bottle and was saturated with the vapour of the ether and the expired air necessarily passed to the atmosphere.[6]

He then proceeded to try it out and inhale ether himself with the assistance of his friend and former pupil, surgeon Alex McDonnell.

> I rendered myself insensible for some seconds, five or six times – and the following observations were made by Mr Mc Donnell on myself. The pupils dilated on every occasion. My pulse rose inconsiderably at the beginning of each inhalation and fell to the natural standard on the approach of insensibility. Its force was not sensibly affected. My complexion was rather raised each time and, on one occasion only, my lips became blue – At the moment of insensibility, I had the feeling of a profound stun, as if from a heavy blow on the head, but without any sense of blow and without pain – Half an hour after my experiments no sensible effects remained.[6]

He had decided to operate on one of his patients, a healthy 18-year-old girl called Mary Kane from near Drogheda who had developed suppurative arthritis of the elbow after getting a thorn in it whilst collecting firewood. The thorn had punctured the arm near the elbow and must have entered the joint. The joint had become inflamed and she had had it treated locally. The treatment had included the application of turpentine, bluestone and some green ointment, which MacDonnell felt had made things worse. Two weeks after the accident, she was referred to the Richmond Hospital. By then she had considerable pain in the elbow and had a large ulcer over the joint with a profuse discharge. A probe could be passed into the joint. Over the following four weeks, she became progressively emaciated, had severe bowel problems and developed a sacral ulcer, as she could only lie supine. On 31 December, MacDonnell decided that she needed an amputation to save her life and that he would perform the operation on the following day.

On Friday morning, 1 January 1847, the anaesthetic was administered but failed on the first attempt. However, they were successful the second time and proceeded with the amputation. (In his report MacDonnell states that 'we succeeded in establishing complete insensibility' so it's not clear who exactly gave the ether.) Mr Carmichael, Dr Adams, Mr Hamilton and Dr Hutton assisted him. Several physicians and the class of the Richmond Hospital witnessed the procedure.

Twice before the dressing of the wound was completed the patient gave evidence of suffering, just at the moment of finishing the division of the muscles and again at the time of tying one of the arteries. Her own evidence is clear and positive, that she had no unpleasant sensation from the inhalation, and that, till, as she says, she 'saw me put a thread on her arm' she felt nothing.[6]

Surgeons Tufnell and Brabazon, who noted her pulse rate and eye signs, monitored the patient throughout the procedure. She was a little tachycardic (a fast heart rate) when she came into the theatre with a pulse-rate of 132 but this settled down to 120 when she inhaled the gas; it decreased further to 102 when surgery commenced but rose again to 144 during sawing of the bone. It then peaked at 160 and dropped to 144 during ligature of the blood vessels. Her pupils

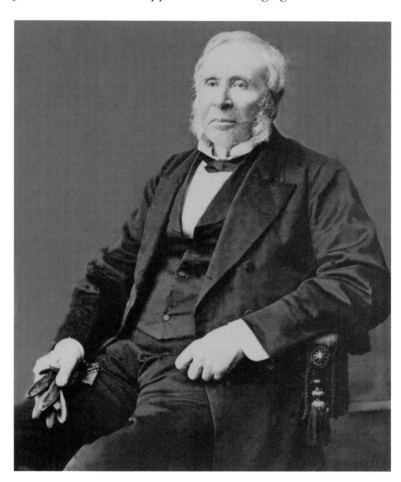

John MacDonnell. Courtesy of the Royal College of Surgeons in Ireland.

17

remained dilated at all times during inhalation of the vapour. As the wound was being closed, the surgeons noted that the muscles were quite relaxed which facilitated the identification of small bleeding arteries. MacDonnell also realised that once the patient started to breathe room air, the anaesthetic started to wear off and he surmised that the vapour could be given for longer periods by allowing intermittent breathing of atmospheric air alternately with the ether vapour.[6]

MacDonnell wrote up his case report over the weekend and pressurised Arthur Jacob, the editor of *The Dublin Medical Press* to delay the print run so that his account could be published in the 6 January issue.[7]

He declared:

> I regard this discovery as one of the most important of the century. It will rank with vaccination and other of the greatest benefits that medical science has bestowed upon man. It adds to the long list of those benefits, and establishes another claim, in favour of that science, upon the respect and gratitude of mankind. It offers an occasion beyond measure more worthy of Te Deums in Christian cathedrals and for thanksgiving to the Author and Giver of all good than all the victories of fire and sword have ever achieved.[6]

In an addendum dated 3 January, he noted that his own patient had made a good recovery from the procedure with no ill effects from the inhalation of the vapour.

References

1   Bigelow H.J., 'Insensibility during surgical operations produced by inhalation', *Boston Medical and Surgical Journal*, 1846, 35, pp. 309–17.

2   Ellis R.H., 'The introduction of ether anaesthesia to Great Britain', *Anaesthesia*, 1976, 31, pp. 766–77.

3   Sykes W.S., *Essays on the First Hundred Years of Anaesthesia*, London: E&S Livingstone Ltd, 1960, p. 60.

4   Haridas R.P., 'The etymology and use of the word "anaesthesia": Oliver Wendell Holmes "letter to W.G. Morton"', *Anaesthesia and Intensive Care*, 2016, 44, p. 40.

5   Forbes J., 'On a New Means of Rendering Surgical Operations Painless', *British and Foreign Medical Review*, 1847, 23, pp. 309–12.

6   MacDonnell J. (letter), 'Amputation of the Arm, Performed at the Richmond Hospital, without Pain' (1847), *Dublin Medical Press*, 17, pp. 8–9.

7   Widdess J.D.H., 'The introduction of ether and chloroform to Dublin', *Irish Journal of Medical Science*, 1946, 21, p. 65.

Chapter 3

The Medical and Lay Press, 1847

Declan Warde

There were both morning and evening editions of *The Pilot*, a Dublin newspaper, published on 1 January 1847. The latter contained a brief report of the momentous event that had taken place in the city earlier that day:

> This day an important operation was performed in the Richmond Hospital – amputation of the arm of a female without the slightest pain, the pain first being rendered insensible by inhaling the vapours of ether. The only sign of sensibility to pain was whilst the operator was tying up the arteries. The patient, on recovery, stated that she had not been sensible to the slightest pain, and had no recollection whatever of the operation.[1]

IMPORTANT OPERATION—AMPUTATION WITHOUT PAIN.

This day (Friday) an important operation was performed in the Richmond Hospital—amputation of the arm of a female without the slightest pain, the patient being first rendered insensible by inhaling the vapours of ether. The only sign of sensibility to pain was whilst the operator was tying up the arteries. The patient, on recovering, stated that she had not been sensible to the slightest pain, and had no recollection whatever of the operation.

Report in The Pilot, *1 January 1847, of the first administration of a general anaesthetic in Ireland.*

The Freeman's Journal and *The Dublin Evening Packet and Correspondent* reprinted this piece on 2 January, a day on which at least six Irish newspapers included a *Medical Times* report of the lower limb amputation carried out in London by Robert Liston on 21 December of the previous year.

A more detailed account of the New Year's Day operation in the Richmond Hospital under the heading 'Triumph of Science' appeared on 5 January in *The Freeman's Journal*. The article ended, 'We cannot conclude our notice of this interesting and constructive case without congratulating Mr MacDonnell on the new triumph this operation adds to an already remarkably successful personal career'.[2]

By the time MacDonnell's letter to the *Dublin Medical Press* was published,[3] the lay press was awash with stories concerning painless surgery, some of which dealt with the subject with less gravitas than might perhaps have been expected in Victorian times. For example, on 6 January, *The Cork Examiner* reprinted the following extract from the *Liverpool Albion*:

> The Lancet and all the medical publications of today are plethoric with disquisitions on the recent discovery of a mode of performing operations without pain, whereby teeth can be extracted and limbs lopped off while the patient is in a state of happy unconsciousness. No doubt the head might be removed in the same way, but there is no instance of such occurrence having taken place, nor indeed would there be any necessity to record it if it had ...[4]

One week later, the *Dublin Medical Press* published a letter dated 1 January from **Thomas Jolliffe Tufnell (1809–1885)**, surgeon to the Dublin Military Prison and the City of Dublin Hospital. He had been present when MacDonnell operated on Mary Kane and described the effects of inhaled ether in four male patients, the first and third of whom underwent dental extractions:

> Dr MacDonnell having kindly lent me his apparatus, I proceeded to try the effects on four different individuals in the presence of Dr Bellingham ... Idiosyncrasy of patient appears to govern effect, I would therefore advise in every case, where practicable that prior to operation, the patient should be placed under the influence of ether to note its effect ... The depression of pulse is

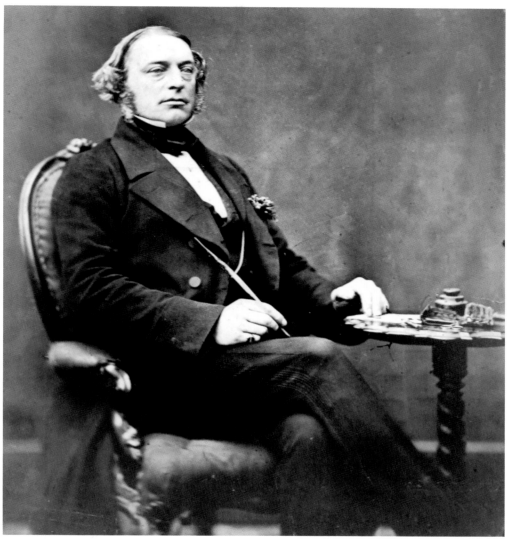

Photograph of the surgeon Thomas Jolliffe Tufnell, who was present when John MacDonnell operated on Mary Kane. Reproduced by kind permission of the Royal College of Physicians of Ireland (MPS/6/1).

evidently owing to reflex action on the heart, which resumes its natural standard on the brain receiving purer blood when the bottle is removed from the mouth.[5]

In the interim, on 9 January, he had spoken concerning the same four anaesthetics at a meeting of the Surgical Society of Ireland. However, the information provided by him there was somewhat at variance with that contained

21

in his letter to the *Dublin Medical Press*. He indicated that the first and third patients were in fact one and the same; in other words, two dental extractions were carried out under separate anaesthetics on the same man. He said that after he had removed the first tooth, six minutes had elapsed since the ether administration and the patient was not completely insensible. He allowed the man to recover, and a short time later anaesthetised him again before removing the second. He remarked, referring to the first anaesthetic, 'This being the first experiment, I was not willing to push it further'. Tufnell stated that two of the patients concerned were dragoons (mounted infantrymen). It is doubtful that they would have been staff members at the prison, and the likelihood is that they were military prisoners.[6]

What was probably the first use of anaesthetic ether on the island of Ireland, outside Dublin, was referred to in a report contained in the *Cork Examiner* of 15 January:

> William Shea, a patient in the North Infirmary, had his great toe removed by Dr Howe, Wednesday, in presence of a number of the most eminent of the faculty of this city, he (the patient) being at the time under the influence of Sulphuric Ether. During this severe operation he did not evince the slightest symptom of pain, and was not conscious of its being performed for fully twenty minutes after the wound was dressed and bandaged.[7]

Dr George Howe had a practice in Bridge Street, Cork and was surgeon to the North Infirmary. He had graduated MD from the University of Edinburgh in 1819 and was also a licentiate of the Royal College of Surgeons in Ireland.

One week later, on 22 January, *The Belfast News-Letter* described ether's use in the management of the victim of an industrial accident in the city:

> The extraordinary discovery of the anodyne properties of the fumes of sulphuric ether … were employed with some success in the Surgical Hospital of this town. On yesterday, it was considered necessary to amputate a young woman's arm in order to save her life, her hand having been shattered a few weeks ago by the machinery in Mr Ewart's factory. The medical attendants succeeded in throwing the patient into a kind of trance, by means of the vapour of sulphuric ether; but owing to the imperfect

apparatus used on this occasion, she could not be made altogether insensible. However the pain she experienced was not acute; and her only intelligence of the operation was when the bone was being sawed through. We understand that the ether will be employed in another case today; and as the apparatus will be made more perfect, every hope of the success of the experiment is confidently entertained.[8]

The newspaper did not provide the names of the medical attendants but it is likely that the ether was administered by Dr Horatio Stewart for surgeon Alexander Gordon who later became the first professor of surgery at Queen's College Belfast.[9]

The *Dublin Medical Press* of 20 January contained an editorial comment to the effect that ether had by then been used in hundreds of operations with no fatal or even alarming result. The writer concluded by remarking, in a clear reference to an attempt that had, by then, been made by William Thomas Green Morton to patent the sulphuric ether preparation used by him as 'Letheon':

An attempt is being made to restrict the use of this agent by patent. We are convinced that this never can be effected except to secure the invention of some particular inhaler. We wish the discoverer may have every legitimate advantage to which he is entitled, but any attempt to monopolize medicinal remedies must be resisted.[10]

The following page of the same issue included an advertisement for an 'Instrument for the Inhalation of Ether' from a Dublin manufacturer.

The instrument, constructed by Mr J. Millikin of Dublin had been exhibited at the 9 January meeting of the Surgical Society of Ireland, and four students in attendance volunteered to try the effects of inhaled ether on themselves. Two of the four could not bring themselves to inhale for sufficiently long to be affected, but the remaining two (Messrs Halahan and Arthur) persevered until brought under the vapour's influence.[11] At the following meeting, held on 23 January, Tufnell read the report of a committee appointed by the council of the society, consisting of MacDonnell, O'Bryen Bellingham (surgeon to St Vincent's Hospital) and himself on the phenomena exhibited two weeks earlier. It included the following recommendations:

TO THE MEDICAL PROFESSION.

GENTLEMEN— I beg to submit to your notice the instrument constructed by me for the Inhalation of Ether, examined and approved of by the Committee appointed by the Council of the College, and exhibited at the Surgical Society, and beg respectfully to refer to Dr. Colles, Dr. Jameson, and Dr. Orr, who severally used it in painless operations in their respective hospitals.

I am, gentlemen, your very obedient servant,

J. MILLIKIN,

Surgical Instrument-maker to the College of Surgeons, 1 St. Andrew-street, Dublin.

1. That when practicable, therefore, a trial should be made prior to operation.
2. That where there is reason to apprehend any derangement of the cerebral circulation or organic disease of the heart, it should be employed with the greatest caution.
3. That the lungs being primarily influenced, and much irritation in the air passages sometimes produced, as evinced by the frequent cough, in persons labouring under diseases of the lungs it might be injurious.
4. That having as yet had no opportunity to conduct experiments in lower animals, it is impossible for your committee to say with what safety or to what extent the inhalation might be carried and the effect reproduced after partial restoration to consciousness.
5. That the operations most fitted for its employment were those where large and painful incisions have to be made as in amputation – cases that can speedily be terminated.[12]

Contributions to the *Dublin Medical Press* came not only from local practitioners, but also from further afield. The issue of 27 January included a letter from James Robinson in London who provided guidance, based on the appearance of the patient, of when, in his opinion, was the proper time to commence operating on those who are under ether's influence:

> Gentlemen, Having now administered the vapour of ether for the purpose of rendering surgical operations painless in a great number of cases ... permit me, if not encroaching too much on your valuable columns, briefly to state the appearance of the patient when under the influence of the vapour, that indicates the proper time for the operation to commence ...

He went on to describe his induction technique and also, for lengthy operations, a method of having the patient inhale atmospheric air and the vapour of ether alternately, at intervals of half a minute.[13]

The first reference to what is now termed ether anaesthesia to appear in *The Dublin Quarterly Journal of Medical Science* (now *The Irish Journal of Medical Science*) was in a detailed account, extending to almost 2,000 words, which appeared in the February 1847 issue and was written by the editor at the time **William Robert Wills Wilde (1815–1876)**. A native of County Roscommon, Wilde graduated in 1837 from the Royal College of Surgeons in Ireland. He became a noted otolaryngologist and ophthalmologist who, apart from his medical writings, was the author of significant works on archaeology and folklore. He edited the Irish census for several decades and made many valuable observations on population and disease. He was father to the poet and playwright Oscar Wilde (1854–1900) and was knighted in 1864, principally for his work in connection with the census.[14]

Wilde wrote that since the publication of the previous issue of the journal, a most important and valuable discovery had been made, namely the use of the vapour of sulphuric ether for the purpose of rendering patients insensible to pain during surgical operations. He continued by referring to Morton's public demonstration of the use of the agent in Boston and the communication of the facts to Great Britain. He also reported that, by the time of writing, ether had been employed with success by a number of Dublin surgeons. He went into some detail concerning the mode of administration and its effects during induction of and recovery from anaesthesia. He specifically stated that inhalation of ether could result in irregular action of the heart and that blood drawn during the state of insensibility was darker than natural. He advised against its use in certain types of surgery, for example operations on the globe of the eye, considering that the

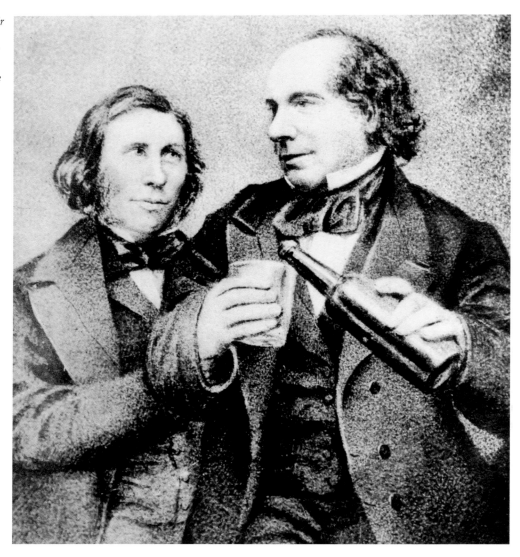

Photograph of Sir William Wilde (on left) relaxing with Dr William Stokes of Cheyne –Stokes respiration and Stokes –Adams attack fame. Reproduced by kind permission of the Royal College of Physicians of Ireland (PDH/6/2/11).

involuntary struggle which often occurs as the effects of the agent wear off might prove very hazardous, perhaps at the most critical moment. He cautioned that it was possible that accidents would occur in the inhalation of ether, and wrote that when they did, 'the present rage for its application may receive a check'. Its ultimate, perhaps persistent, consequences on the constitution had not, in Wilde's opinion, yet been tested, neither had its value in relieving pain and suffering induced by disease.[15]

Reports in the *Dublin Medical Press* during the same month referred to the potential use of ether in order to cause insensibility, particularly in females, for criminal purposes and also, citing a report from France, pointing out the inherent danger of performing operations under candlelight since ether is explosive.

Returning to the lay press, the 12 February 1847 edition of the *Anglo-Celt*, a newspaper primarily concerned with events occurring in County Cavan, contained what can only be assumed to be a fictitious account of the use of inhaled ether by persons other than qualified medical practitioners:

> We understand that the inhalation of ether has been resorted to professionally, by various pork-butchers with great success. The chief difficulty they have experienced has consisted in the opposition of the patient; but when the natural obstinacy of the pig has been overcome, and he has been persuaded to inhale the ether, he has been killed with comfort to himself, and, without disturbance to the neighbourhood.[16]

During March 1847, reports emerged from England of the postoperative deaths of two patients following ether anaesthetics. In the case of the first patient to die, William Herbert, it was the operating surgeon who attributed his patient's demise to the anaesthetic agent. This was despite the fact that Mr Herbert did not expire until 50 hours after the operation (lithotomy) had been completed, the autopsy findings were inconclusive and there was no inquest.[17] The second patient, Ann Parkinson, died 40 hours after surgery. An inquest was held into her death with the jury concluding that:

> the deceased ... died from the effects of the vapour of ether, inhaled by her for the purpose of alleviating pain during the removal of a tumour from her left thigh, and not from the effect of the operation, or from any other cause.[18]

The two deaths were widely reported; the Irish publications in which accounts soon appeared included the *Dublin Medical Press*, *The Freeman's Journal*, and *Derry Journal*. Although there had been no other fatalities attributed to ether, William Wilde wrote in the May edition of the *Dublin Quarterly Journal of Medical Science*:

We regret to say, that our fears with respect to the general employment of this agent, contained in our last Number have, in several instances, been verified. Several deaths, caused either directly or hastened by the inhalation of the vapour of sulphuric ether, have lately been recorded and the journals that were at first loudest in its praise have recently assumed a very cautious tone on the subject.[19]

The fatalities caused the *Medical Times* to ask if 'the great discovery of the age' should be abandoned. It claimed that there had been numerous less serious 'accidents' which had caused 'distrust and suspicion' of the agent in England. While it remained in use for major operations in large medical centres like London and Edinburgh, usage in other places declined. It would be fair to say that its abandonment was, in many instances, because of the practical difficulty of inducing insensibility without struggling or excitement, rather than for safety reasons.[20]

Dr John Snow (1813–1858), soon to be regarded as the foremost anaesthetist of the day and voted 'greatest doctor of all time' by readers of the British publication *Hospital Doctor* in 2003,[21] believed that Mrs Parkinson died from haemorrhage and while he did not express a view as to the precise cause of Mr Herbert's demise, it is clear that he did not accept that ether was responsible.[22] He was supported some years later in his opinions on both deaths by a committee of the Boston Society for Medical Improvement, appointed to investigate reported deaths from ether anaesthesia up to June 1861, which concluded that each occurred as a consequence of 'shock and exhaustion'.[23]

The *Kerry Evening Post* of 30 June 1847 reported the case of a child aged just two years on whom, three days earlier, the surgeon Francis Crumpe (1794 – 1877) had operated for talipes (club foot) at the Kerry County Infirmary in Tralee. It had been more difficult to bring the young patient under ether's influence than had been the case for two adults who had undergone surgery in the infirmary on the same day. The child also took longer than the adults to recover consciousness following the anaesthetic.[24] An extensive English-language literature review has not revealed the existence of any earlier published reports of the administration of general anaesthetics, in Ireland or overseas, to children aged two years or less.

Medical practitioners searched for an alternative to ether which would be both easier to administer and more reliable in its action. In early November 1847, **James Young Simpson (1811–1870)**, professor of midwifery at the University of

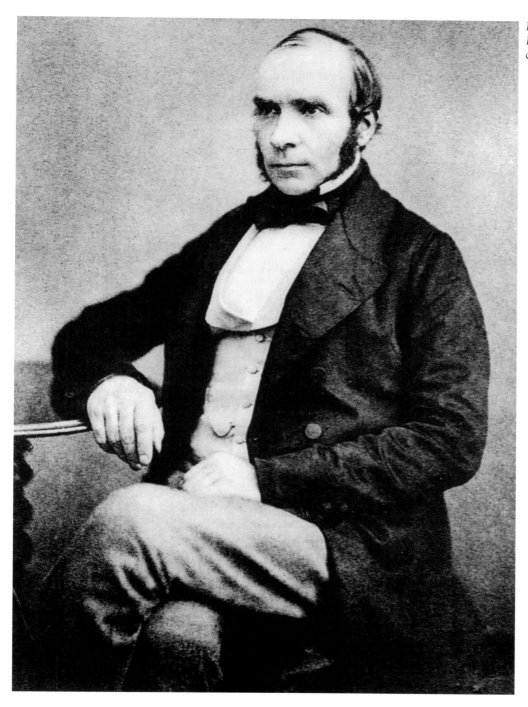

Photograph of Dr John Snow c.1857.

Photograph of Professor Sir James Young Simpson (1811 – 70). Courtesy of NIH Digital Collections.

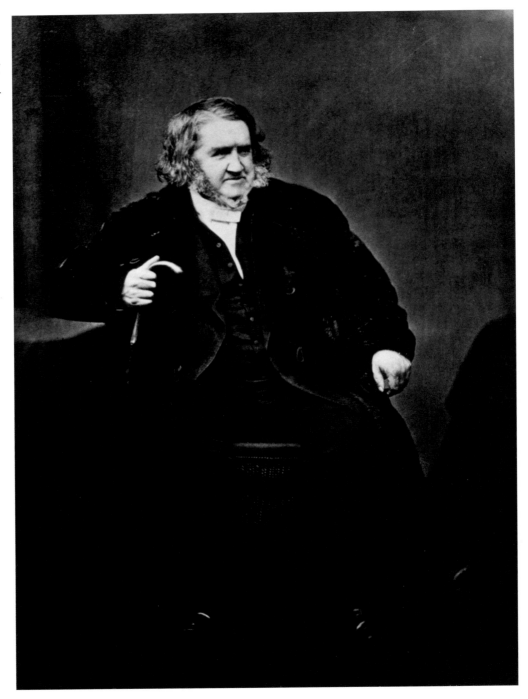

Edinburgh, first used chloroform in anaesthetic practice and claimed for it the following advantages over sulphuric ether: (i) a lesser quantity of anaesthetic agent was required, (ii) its action was much more rapid and complete, and generally more persistent, (iii) inhalation was more agreeable and pleasant than when ether was used. Simpson also believed that chloroform would prove to be less expensive to use than ether.[25]

News of his use of the agent reached Ireland quickly, with *The Freeman's Journal* of 19 November expressing the view that an anaesthetic agent far more effective than ether had been discovered and that its advantages were so varied and palpable that the latter may be considered as already superseded.[26]

The exact date on which inhaled chloroform was first used to produce surgical anaesthesia in Ireland is uncertain but it was probably on 24 November 1847 in Cork. On that date, *The Cork Examiner* had reprinted a report from *The Scotsman* newspaper on Simpson's use of the agent.[27] Three days later, *The Southern Reporter* and *Cork Commercial Courier* advised:

> On Wednesday the effect of this newly discovered remedy was tested at the North Infirmary, in two cases of amputation of the fingers. The medicine was prepared and administered by Dr Grattan, in the presence of the principal medical men of the city. The first case was a sailor, a stout plethoric man … The surgeon was Dr Howe in both cases.[28]

It seems reasonable to speculate that one or both of the doctors involved had read *The Cork Examiner* item of Wednesday 24 November and that it was agreed between them that chloroform would be used later that day. **Nicholas Grattan (c. 1808–1869)**, who administered the anaesthetic, had become a member of the Royal College of Surgeons, England in 1831 and would later be one of the first presidents of the County and City of Cork Medical and Surgical Society.

The *Dublin Medical Press* of 15 December 1847 carried a report of a Surgical Society of Ireland meeting held 11 days earlier at which a number of Dublin medical men spoke of their use of chloroform over the preceding few days. **Thomas Byrne**, external surgeon to the Westmoreland Lock Hospital on Townsend Street, considered ether to be an unsatisfactory agent for suspending consciousness in surgical operations; it succeeded in some cases only while in all there was a phase of excitement of shorter or longer duration. In the use of chloroform, he believed there was no stage of excitement, or it would be very limited; his experience of the newer agent led him to conclude that it would, in all cases, be preferred to ether. Over the previous ten days, beginning on 25 November, he had the opportunity of trying chloroform in five or six cases. In the first two, the effect was unsatisfactory but Byrne believed that this was because the chloroform had been hurriedly prepared. In the third case, a woman who was to undergo surgery on warty excrescences extending from the pubes to the coccyx, it worked well, although a second application was required during the surgery. The agent was satisfactory in the remaining two patients, who were described by Byrne as 'amateur performers' because they were not undergoing surgery.

Byrne's method of administering chloroform was by taking a sponge, cutting it into a conical shape of about six inches in length, with the base slightly excavated, then taking a towel, folding it two or three times on itself, holding it to the fire until it was very hot, warming the sponge, taking hold of it by the apex through the folds of the towel, pouring a drachm of chloroform into the excavated base, and applying the sponge thus adjusted to the nares, the towel at the same time loosely overlapping nose, mouth and part of the cheeks.

Michael Stapleton, a surgeon at the Charitable Infirmary, Jervis Street stated that he had tried chloroform in some cases with mixed results while **John Hamilton** of the Richmond Hospital had found it to be very satisfactory. **Thomas Mitchell**, master of the South East Lying-in Hospital on Cumberland Street described its use during labour in two patients, on 30 November and 2 December 1847, one with good results, the other less so. However, he commented that in the case of the patient in whom chloroform's action was not very satisfactory, that he did not think that she was best suited to its employment, as she was very excited and surrounded by a class of pupils – two conditions which, in Mitchell's opinion, were very unfavourable to its satisfactory exhibition.[29] Alexander Tyler and Robert Shekleton, working in the Anglesey (Bishop Street) and Rotunda (Rutland Square) Lying-in Hospitals respectively, had also used chloroform in midwifery prior to the meeting.[30]

Neither the pharmaceutical suppliers nor the publishing industry of the time were slow to appreciate the commercial opportunities offered by the introduction of chloroform, with an advertisement for the agent appearing in the same (15 December) issue of the *Dublin Medical Press* and one for pamphlets authored by Simpson, at a cost of sixpence each, just two weeks later.

However, the general enthusiasm with which the agent's early use was

CHLOROFORM OR PERCHLORIDE OF FORMYLE, (according to DUMAS' Formula, as recommended by Professor SIMPSON), prepared by

BEWLEY AND EVANS,

PHARMACEUTICAL CHEMISTS AND APOTHECARIES, 3, LOWER SACKVILLE-STREET, DUBLIN.

Advertisement for chloroform. Dublin Medical Press, 15 December 1847.

PROFESSOR SIMPSON'S PAMPHLETS ON CHLOROFORM.

Now published, price 6d. each, or by post 8d.,

I.

ANSWER to the RELIGIOUS OBJECTIONS urged against the Employment of ANÆSTHETIC AGENTS in SURGERY and MIDWIFERY.

By J. Y. SIMPSON, M.D., F.R.S.E., Professor of Midwifery in the University of Edinburgh.

II.

REMARKS on the SUPERINDUCTION of ANÆSTHESIA in NATURAL and MORBID PARTURITION. With Illustrative Cases.

III.

ACCOUNT of a NEW ANÆSTHETIC AGENT to supersede SULPHURIC ETHER in SURGERY and MIDWIFERY. *Third Thousand.*

Edinburgh: Sutherland and Knox. London: Samuel Highley. Sold by all Booksellers.

Advertisement for pamphlets authored by James Young Simpson. Dublin Medical Press, 29 December 1847.

greeted by the Irish medical community may have been tempered somewhat at the end of the year by a report in the *Dublin Medical Press* of 29 December that had first appeared in *The Medical Gazette*:

... The patient, a boy aged 11 years, undergoing division of the flexor tendons of the knee joint in Guy's Hospital, London, gave great concern because of feebleness of pulse etc., the symptoms of collapse being extreme. Ammonia was employed, he gave two or three deep inspirations, but it was more than 15 minutes before he was considered to be out of danger.[31]

Many decades were to elapse before the inherent dangers associated with chloroform anaesthesia were fully understood.

From the administration of the first ether anaesthetic in the country on New Year's Day 1847 to the initial indication in late December that the inhalation of chloroform vapour might not be as safe as was previously believed, the Irish medical and lay press fulfilled its role in 'spreading the news' during what was a seminal year for Irish anaesthesia.

References

1   'Important Operation – Amputation without Pain', *Pilot* (evening edition), 1 January 1847, p. 1.
2   'Triumph of Science', *The Freeman's Journal*, 5 January 1847, p. 2.
3   MacDonnell J., 'Amputation of the arm, performed at the Richmond Hospital, without pain', *Dublin Medical Press*, 1847, 17, pp. 8–9.
4   'Metropolitan Gossip', *Cork Examiner*, 6 January 1847, p. 2.
5   Tufnell J., 'Illustrating the effects of inhalation of sulphuric ether vapour', *Dublin Medical Press*, 1847, 17, p. 25.
6   'Surgical Society of Ireland – January 9', *Dublin Medical Press*, 1847, 17, pp. 71–5.
7   'Amputation of the Great Toe – Vapour of Sulphuric Ether', *Cork Examiner*, 15 January 1847, p. 2.
8   'Important use of Sulphuric Ether', *The Belfast News-Letter*, 22 January 1847, p. 2.
9   Fee H., 'Clouds of unknowing', *Ulster Medical Journal*, 2009, 78, pp. 146–56.
10 'Editorial. The etherisation for surgical operations', *Dublin Medical Press*, 1847, 17, p. 47.
11 'Minutes of the meeting of The Surgical Society of Ireland held on January 9th 1847', RCSI/MS/SURG/01, Royal College of Surgeons in Ireland.
12 'Surgical Society of Ireland – January 23', *Dublin Medical Press*, 1847, 17, pp. 89–91.
13 Robinson J., 'Inhalation of ether in surgical operations', *Dublin Medical Press*, 1847, 17, p. 57.
14 Lyons J.B., 'Wilde, Sir William Robert Wills' in *Dictionary of Irish Biography*, vol. 9, Staines–Z, Cambridge: Royal Irish Academy and Cambridge University Press, 2009, pp. 936–7.
15 Wilde W.R.W., 'The employment of the vapour of sulphuric ether as a means of rendering surgical operations painless', *Dublin Quarterly Journal of Medical Science*, 1847, 3, pp. 276–80.
16 'The Progress of Ether', *Anglo-Celt*, 12 February 1847, p. 4.

17 Nunn R.S., 'Operation for stone in the bladder', *The Lancet*, 1847, 1, p. 343.

18 'Fatal operation under the influence of ether', *The Lancet*, 1847, 1, pp. 340–2.

19 Wilde W.R.W., 'The ether inhalation', *Dublin Quarterly Journal of Medical Science*, 1847, 3, p. 554.

20 Snow S.J., *Operations without Pain*, Basingstoke: Palgrave Macmillan, 2006, pp. 61–2.

21 *Durham University: Our History*, available at dur.ac.uk/johnsnow.college/aboutthecollege/ourstory/ (accessed 16 January 2021).

22 Snow J., *On Chloroform and other Anæsthetics: Their Action and Administration*, London: Churchill, 1858, pp. 365–8.

23 'Report of a Committee of the Boston Society for Medical Improvement, on the Alleged Dangers which Accompany the Inhalation of the Vapor of Sulphuric Ether', *Boston Medical and Surgical Journal*, 1861, 65, pp. 229–54.

24 'Ether in surgical operations', *Kerry Evening Post*, 30 June 1847.

25 Simpson J.Y., *Account of a New Anæsthetic Agent as a Substitute for Sulphuric Ether in Surgery and Midwifery*, Edinburgh: Sutherland and Knox, 1847.

26 'Ether Superseded – New Anæsthetic Agent', *The Freeman's Journal*, 19 November 1847, p. 3.

27 'Substitute for Ether in Surgical Operations', *Cork Examiner*, 24 November 1847, p. 4.

28 'Trial of Chloroform in Cork', *Southern Reporter and Cork Commercial Courier*, 27 November 1847, p. 4.

29 'Surgical Society of Ireland – Saturday, December 4th', *Dublin Medical Press*, 1847, 18, pp. 370–2.

30 Loughrey J.P.R., Bowen M.P. and Thornton P.C., 'Early inhalational obstetric anaesthesia in Ireland (abstract)', *Journal of Anesthesia History*, 2018, 4, p. 69.

31 'Operation under the influence of chloroform (by Dr William Gull, from *Medical Gazette*)', *Dublin Medical Press*, 1847, 18, p. 408.

Chapter 4

Chloroform's Apogee

Declan Warde

The ease of use and apparent safety of chloroform led to its widespread adoption in many countries within weeks, and as elsewhere, Irish practitioners in centres large and small were soon reporting their own, sometimes very limited, experience with the new agent. One such, Dr John Vereker Bindon, working in the village of Moneygall, County Offaly used it successfully in the delivery of one baby and wrote:

> I consider the use of chloroform in labour of the greatest benefit to suffering women. And I have no doubt of its safety both to the mother and child; it appears wonderfully to cause relaxation of the passages, and at the same time to expedite delivery.[1]

Moneygall is perhaps best known nowadays as the birthplace and childhood home of Falmouth Kearney who emigrated to North America in 1850 and was the maternal great-great-great grandfather of Barack Obama, 44th president of the United States of America.

The first death attributed to chloroform anaesthesia occurred near Newcastle-upon-Tyne, England on 28 January 1848. The patient, Hannah Greener, was a healthy girl aged 15 years who was about to have a toenail removed. The corresponding nail on her other foot had been uneventfully excised three months earlier after she had inhaled sulphuric ether.[2] She died within three minutes or so of being administered chloroform. Various authors subsequently ascribed her death to chloroform overdose, to aspiration of water and brandy used in attempts to resuscitate her, or to some combination of complications that will never be determined. However, given our present state of knowledge, the sudden onset of a fatal arrhythmia appears to provide the most likely explanation.[3]

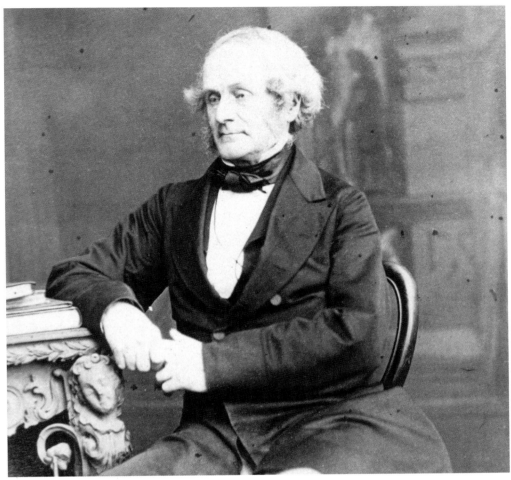

Photograph of Edward William Murphy, Dublin graduate and later professor of midwifery, University College and Hospital, London. Courtesy of NIH Digital Collections.

Hannah Greener's demise, and others that followed, did little if anything to affect the popularity of chloroform among both medical practitioners and patients. It was believed that all would be well if reasonable care was taken in patient selection and the administration of the agent. Studies addressing the relative safety of different medicinal products were almost unheard of at the time; as chloroform was easier to use than ether, it is not surprising that the 'older' drug was, to all intents and purposes, abandoned in most places within a couple of months. One exception was the northeastern part of the United States of America, where ether continued to be widely used.

The most prolific Irish writer on chloroform in the first few years following its introduction was **Edward William Murphy (1802–1877)**, who was born in

Dublin in 1802. He obtained a licentiate of the Royal College of Surgeons in Ireland (LRCSI) in 1827, graduated MB from Trinity College Dublin and was awarded the Fellowship of the Royal College of Surgeons in Ireland (FRCSI) in 1832; he became MD (Trinity) in 1853. After qualifying, he devoted himself to midwifery, and in or about the year 1830, became assistant physician to the Dublin Lying-in Hospital (now the Rotunda Hospital). He relocated to London in 1840 and within two years, was appointed as professor of midwifery in University College and Hospital, serving until 1865.

John Snow administered chloroform on 24 November and 2 December 1847 to two patients of Murphy's who were in protracted labour and required instrumental delivery. The Dubliner first used it himself on 17 December of the same year, on a patient of another doctor who had called him for assistance, using, in his own words:

> an inhaler of very simple construction, contrived by Messrs Stevens and Pratt of Gower Street. A small circular tin box, to which a mouthpiece like a speaking trumpet was attached, contained a piece of sponge. Behind the mouthpiece a tin plate was interposed, leaving a small fissure below for the vapour of chloroform to be drawn into the mouth. The expired air passed through an opening in the upper part of the mouthpiece and atmospheric air entered through longitudinal fissures in the lid of the box beneath which a small piece of cloth was placed. Thus the patient inhaled chloroform by the mouth. After one or two inspirations the nostrils were closed by the fingers until the effect of chloroform was observable in the patient, when they were allowed to remain open. The admission of atmospheric air in this way prevented so rapid an action of the vapour as would otherwise take place. Its influence was less powerful than if the chloroform alone were inspired and yet was quite sufficient to accomplish the desired object – relief from pain. The writer did not observe in any of the cases so given, the exciting effects produced by æther ...[4]

The inhaler became known as Murphy's Chloroform Inhaler. It was a neat, compact piece of apparatus, one of the first to appear as an alternative to the use of the 'corner of a towel' advocated by Simpson. Its efficiency cannot have been

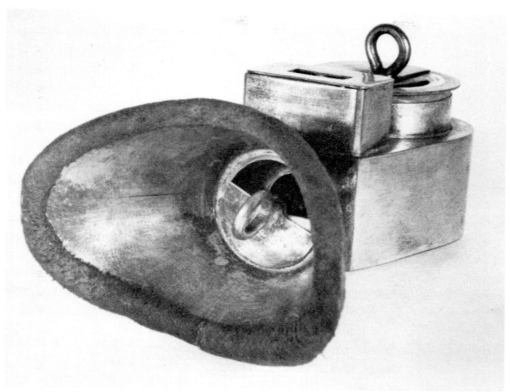

Murphy's Chloroform Inhaler, 1850. Reproduced from Bryn Thomas K. The Development of Anaesthetic Apparatus: A History Based on the Charles King Collection of the Association of Anaesthetists of Great Britain and Ireland, Blackwell, 1975.

high, since the amount of chloroform allowed was very small and air was admitted freely.[5]

Murphy became a firm advocate of the use of chloroform in midwifery, either for the purposes of providing pain relief or for inducing loss of consciousness when considered necessary. His first two pamphlets on the subject were published in 1848 and 1850.[4,6] A third, containing a description of an improved version of his inhaler, followed five years later. Referring to chloroform, he wrote, 'The practitioner who ventures upon its use will soon be satisfied of its great advantage, not only in very severe cases, but even in many of the ordinary cases of natural labour'.[7] John Snow recognised Murphy's early role in the provision of labour analgesia when he declared in *On Chloroform and Other Anæsthetics*, published posthumously, 'Drs Murphy and Dr Ridge were, I believe, amongst the first to state that relief from pain may be afforded in obstetric cases without removing the consciousness of the patient; and I soon observed the same circumstance'.[8]

Not all Irish obstetricians shared Murphy's enthusiasm for the use of chloroform. **William Fetherston Montgomery (*c.* 1797–1859)**, first professor of midwifery at the School of Physic in Trinity College Dublin, mindful of the fact that deaths associated with chloroform anaesthesia were by then being reported on a regular basis, wrote in May 1849 concerning the administration of the agent to women in natural labour that, 'the subject had been pressed, or rather forced, not only on the profession, but the public, with an overweaning zeal, quite unparalleled ...'. He stated that those medical men who had hesitated about, or rejected the indiscriminate use of chloroform in natural labour, had been portrayed as deficient in energy, or in feeling and humanity. He cautioned against its use in such a manner, believing that it should be reserved for such situations as instrumental delivery or the removal of a retained placenta.[9]

Almost 50 years later, Montgomery's opposition to the routine use of anaesthetic agents to relieve the pain of labour had not been forgotten in Scotland, where the practice had been introduced. In July 1897, the *Dublin Journal of Medical Science* reported on an inaugural address delivered earlier in the year by Prof. Alexander Russell Simpson, president of the Glasgow Obstetrical and Gynaecological Society and subsequently published in the *Glasgow Medical Journal*. Simpson was a nephew of James Young Simpson and had succeeded his uncle as professor of midwifery in Edinburgh. He had stated, when speaking on the struggle for and against the use of anaesthetics in midwifery:

> Dr Montgomery, the then chief of the great Dublin school of midwifery, wrote during the session a letter to Edinburgh in which he said, 'I do not believe that anyone in Dublin has as yet used ether in midwifery; the feeling is very strong against its use in ordinary cases, and merely to avert the ordinary amount of pain which the Almighty has seen fit – and most wisely we cannot doubt – to allot to natural labour, and in this feeling I heartily and entirely concur'. Dr Matthews Duncan (junior assistant to Prof. Simpson) marked the following alternative reading, which well-showed the absurdity of Montgomery's train of reasoning:– 'I do not believe that anyone in Dublin has as yet used a carriage in locomotion; the feeling is very strong against its use in ordinary progression, and merely to avert the ordinary amount of fatigue which the Almighty has seen fit – and most wisely we cannot

doubt – to allot to natural walking, and in this feeling I heartily and entirely concur![10, 11]

Dr John Denham, ex-assistant physician to the Dublin Lying-in Hospital, read a paper on the use of chloroform in 56 cases of labour at meetings of the Dublin Obstetrical Society held in January and March 1849.[12] He began by outlining 15 cases of natural labour in which chloroform was given and concluded that it was applicable in many instances, useless in some and injurious, in terms of slowing or stopping labour, in a few. Where preternatural labours were concerned, especially those where turning was required, he believed the agent to be highly useful, and also for instrumental delivery using forceps for live infants or the crotchet hook in the case of those who had died during labour. Although Denham had presented his paper early in the year, the fact that it was not published until August 1849 afforded him the opportunity to respond to the comments made by Montgomery in May. He wrote:

> From what I have seen of chloroform, I do not think that its use should be so restricted as Dr. Montgomery, in his valuable paper lately published in this Journal, would have us believe; nor have I witnessed the fearful results so graphically described by him as likely to follow from its use. Whilst I admit that some of the advocates for chloroform have been too lavish of their praise, on the other hand I think that those opposed to it have been too unsparing in their censure.[12]

In his original paper on chloroform anaesthesia, James Young Simpson had opined:

> When used for surgical purposes, perhaps it will be found to be most easily given upon a handkerchief, gathered up into a cup-like form in the hand of the exhibitor, and with the open end of the cup placed over the nose and mouth of the patient.[13]

His view had not changed when writing in the *Dublin Medical Press* in 1849: 'In administering chloroform in obstetric practice, I have always used the handkerchief as the simplest and best practice'.[14]

John Snow, on the other hand, believed that some chloroform deaths could be attributed to this mode of administration. In 1849, he wrote:

> It must be sufficiently evident from these considerations that
> unless some means were used for regulating the strength of the
> vapour, fatal accidents would be liable to occur from the
> employment of chloroform. Unfortunately, Dr Simpson, to whom
> we are indebted for its introduction, recommended it to be used
> in a handkerchief and even held it out to be one of the advantages
> of the new anaesthetic, that it did not require any apparatus. This
> advice, coming from so high a quarter, could not fail to meet with
> numerous followers; and to this circumstance many of the
> accidents that have occurred must, in my opinion, be partly
> attributed.[15]

At that time, **Christopher Fleming (1800–1880)**, a future president of the
Royal College of Surgeons in Ireland, was surgeon to the Netterville Hospital and
Dispensary, Blackhall Street, Dublin; he was appointed surgeon to the Richmond
Hospital in 1851 where his initial role was, in fact, to give anaesthetics.[16] Fleming
regarded the administration of chloroform by handkerchief as a reckless practice
and in late 1850, described a simple apparatus consisting of a glass capsule, stopper
bottle and sponge, which he had been using for two years with excellent results.[17]

On 25 January 1851, he delivered a comprehensive paper to the Surgical
Society of Ireland with the title 'On the Application of Anæsthetic Remedies to
Surgical Purposes'. In it, he referred, rather obliquely, to what was, to his
knowledge, the only death associated with anaesthesia in the country up to that
time

> The Infirmary surgeons throughout Ireland, and other surgeons
> in their respective localities, have been, with very few exceptions,
> the earliest in the field in the adoption of anæsthetic surgery, and
> the judicious selection of their cases, and cautious and restricted
> use of the agent, are proved incontestably by the fact, that only
> one occurrence has taken place, and that, very recently, where
> fatal consequences were attributable (though by no means
> satisfactorily chargeable) to the remedy, and that, it is worthy of
> observation, occurred in the hands of one of the most respected,
> the most careful, and the most talented, of their body.[18]

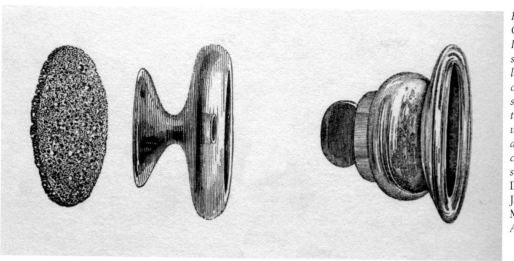

Fleming's Chloroform Inhaler (1850) showing on the left, the tubular capsule and sponge and, on the right, a lateral view of the long diameter of the capsule and stopper bottle. Dublin Quarterly Journal of Medical Science, *August 1851.*

He stressed the need for any person providing anaesthesia to have adequate knowledge of both the agent used and the patient's preoperative condition, and made it clear that chloroform had completely supplanted ether as the agent of choice:

> … certain rules must guide the surgeon, which should be observed as rigidly as the performance of his varied operations, in order that he may be prepared to meet any contingency. He should have a clear and distinct knowledge of the agent to be employed, and be fully satisfied of its purity – he should have a simple apparatus for its administration – he should consider the actual condition of the patient, as to the state of his health and strength at the time of exhibition – and selecting a proper position, free from constriction of any kind, he should have at hand remedies to counteract any injurious effects which may supervene … Chloroform, the agent at present in use for anæsthetic purposes, is familiar by name to all. It has now borne the test of more than three years experience … The advantages which this agent possesses over that first suggested, it is unnecessary for me here to specify.

In acknowledging the fact that the level of knowledge at the time concerning anaesthesia was in its infancy, he remarked:

> I yet contemplate the adoption of anæsthesia in every instance
> with anxiety, and I hence deprecate it unless the serious nature of
> the case demands it. I am strongly opposed to it in trifling, passing
> operations. I am favourable to it in all severe operative
> proceedings, with the exceptions I have noted, and with the
> precautions I have specified.[18]

Fleming's knowledge of what appears to have been the first anaesthetic death
in Ireland was obtained from a comprehensive letter written to him earlier in
January by **George Roe**, surgeon and physician to the County Cavan Infirmary
and County Gaol; it was published in full two months later.[19]
Roe wrote concerning a young man, James Jones:

> At his own request I consented to amputate the leg on the 20th
> of September, having promised I would give him something to
> numb and take away the pain of the operation ... He was
> cheerful, and appeared to be firm and courageous, but when
> placed on the table, the heart's action was very quick and weak,
> but he did not appear faintish, or more pale than usual. I then
> saw Mr Nalty, the apothecary, measure one drachm of
> chloroform ... and pour it upon a little folded lint, which was
> placed in an oval, hollowed sponge, held in the hand with a small
> towel. Recollecting I had used this chloroform in another case,
> and finding some little delay in producing the anæsthetic effects
> and supposing the strength of the chloroform might be a little
> weakened as the bottle had not been kept very closely stopped, I
> directed Mr Nalty to add thirty drops more to that already put
> on the lint. I then applied the sponge &c to the patient's nose,
> directing him to keep his mouth shut. I then gave up the towel
> &c to Dr Halpin, who was at the opposite side of the table, while
> I went to prepare myself for the operation ... I was examining the
> state of the circulation in the tibial arteries ... which could not
> have occupied one minute ... when Dr Halpin told me the
> anæsthetic effects were produced. This struck me as being
> unusually quick and sudden, and on removing the towel from the

face we saw a slight convulsive action of the left eyelid, and the lids partially open, and a small quantity of saliva (frothy) at the mouth. I felt rather uneasy, but not much alarmed, as Dr Halpin said he had seen such symptoms from the effect of chloroform, but which I had not met with; and on a more minute and instant examination of the heart, the eyes, muscles of the limbs &c, we found him dead. Every means within our reach were resorted to, to try and restore animation … without the least effect. I lament I had no means of making or procuring oxygen gas, and unfortunately my little portable galvanic apparatus was not then in order or ready for use; so that we had the sad and painful spectacle of our patient killed, as if by a stroke of lightning, in less than one minute, before our eyes.[19]

Dr Roe went on to outline other cases in which he had used chloroform without ill-effect, and was anxious to know in what way he might have erred, and what was the cause of his misfortune in the death of his patient. He continued:

When we hear the very indiscriminate, and I would almost say the unjustifiable use made of chloroform made by every description of practitioner, it is scarcely a matter of surprise that much more mischief is not done; yet the medical records and other public journals furnish proofs enough of its great and fatal danger, sufficient to warn the young and inexperienced from using without due care and knowledge such a remedy, and one possessing such awful power over human life. I wish I could say that all the medical records of its use and advantages had been given with that facility, truth and honesty, which such a subject requires. It is not by the relation of a number of successful cases, however great, that the laws and rules which should regulate its exhibition, can be laid down or ascertained. We ought to have a faithful account and record of the unsuccessful, dangerous and fatal cases in which it has been employed; and I fear many who have extolled its use and benefits, have most unjustly and unworthily suppressed its dangers, bad effects, and even fatality in their own hands … I presume that I am now writing to a great admirer and a warm advocate for the use of chloroform, and if so, I hope you will give some general rules and instructions by which its good effects may be attained and regulated, without the risk and dangers of its disagreeable or fatal consequences ... I cannot conclude this letter ... without expressing very deep regret that it was not in my power to procure a post-mortem examination in this case, although with that view I entreated – indeed insisted upon an inquest being held upon the body.

However, only a partial inquest was held, as the deceased's family and friends did not wish it to proceed further. A jury verdict was brought in as follows: 'That the above-named James Jones came by his death in consequence of the administration of chloroform, applied at his own request, and in the usual manner, without any blame being attributable to the medical gentlemen who applied it'.[19]

Professor Richard Clarke's masterly history of the Royal Victoria Hospital in Belfast provides an interesting insight into early anaesthesia at what was known in the mid-nineteenth century as the General Hospital.[20] Other than brief newspaper accounts, there are no surviving records of the initial experience with either ether or chloroform there, the first mention of anaesthesia being in the surgical part of the annual report covering the period 1 April 1849 to 31 March 1850:

42 surgical operations have been performed, several of them under the influence of chloroform. The facts in reference to this agent are not yet sufficiently numerous to enable us to recommend or condemn its general use. It is, perhaps, only right, that we should take this opportunity of stating that it requires great caution and considerable experience to render its operation safe.

Subsequent reports became increasingly positive about the use of chloroform with that for 1851 stating:

The use of chloroform, which tends so much to allay the sufferings of the patient during an operation, has been more generally adopted than formerly, and with decided success, no injurious effects having, in any case, remitted from its employment in this establishment.

The sum of £1 4s 0d. had been spent on the agent during the 17 months ending 5 September 1851. One year later, it was observed:

> Chloroform, we may remark, has continued to be used in almost every surgical operation, with the happiest effect in the alleviation of human suffering, and it is very satisfying to report that in no case has the least unpleasant effect followed its use.

Eighty-five operations had been performed during the year, the largest group being amputations. The 1853 report stated:

> Chloroform has been administered to the patients, when practicable, and with the most satisfactory results in alleviating both mental dread and physical pain; and it is our duty to put it in record, that, during the several years it has been exhibited in this institution, no accident whatever or evil has followed its administration.

Comments in the reports for the remainder of the decade were also favourable and 'No untoward symptom was manifest'.[20]

Chloroform was by now being used with apparent success, both in Ireland and elsewhere, in the management of various conditions including tetanus, delirium tremens and severe rheumatism. Others were experimenting with its use as a local anaesthetic. Simpson, in addition to carrying out animal experiments, rubbed chloroform on his own painful gums, found it to be effective and believed it to be of potential benefit to dentists. It was also used to relieve postoperative pain, by direct application to limb stumps remaining after amputation, and was incorporated into many lotions and ointments used in painful conditions.[21-24]

In late 1853, **Dr Samuel Little Hardy (1815–1868)**, physician to the Institution for the Diseases of Children in Pitt Street, Dublin and ex-assistant physician to the Rotunda Lying-in Hospital, wrote:

> That chloroform may be used with very great benefit to the patient without being inhaled, and so as to cause relief from suffering much more quickly than it does when applied in the

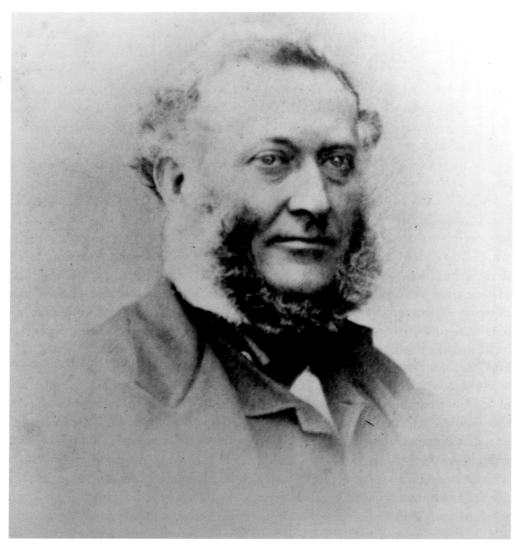

liquid form, or in ointment or liniment, I have endeavoured to prove by the local application of the vapour by means of an apparatus suited to the purpose.

He went on to describe his apparatus, which produced a vapour spray, and stated that the technique devised by him seemed particularly suited to affections of the uterine system, including carcinoma, which were frequently very painful and for

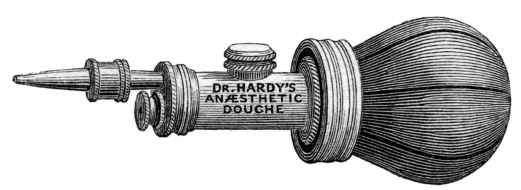

Hardy's device for the local application of chloroform vapour, Dublin Quarterly Journal of Medical Science, *November 1853.*

which 'the evil effects of opium prevented its more frequent use'. He had found that in every instance in which pain was removed by local application of the vapour, there was no return for several hours. He described the case histories and usage of chloroform in this manner in a number of his patients and the beneficial effects obtained, and concluded that: (i) in many diseases attended with pain, the local application of the vapour of chloroform frequently acted as quickly in affording immunity from suffering as though inhaled; (ii) that the vapour applied locally was not attended with any unpleasant effects (save the sensation of more or less heat) and (iii) that as a remedy, its local application was preferable to the use of opium and most narcotics in spasmodic and painful affections, particularly of the uterine system.[25]

Hardy's apparatus and technique were popular for some years not only in Ireland but also in a number of other European countries, including Denmark, Germany and especially France, where they were employed not only in the management of uterine afflictions but also prior to surgery for various superficial lesions such as abscesses and skin tumours. They were never widely used in England, perhaps at least in part because John Snow was not an enthusiast.

One of the more regular and sometimes controversial contributors in the mid-nineteenth century to both medical meetings and the scientific literature where anaesthesia, and in particular the relative safety of different anaesthetic agents, were discussed was **Dr Charles Kidd**. Born in Limerick to Thomas and Rebecca Kidd in 1816, he became a Licentiate of Apothecaries Hall, Dublin (LAH) in 1839 and a member of the Royal College of Surgeons in London (MRCS) the same year. He was awarded MD by the University of Glasgow in

1845. After qualifying, Kidd worked for some years in County Clare and *The Freeman's Journal* of 7 May 1846 made reference to his good work in attending the sick poor of the parish of Doonass during the Great Famine.[26]

By August 1848, the first of a number of items by him in the *Medical Times* was published. Commissioned by the publication, he travelled extensively in Europe, often reporting on either outbreaks of disease or medical innovations in the continental cities he visited. He was based in London from 1850 onwards, serving as hospital reporter for *The Lancet* and other journals while also running his own medical practice.

In July of that year, he wrote, apparently for the first time, on an anaesthetic subject – the sudden death in Guy's Hospital following the inhalation of chloroform of a healthy young policeman scheduled to undergo surgery on a finger.[27] The majority of his subsequent papers focused on anaesthesia – he was a proponent of chloroform and frequently offered his opinion as to the specific cause of death in cases where the agent had been employed.

Kidd's initial contribution to the Irish medical literature appears to have been in June 1858, when he wrote in a letter to the *Dublin Medical Press*:

> I have now carefully examined about eleven thousand applications of chloroform in private practice and in the hospitals, chiefly as to heart and pulse. I carefully examined, in this interval, the post-mortem revelations in four deaths from chloroform occurring in the hospitals (the only four, in fact, I could make out), though I may say I lived continuously in London hospitals for the last nine years, watching such cases, yet all the evidence I have been able to accumulate is that chloroform is rather in favour of patients with diseased heart than a cause of death.[28]

The letter was written three days after the death of John Snow. Kidd briefly mentioned the great man's passing, '… poor Dr Snow, whose loss to science I unfeignedly regret'. While most of the 11,000 'applications' of chloroform referred to by him were in patients anaesthetised by others, he did also have an anaesthetic practice of his own, though the precise extent of his work in this area is unclear.

Just two weeks later, in the same journal, he described what he referred to as 'four well-marked stages of Chloroformisation marked out by Nature'.[29] This was not, however, the first such attempt to define levels of the depth of anaesthesia, as Snow had also done so in his first book, published in 1847.[30] In September 1858, Kidd provided for *Dublin Medical Press* readers a detailed account of his views on the approach to be taken by the chloroform administrator when caring for an adult patient about to undergo a capital operation such as amputation of a lower extremity. He referred, among other matters, to the advisability of preoperative fasting, the fact that a patient could take chloroform without incident a number of times and yet die on a later occasion, and recommended having a portable galvanic chain or battery for resuscitation in one's pocket, also a supply of smelling salts, cold water etc.[31]

ON

ÆTHER

AND

CHLOROFORM

AS ANÆSTHETICS.

BEING THE RESULT OF ABOUT 11,000 ADMINISTRATIONS OF THESE AGENTS PERSONALLY STUDIED IN THE HOSPITALS OF LONDON, PARIS, ETC., DURING THE LAST TEN YEARS.

BY CHARLES KIDD, M.D.,

MEMBER OF THE ROYAL COLLEGE OF SURGEONS, ENGLAND; FELLOW OF THE SURGICAL SOCIETY, IRELAND, AND OTHER SOCIETIES, ETC.

[Second Edition.]

LONDON:

RENSHAW, 356 STRAND.

1858.

Title page of Dr Charles Kidd's 1858 book On Æther and Chloroform as Anæsthetics.

Before the end of the year, the periodical contained an anonymous review of his book *On Æther and Chloroform*, which had been published earlier in 1858.[32] The reviewer was positive in his comments, and strongly recommended Kidd's book, the first on the subject of anaesthesia by an Irish-born author.

Another unidentified writer was not so complimentary, however. He reviewed three works for the February 1859 issue of the *Dublin Quarterly Journal of Medical Science* – Kidd's book, and also *On Chloroform and Other Anaesthetics* by John Snow, and *On Chloroform and its Safe Administration* by William Martin Coates, surgeon to Salisbury Infirmary in Wiltshire. Referring to what later came to be regarded as Snow's masterpiece, first published a few months after the author's death, he wrote of 'a work which may truly be styled

Dr Snow's legacy to his sorrowing professional brethren'. The writer also commented positively on Coates' effort. In contrast, his opinions, transcribed in part below, of both Charles Kidd and his book were entirely negative:

> At Dr Snow's decease, that there should have been aspirants to fill the position he had so long and so honourably occupied was natural; and that these candidates should put forward their claim by trying, in some way or other, to prove their competency, was also to be expected. We presume it was with some such views that the author of the brochure which stands second on our list strung together various papers that had already appeared in some of our medical journals and rushed into print with his work 'On Æther and Chloroform', announcing it as the second edition, though when or where the first edition appeared seems to be an enigma that it would require an Œdipus to solve; dubbing himself, amongst his other qualifications, a 'Fellow of the Surgical Society, Ireland'. Now though we have been for many years an humble **member** of that distinguished Society; we still must plead our utter ignorance of that high-sounding title of 'Fellow': that there are such persons as Fellows of the Royal College of Surgeons in Ireland we know to our cost; but **Fellow** of the Surgical Society, we must again repeat, is a title that up to the appearance of Dr Kidd's book, we had never before heard of; however, we can only say that we live and learn.
>
> We never remember opening a work of its pretensions in which such a variety of topics have been introduced as the one under consideration ... We verily believe that, were the title-page removed, and the book itself placed in the hands of any of our readers, he would be puzzled to determine on what subject it was written. Such a variety of topics are introduced.[33]

Kidd's reaction to the reviewer's comments is not known. In his preface, he had described the book as 'a metamorphosed chrysalis of a former edition of a smaller work of the same kind'; it may be that it was originally published as a pamphlet. In later publications, he referred to himself as an associate member of the Surgical Society of Ireland rather than as a fellow. He was not deterred from producing a further book, in 1859, titled *A Manual of Anæsthetics, Theoretical and Practical (New Edition)*; once again, its provenance, where the existence of an earlier edition is concerned, is unclear – in many respects this far more substantial work represented a second (or third!) version of *On Æther and Chloroform*.

References

1   Bindon J.V., 'Chloroform in midwifery practice', *Dublin Medical Press*, 1848, 472, p. 35.
2   Duncum B.M., *The Development of Inhalation Anaesthesia*, London: Oxford University Press, 1947, p. 195.
3   Knight P.R. and Bacon D.R., 'An unexplained death: Hannah Greener and chloroform', *Anesthesiology*, 2002, 96, pp. 1250–3.
4   Murphy E.W., *Chloroform in the Practice of Midwifery*, London: Taylor and Walton, 1848, p. 14.
5   Bryn Thomas K., *The Development of Anaesthetic Apparatus*, Oxford: Blackwell, 1975, pp. 65–6.
6   Murphy E.W., *Further Observations on Chloroform in the Practice of Midwifery*, London: Taylor, Walton and Maberly, 1850.
7   Murphy E.W., *Chloroform; Its Properties and Safety in Childbirth*, London: Walton and Maberly, 1855, p. 71.
8   Snow J., *On Chloroform and Other Anæsthetics: Their Action and Administration*, London: Churchill, 1858, p. 318.
9   Montgomery W.F., 'Objection to the indiscriminate use of anæsthetic agents', *Dublin Quarterly Journal of Medical Science*, 1849, 7, pp. 321–40.
10 Simpson A.R., 'Inaugural Address to the Glasgow Obstetrical and Gynaecological Society: The Jubilee of Anæsthetic Midwifery', *Glasgow Medical Journal*, 1897, 47, pp. 161–87.
11 'The Jubilee of Anæsthetic Midwifery', *Dublin Journal of Medical Science*, 1897, 104, pp. 91–2.
12 Denham J., 'A report upon the use of chloroform in fifty-six cases of labour occurring in the Dublin Lying-in Hospital', *Dublin Quarterly Journal of Medical Science*, 1849, 8, pp. 107–42.
13 Simpson J.Y., *Account of a New Anæsthetic Agent as a Substitute for Sulphuric Ether in Surgery and Midwifery*, Edinburgh: Sutherland and Knox, 1847, pp. 10–11.
14 Simpson J.Y., 'Chloroform in midwifery practice', *Dublin Medical Press*, 1849, 21, pp. 22–3.
15 Snow J., 'On the fatal cases of inhalation of chloroform', *Edinburgh Medical and Surgical Journal*, 1849, 72, pp. 75–89.
16 O'Brien E., 'Of Vagabonds, Strolling Beggars and Sturdy Women' in E. O'Brien, L. Browne and K. O'Malley (eds), *The House of Industry Hospitals 1772–1987*, Dublin: Anniversary Press, 1988, p. 56.
17 Fleming C., 'On a simple apparatus for the inhalation of chloroform', *Dublin Medical Press*, 1850, 24, p. 292.
18 Fleming C., 'On the application of anæsthetic remedies to surgical purposes', *Dublin Medical Press*, 1851, 25, pp. 161–8.
19 Roe G., 'Fatal effects attributed to chloroform', *Dublin Medical Press*, 1851, 25, pp. 195–7.

20 Clarke R.S.J., *The Royal Victoria Hospital Belfast: A History 1797–1997*, Belfast: Blackstaff, 1997, pp. 35–6.

21 Banks J.T., 'Case of tetanus; chloroform inhalations; recovery', *Dublin Quarterly Journal of Medical Science*, 1852, 13, p. 225.

22 Butcher G.H., 'On the internal administration of chloroform in delirium tremens', *Dublin Quarterly Journal of Medical Science*, 1852, 14, pp. 227–30.

23 Kirby J., 'Miscellaneous cases and observations in the practice of medicine', *Dublin Medical Press*, 1853, 29, pp. 161–4.

24 Stratmann L., *Chloroform, the Quest for Oblivion*, Stroud: Sutton, 2003, pp. 83–4.

25 Hardy S.L., 'On the local application of the vapour of chloroform in the treatment of various diseases, especially those of the uterine organs; with the description of an apparatus invented for this purpose', *Dublin Quarterly Journal of Medical Science*, 1853, 16, pp. 306–18.

26 'State of the South – Famine', *The Freeman's Journal*, 7 May 1846, p. 2.

27 Kidd C., 'Chloroform', *Medical Times*, 1850, 22, p. 63.

28 Kidd C., 'The chloroform controversy', *Dublin Medical Press*, 1858, 39, p. 410.

29 Kidd C., 'Stages of chloroform', *Dublin Medical Press*, 1858, 40, p. 29.

30 Snow J., *On the Inhalation of the Vapour of Ether*, Churchill: London, 1847, pp. 1–14.

31 Kidd C., 'Dr. Kidd on chloroform', *Dublin Medical Press*, 1858, 40, pp. 184–5.

32 Anonymous, 'Review of Kidd C. On Æther and Chloroform as Anæsthetics. Renshaw: London, 1858', *Dublin Medical Press*, 1858, 40, p. 280.

33 Anonymous, 'Reviews of Snow J. On Chloroform and other Anæsthetics: Their Action and Administration. Churchill: London: 1858, Kidd C. On Æther and Chloroform as Anæsthetics. Renshaw: London, 1858 and Coates WM. On Chloroform and its Safe Administration. Walton and Maberly: London, 1858', *Dublin Quarterly Journal of Medical Science*, 1859, 27, pp. 207–17.

Chapter 5

Early Safety Concerns:
Two Committees

Declan Warde

While driving his phaeton in July 1861, **Francis Rynd** (1801–1861), surgeon to the city's Meath Hospital since 1836, was involved in a minor accident in Clontarf, Dublin. Although the pedestrian involved was unhurt, an altercation ensued; Rynd suffered a heart attack shortly afterwards and died.[1]

In June 1844, using an instrument in the form of a trocar and cannula which had been designed by him specifically for the purpose, he had introduced 15 grains of a morphine solution to the supraorbital nerve, and along the courses of the temporal, malar and buccal nerves, of a female patient suffering from chronic facial pain. The pain ceased immediately and the lady appears to have made a complete recovery.[2] Rynd's appliance caused the fluid to enter the tissues by gravity and it is now considered to have been the first hollow-bore needle.

He did not publish a detailed illustrated account of his instrument until shortly before his death,[3] with the result that much of the credit for early hypodermic injections went to Charles Pravaz (Paris) and Alexander Wood (Edinburgh) who, in 1853, had independently developed syringes with needles fine enough to pierce the skin. Francis Rynd could not have foreseen, at the time of his 1844 invention, that its use would, in one form or another, become an indispensable part of the everyday practice of a new medical specialty, anaesthesia, that was still awaiting discovery.

Debate over the relative safety of ether and chloroform continued into the 1860s and for some decades afterwards. Charles Kidd was of the view that ether was nowhere near as safe as it was held out to be and that deaths associated with its use were far more common than was generally believed.[4]

Differences of opinion also persisted as to the value of chloroform in labour. **Richard Doherty**, professor of midwifery for almost 30 years at Queen's College Galway (now the National University of Ireland Galway) wrote in a letter to Kidd:

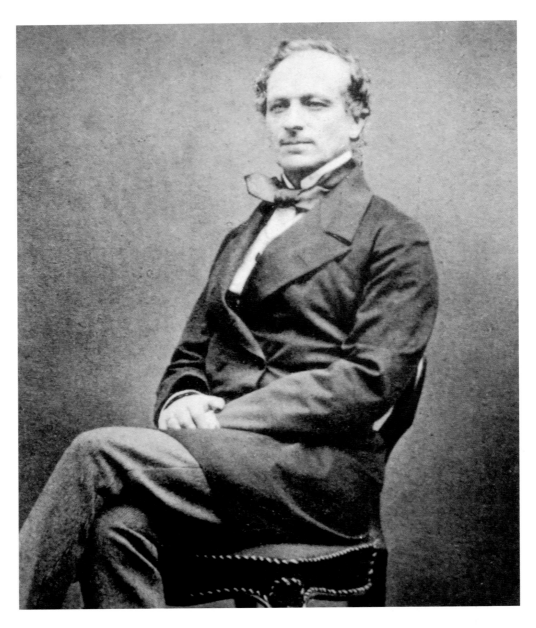

Photograph of Francis Rynd, surgeon to the Meath Hospital, Dublin. Wellcome Collection.

I don't think it justifiable, under such circumstances, to add the risk, slight as it may be, which chloroform produces, to the ordinary risks of labour; but there are many cases, usually termed natural, in which its administration is of great benefit to the

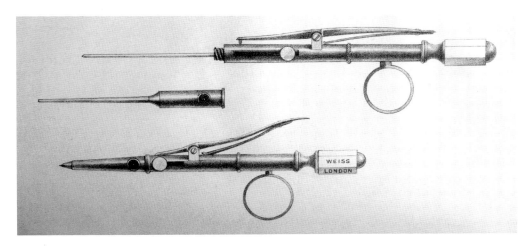

Francis Rynd's hollow-bore device for the subcutaneous introduction of fluid. Dublin Quarterly Journal of Medical Science, *August 1861.*

patient – 1stly, when the dilatation of the os is very painful; and 2ndly, when the latter portion of the second stage is attended with great suffering and excessive uterine action.[5]

Doherty expressed the view that, in the first group, it was not necessary to induce stupor, that small doses of chloroform, usually self-administered using a modified version of Snow's inhaler, were sufficient to render the pain bearable. He believed that when the expulsive stage of labour was attended with agonising and powerful efforts, chloroform offered many benefits. However, in these cases, he found it necessary to carry its effects further and took over administration himself, but still avoided proceeding as far as insensibility if possible.

He wrote that in his experience with chloroform in 150 midwifery patients in what nowadays might be termed 'difficult' labour, there had been no serious after-effects, nor had there been any patients in which the necessity for instrumental delivery could be attributed to the agent's use. On the contrary, he was of the view that some cases would ultimately have become instrumental from exhaustion if the pain of the first stage had not been assuaged by chloroform.

Dr Robert Johns, visiting accoucheur to the Coombe Lying-in Hospital, Dublin had a very different opinion to that of Doherty where the use of chloroform in parturition was concerned: 'I am firmly convinced that chloroform, when inhaled during labour, very fruitfully predisposes to haemorrhage, puerperal inflammation, chest affections, and to other diseases detrimental to health and life, which it aggravates if given during their presence'.[6] He quoted figures from the Coombe and many international sources in support of his argument and also stated that chloroform on occasion caused uterine contractions to be impaired or indeed to cease altogether. He claimed that he was aware of at least two deaths during labour in Scotland that were attributable to the agent but had not been made public. He concluded: 'I think I have now demonstrated that chloroform inhalation is far from being a safe remedy in childbed, and should not then be employed', childbed being an archaic term for childbirth.

The debate filled many journal pages at the time. Among the contributors was, not surprisingly, Kidd himself. He complained that Johns had carefully compiled everything ever alleged *against* chloroform but had not stated what the authors quoted by him (Johns) may have said in favour of it. He claimed, moreover, that on occasion, the Dublin-based writer had referred to views opposing the use of chloroform in midwifery held by certain practitioners some years previously, that these had altered by the time of writing, but that the change of opinion was not reflected in Johns' paper. He also poured scorn on the writer's use of statistics, suggesting that the figures quoted by him were meaningless.[7] Over a year after the publication of Johns' paper, by which time he had died, his claims regarding the use of chloroform in labour were also comprehensively rebutted by Dr Edward Sinclair, vice president of the Royal College of Physicians of Ireland.[8]

The first formal investigation into the safety of an anaesthetic agent was carried out by a committee of the Boston Society for Medical Improvement. The society, a grouping of elite Boston physicians, had been established in 1828 for 'the cultivation of confidence and good feeling between members of the profession, the eliciting and imparting of information upon the different branches of medical science and the establishment of a Museum and Library of Pathological Anatomy'. The committee's report, published in October 1861, was titled 'Report of a Committee of the Boston Society for Medical Improvement, on the Alleged Dangers which Accompany the Inhalation of the Vapor of Sulphuric Ether'.[9]

Its conclusions are abbreviated and paraphrased below:

(i) All anæsthetics are depressing agents. No anæsthetic should be used carelessly, nor can it be administered without risk by an incompetent person.
(ii) It is widely conceded that sulphuric ether is safer than any other anæsthetic.
(iii) Proper precautions being taken, sulphuric ether will produce entire insensibility in all cases, and no anæsthetic requires so few precautions in its use.

THE

BOSTON MEDICAL AND SURGICAL JOURNAL.

VOL. LXV.   THURSDAY, OCTOBER 24, 1861.   No. 12.

REPORT OF A COMMITTEE OF THE BOSTON SOCIETY FOR MEDI-
CAL IMPROVEMENT, ON THE ALLEGED DANGERS WHICH
ACCOMPANY THE INHALATION OF THE VAPOR
OF SULPHURIC ETHER.

[Read before the Boston Society for Medical Improvement, October 14th, 1861, and communicated for the
Boston Medical and Surgical Journal.]

*Report of the
first formal
investigation into
the safety of an
anaesthetic agent.*

(iv) Of the whole number of alleged deaths in the United States and Europe from sulphuric ether anæsthesia (41) there is no case which cannot be explained on some other ground equally plausible, or in which, if it were possible to repeat the experiment, insensibility could not be produced and death avoided. This cannot be said of chloroform.

(v) The advantages of chloroform are exclusively those of convenience.

The *Dublin Medical Press* of 4 December 1861 contained a summary of the Boston report.[10] The author of an accompanying editorial, no doubt cognisant of the fact that the first public demonstration of ether anaesthesia had taken place in Boston and also that the agent remained popular in the northeastern United States, included a comment to the effect that the committee's statements in support of ether sounded more like those of an advocate than the verdict of an impartial jury. However, the writer did also point out that some of the arguments made in the agent's favour were apparently incontrovertible.[11] Coincidentally, there were reports in the same issue of three deaths from chloroform, two in England (both at induction of anaesthesia) and the third in Londonderry (as a result of chloroform abuse).

Following the introduction of general anaesthesia, the number of patients undergoing surgery gradually increased. However, deaths attributed to chloroform had become an increasing cause for concern, particularly as there was no agreement among doctors as to precisely why they occurred. By 1863, it was apparent in the United Kingdom that despite preoperative checks of the

59

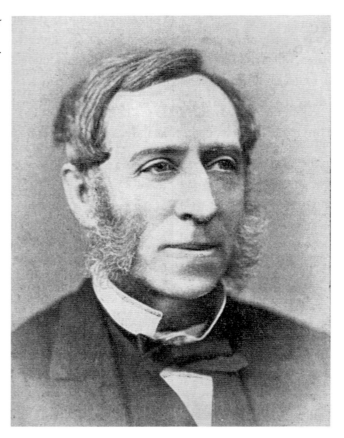

Photograph of Sir Richard Quain (1816 – 98) by G. Jerrard, 1881. Wellcome Collection.

patient's condition and every variation in administration, such fatalities were still occurring with alarming frequency. Early confidence that children were in some way immune had been shattered by a number of sudden deaths that were similar to those in adults.

The medical profession was anxious for official guidance, and London's Royal Medical and Chirurgical Society, later to merge with many other specialist societies to form the Royal Society of Medicine, established a committee whose objects were to inquire into the use of chloroform by inhalation, and its results: (i) in the treatment of internal diseases, such as tetanus, delirium tremens, asthma, epilepsy and infantile convulsions; (ii) in surgical operations and (iii) in obstetric practice, and in particular, 'to give their anxious attention to devise means for obviating such accidents'. The committee membership included some of the most prominent English and Scottish physicians and surgeons of the day and one Irishman, **Dr (later Sir) Richard Quain (1816–1898)**. He was born in Mallow,

County Cork, received his early medical education while apprenticed to a surgeon-apothecary in Limerick and later enrolled in medicine in University College, London from which he graduated with honours in 1840. He became physician to the Brompton Hospital, London in 1855, where he worked for the remainder of his career; he was appointed physician-extraordinary to Queen Victoria in 1890.[12–14]

The committee found that the energy with which chloroform acts and the extent to which it depresses the force of the heart's action rendered it necessary to exercise great caution in its administration and suggested the expediency of searching for other less objectionable anaesthetics. It considered ether to be slow and uncertain in its action, though capable of producing the requisite insensibility, and less dangerous in its operation than chloroform. On the whole, however, it concurred with the general opinion which in the United Kingdom had led to the disuse of ether as an inconvenient anaesthetic when used alone and suggested that it might be preferable to employ it mixed with alcohol and chloroform – the so-called A.C.E. mixture, popular at the time in some parts of continental Europe. In its rules for the administration of chloroform, the committee stated that apparatus was not essential to safety if due care was taken. It considered free admission of air with the anaesthetic to be the one thing necessary, and as long as this was guaranteed, any apparatus could be used.[15] The report, when published, was considered to be a disappointment. It did not provide the degree of clarity for which doctors had hoped, and such suggestions as it did make were immediately challenged by, amongst others, Charles Kidd who, although he had not been a member, had been called in to the committee in an advisory capacity.[11,13]

In April 1863, the *Dublin Medical Press* published a letter from Kidd in which he described what he referred to as 'a most important instance of recovery from chloroform death (so to call it), the first case in which this form and manner of electricity has been used in the human subject'.[16] He was referring to the case of a middle-aged lady who had been undergoing perineal surgery in London. There had been initial difficulty in anaesthetising her, both chloroform and sulphuric ether being used; she was clearly feeling pain when the surgery commenced so that more chloroform was given. Kidd wrote:

> I did not exactly administer the chloroform myself, but in the institution referred to I am accustomed every week to assist other administrators. I watch the pulse and respiration, and general

state of the patient, while the house-surgeon or other gives the chloroform, and thus very great security against accidents is insured.

Half-way through the operation, Kidd noticed that the pulse had stopped:

> A little cold water restored the cardiac action for a minute or two, the sutures were put in but there was no rally of the patient; respiration and pulse were both stopped and the face quickly assumed the ghastly aspect of death. The tongue was drawn forwards and the patient turned on her side to no effect – it seemed that she was dead.

He had always believed that the 'mischief' in chloroform deaths began with the respiratory muscles and not the heart, and that the imperative was to recommence the action of the diaphragm. He wrote that he rushed across the room, seized an electric battery, pulled a pin out of his necktie, stuck it in the patient's sternomastoid, and quickly applied the 'Faradisation' current; the effect was like magic – there was a moan of suffering each time the current was interrupted and completed; the sternomastoid was violently contracted and respiration well-established in about three minutes. Kidd noted that experiments on the lower animals had proven to be most convincing as to the extreme value of Faradisation through the phrenic nerve as it lies in the neck; the other pole being placed under the floating ribs.

Notwithstanding Faradisation and other resuscitative measures, chloroform deaths continued to occur with Dr Benjamin Ward Richardson of London estimating that their incidence at the time was about 1 in 2,500 anaesthetics.[17] However, relatively few reports appeared in Irish publications. The first from Dublin may have been in late 1865 when the *Medical Press* outlined the case of an elderly man who died while undergoing cataract surgery in the Meath Hospital having been:

> placed under the anæsthetic influence by a clinical student … No arcus senilis existed, nor had any morbid sound been detected on auscultation and as he had already twice been placed under the influence without ill effect, the case must be regarded as one of those untoward occurrences against which it is impossible to guard.[18]

Having unqualified persons administer chloroform was a common practice but not one recommended by John Snow. Following a death in St Bartholomew's Hospital, London, where the anaesthetist had been one of the dressers, he had written in 1852 'The office of administering chloroform should no more be delegated to a dresser than the important operations of surgery'. Nor did he think house surgeons were any more suitable, their time in office being too brief for them to have gained adequate experience. He referred in the same paper to two other London hospitals in which experienced doctors had been appointed over the previous two or three years to administer chloroform.[19] It was not until 1886 that a doctor was appointed to a designated anaesthetic post in any hospital on the island of Ireland (see Chapter 8).

Richardson, who had been a friend and biographer of John Snow, introduced an ether spray device operated by a hand pump in 1866. It was relatively simple, and produced a steady flow of compressed air to allow an even spray of atomised ether to be directed from the nozzle onto a small area of skin, where it immediately vaporised. It quickly became popular for minor surgical or dental procedures but had the disadvantage of causing the instruments and skin to become thickly coated with ice, thus rendering surgery more difficult.[20–22] Samuel Little Hardy's Dublin colleagues quickly pointed out that he had devised an anaesthetic spray a number of years earlier, with Dr Glascott Syme, surgeon to Dr Steevens' Hospital, writing:

> Dr Hardy many years ago drew attention to the production of local anæsthesia by means of the vapour of chloroform directed in a fine stream on the part affected. In many cases the result was most satisfactory, as in facial neuralgia and toothache; but gradually this method fell into disuse, probably from too much having been expected from it from the outset.[23]

Shortly afterwards, the editor of the *Dublin Medical Press and Circular* commented:

> The credit of the first suggestion as to the local application of anæsthetic vapour undoubtedly is due to Dr Hardy of Dublin … by the use of which he hoped to obtain a condition of local anæsthesia without the inhalation of ether or chloroform.[24]

Amongst those who corresponded with the publication on the matter was Dr Frank Jeffrey Davys who practised in Swords, County Dublin.[25] Over 100 years later, his grandson Geoffrey Raymond Davys (see Chapter 24) would become the third dean of the Faculty of Anaesthetists, RCSI.

References

1 Gregory R., 'Neuralgia – introduction of fluid to the nerve (by Mr Rynd)', *Dublin Medical Press*, 1845, 13, pp. 167–8.
2 Rynd F., 'Description of an instrument for the subcutaneous introduction of fluids in affections of the nerves', *Dublin Quarterly Journal of Medical Science*, 1861, 32, p. 13.
3 Andrews H., 'Rynd, Francis', in *Dictionary of Irish Biography*, vol. 8, Patterson–Stagg, Cambridge: Royal Irish Academy and Cambridge University Press, 2009, pp. 707–8.
4 Kidd C., 'The ether and chloroform controversy', *Dublin Medical Press* (New Series), 1861, 3, p. 313.
5 Kidd C., 'Chloroform in midwifery', *Dublin Medical Press* (New Series), 1861, 4, pp. 100–1.
6 Johns R., 'Practical observations on the injurious effects of chloroform inhalation during labour', *Dublin Quarterly Journal of Medical Science*, 1863, 35, pp. 353–65.
7 Kidd C., 'On chloroform in midwifery practice', *Dublin Quarterly Journal of Medical Science*, 1864, 37, pp. 319–29.
8 Sinclair E.B., 'Some observations on the administration of the vapour of chloroform in obstetric practice', *Dublin Quarterly Journal of Medical Science*, 1864, 38, pp. 64–84.
9 'Report of a committee of the Boston Society for Medical Improvement on the alleged dangers which accompany the inhalation of the vapour of sulphuric ether', *Boston Medical and Surgical Journal*, 1861, 65, pp. 229–54.
10 'Ether v. Chloroform (Report of a Committee of the Boston Society for Medical Improvement)', *Dublin Medical Press* (New Series), 1861, 4, pp. 400–2.
11 'Editorial. Ether v. Chloroform', *Dublin Medical Press* (New Series), 1861, 4, p. 399.
12 Stratmann L., *Chloroform: The Quest for Oblivion*, Stroud: Sutton Publishing, 2003, p. 90.
13 'The Chloroform Committee', *British Medical Journal*, 1863, i, p. 69.
14 Duncum B.M., *The Development of Inhalation Anaesthesia*, London: Oxford University Press, 1947, p. 253.
15 'Royal Medical and Chirurgical Society: Abstract of the Report of the Committee on Chloroform', *The Lancet*, 1864, 2, pp. 69–72.
16 Kidd C., 'Chloroform deaths – recovery', *Dublin Medical Press* (New Series), 1863, 7, p. 318.
17 Richardson B.W., 'On general an sthesia and anæsthetics', *British Medical Journal*, 1870, 2, p. 356.
18 'Death from chloroform', *Medical Press* (Second Series), 1865, 12, p. 38.
19 Snow J., 'On the administration of chloroform in the public hospitals', *Medical Times*, 1852, 4, pp. 349–50.
20 Richardson B.W., 'On a new and ready mode of producing local anæsthesia', *Medical Times and Gazette*, 1866, 1, pp. 115–7.
21 Duncum, *The Development*, p. 39.

22   Macdonald A.G., 'A short history of fires and explosions caused by anaesthetic agents', *British Journal of Anaesthesia*, 1994, 72, pp. 710–22.
23   Syme G., 'Dr Richardson's new method of producing local anæsthesia', *Medical Press and Circular*, 1866, 1 NS, pp. 218–9.
24   'Editorial. The priority of invention in local anæsthesia', *Medical Press and Circular*, 1866, 1 NS, p. 327.
25   Davys F.J., 'Richardson's ether spray producer', *Medical Press and Circular*, 1866, 1 NS, p. 651.

Chapter 6

The Introduction of Nitrous Oxide Anaesthesia to Britain and Ireland

Declan Warde

Nitrous oxide, which had been almost completely ignored since Horace Wells' failed January 1845 demonstration in Boston, was re-introduced into American dental anaesthetic practice by Gardner Quincy Colton in 1862.[1] According to Colton, this was not of his own volition. When he was in New Britain, Connecticut to give one of his popular exhibitions, a lady asked him whether he would administer the gas to her while a dentist extracted some teeth. This was done successfully and when Colton returned to the city a year later to give another exhibition, he learned that the dentist, Dr Dunham, had in the meantime used the gas with entire success in over 600 patients. Colton and Dunham, along with a Dr Smith, worked together successfully in New Haven, also in Connecticut, for some time, following which Colton relocated to New York. On arrival there, in association with a number of prominent dentists, he opened an office exclusively for the extraction of teeth, which he named the Colton Dental Association. It was soon imitated in other United States cities and the re-introduction of nitrous oxide was complete.[2]

News of the American revival of the use of the gas in dentistry reached England in late 1863. Samuel Lee Rymer, a London dentist, decided to investigate the matter and carried out a short series of experiments at the National Dental Hospital.[3] He wrote afterwards:

> I have been asked whether I think nitrous oxide will produce all the satisfactory results claimed by Dr. Colton. To this question ... I would not venture to hazard a decided opinion. Nevertheless, I may say, that transient anæsthesia may, in almost all cases, be produced safely by the **proper** inhalation of the gas; by which I mean not only the exhibition of pure nitrous oxide, quickly, but the exercise of some discrimination in allowing its exhibition at

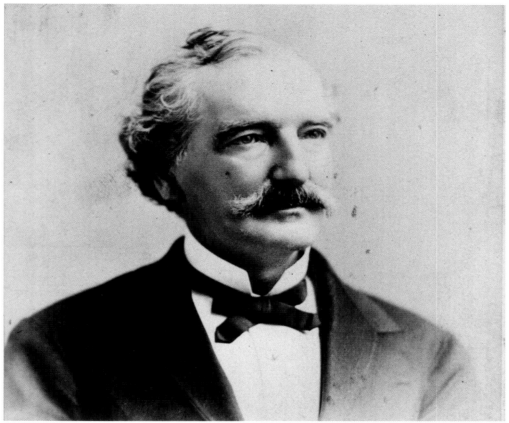

Gardner Quincy Colton 1814 – 98. Photograph by L.C. Perkinson. Courtesy of NIH Digital Collections.

all – thus excluding persons suffering from disease of the vital organs.

He continued:

> Granted that this gas shall be proved generally reliable, what advantages has it ... in Dental Surgery, over chloroform? The reply will be that it has not been found unsafe ... In conclusion I have to add that the uniform success claimed by Dr. Colton is to me a matter of perplexity; for ... I am led to conclude that the action of nitrous oxide varies considerably in different individuals.[4]

Rymer's experiments were not so successful as to induce others to use it and the gas was again forgotten by most practitioners in England.[5,6] They did not, however, escape the attention of Charles Kidd who, in March 1864, wrote to the *Medical Times and Gazette*:

> A great deal has been spoken of and written this year of a new anæsthetic – nitrous oxide – especially among the dentists, where the admirers of balloons and bags for chloroform vapour have been persuaded that this gas is infinitely more safe than chloroform, not one recorded instance of death from the oxide having ever appeared, etc. It is rather clear, I think, that the danger of anæsthetics is pretty much equal for ether, or chloroform, or amylene, or nitrous oxide, or hydrogen, the danger being in the insensibility it produces rather than the agent producing it, the danger being rather in the want of skill in perceiving signs of danger when they come on, and not stopping, than in any fanciful inferiority of this or that anæsthetic to any other. One death has just occurred in a dentist's chair from the administration of nitrous oxide: it was that of a fine young woman, in perfect health, who was induced to have this anæsthetic rather than chloroform.[7]

Kidd did not indicate in which country the alleged death had occurred, nor did he provide any further details.

Colton visited Paris in 1867 and while there, he successfully demonstrated the use of nitrous oxide anaesthesia in dentistry. An American dentist working in the city, Dr T.W. Evans, began to use the gas in his own practice. He travelled to London in March 1868 and gave a series of demonstrations in a number of the city's hospitals.[6] These were attended by leading anaesthetists and dentists, one of whom, Alfred Coleman, later wrote, 'The value of an agent evidently so safe, and so well suited for dental purposes, was only too apparent'. Within a week, Coleman had arranged an apparatus, prepared the gas, and administered it successfully to four patients.[8]

However, opinion in nitrous oxide's favour was far from unanimous. Among those who were yet to be convinced was Benjamin Ward Richardson who, at the time, was president of the Medical Society of London; he commented, at a meeting of the society held shortly after Evans' visit, that the gas had been treated as an unknown, wonderful and perfectly harmless agent whereas, in simple fact, it was one of the best known, least wonderful, and most dangerous of all substances that had been supplied for the production of general anaesthesia.[9] He revised his opinion regarding the safety or otherwise of nitrous oxide shortly afterwards but another assertion of his, that the gas was not a true anaesthetic at all but an asphyxial agent, gained many adherents.[10] Kidd, on the other hand, was more positive than four years earlier:

> ... in this gas (why termed 'laughing' does not well appear) the Dentist has certainly a most extraordinary mode of rendering the Dental patient insensible to the agony of extraction ... That it takes away consciousness of pain is very certain ... The danger or safety of the new nitrous oxide gas depends very much on its modus operandi[11]

Over the following few months, improved and more convenient apparatus for delivery of the gas was devised by both Alfred Coleman and the well-known London anaesthetist **Joseph Thomas Clover (1825–1882)**, while liquid nitrous oxide became available to the medical profession on a large scale. By the end of 1868, the agent was firmly established in place of chloroform for dental work in London and nearly 2,000 successful administrations were reported for the provinces.[12]

The date on which nitrous oxide anaesthesia was first used in Ireland is not known. The earliest report in the Irish medical literature appears to be that contained in a letter written by **Maurice Davies**, a dental surgeon practising in Lower Sackville (now O'Connell) Street, Dublin and published in the *Medical Press and Circular* on 22 December 1869. This was over a year and a half after Evans visited London and referred to the effectiveness of the gas in the provision of anaesthesia for dental surgery. The first sulphuric ether and chloroform anaesthetics in Ireland were administered within two weeks or so of their introduction in England and Scotland respectively; it seems unlikely that nitrous oxide would not also have been employed within a similar timeframe.

Davies wrote concerning the first ten patients, all aged between 19 and 32 years, to whom he had administered the gas prior to extracting teeth. Seven of the procedures were painless, two patients experienced a sensation on dental extraction not amounting to actual pain while one felt the extraction 'in consequence of not being under the influence of the gas'. He described the pulse as accelerated in all at first, and afterwards becoming feeble as the gas took full

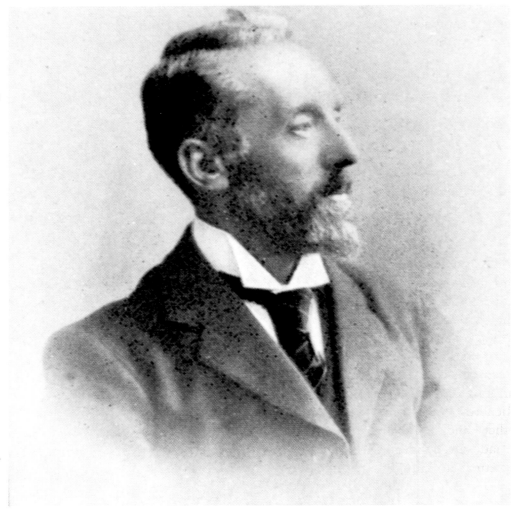

Photograph of Archibald Hamilton Jacob FRCSI, ophthalmologist and editor. Reproduced from Rowlette, R.J. The Medical Press and Circular 1839 – 1939.

effect; two patients showed extreme lividity of features. Recovery was extremely rapid and all were ready to leave the premises within four minutes of the operation being performed. Davies regarded nitrous oxide's advantages as being (i) rapidity of effect, (ii) rapidity of recovery, (iii) fewer disagreeable effects resulting from its administration when compared with other agents and (iv) its tastelessness. Disadvantages were, in some cases, the rapidity of recovery and also the difficulty of preparing and administering it when compared with chloroform.[13]

The editor of the *Medical Press and Circular*, the Dublin-based ophthalmic surgeon **Archibald Hamilton Jacob (1829–1900)**, clearly had some experience, not as positive as that of Davies, of nitrous oxide anaesthesia, for he commented:

> We think it right to say that our experience of nitrous oxide administration by no means confirms that of our correspondent. The anæsthesia is so transitory as to render it unfit for any operation of importance; the appearances of the patients are absolutely frightful and closely resemble those of the last stage of asphyxia, and the agent is by no means free from the objectionable reflex and after-effects of chloroform. The best that can be said of it is that as yet it has not yet been publicly stated to have killed anyone.[13]

Undeterred, Davies continued to advertise painless dentistry facilitated by nitrous oxide in national newspapers; he had begun to do so in late November 1869. Other Irish dentists soon followed his lead, both in using and in advertising their use of the gas and, within a short time, it was being used extensively in dental practice, although apparently not so widely for surgical operations.

Opinions concerning the agent remained polarised at the end of the decade. According to the *Medical Press and Circular* a 'spirited debate' took place at a meeting of the Medical Society of London held in early 1870. Benjamin Ward Richardson still held that nitrous oxide was very unsafe; Charles Kidd, on the other hand, in a complete reversal of his first impressions, stated his belief that it had proved the safest of all anaesthetics, and also that it acted with remarkable quietness in skilful hands.[14]

PAINLESS   DENTISTRY
THE NITROUS OXIDE GAS.
Messrs DAVIES, SURGEON DENTISTS,
10 LOWER SACKVILLE STREET,
(late of 22 North Earl street),
are in daily employment of this most simple, speedy, and successful agent for *Painless Extraction of Teeth*, and all operations pertaining to DENTAL SURGERY.

Advertisement for painless dentistry. Irish Times, *4 March 1870.*

References

1   Duncum B.M., *The Development of Inhalation Anaesthesia*, London: Oxford University Press, 1947, pp. 273–4.
2   Lyman H.M., *Artificial Anæsthesia and Anæsthetics*, New York: Wood, 1881, p. 309.
3   Duncum, *The Development*, p. 277.
4   Rymer S.L., 'Remarks upon the use of nitrous oxide in dental operations', *Dental Review* (NS), 1864, 1, p. 1.
5   Clover J.T., 'On the administration of nitrous oxide', *British Medical Journal*, 1868, 2, pp. 491–2.
6   Duncum, *The Development*, p. 279.
7   Kidd C., 'The new anæsthetic, nitrous oxide', *Medical Times and Gazette*, 1864, 1, p. 301.
8   Coleman A., *Manual of Dental Surgery and Pathology*, London: Smith, Elder, 1881, p. 255.
9   'Medical Annotations. The new anæsthetic (?)', *The Lancet*, 1868, 1, pp. 507–8.
10 Duncum, *The Development*, p. 282.
11 Kidd C., 'Painless dentistry – laughing gas. How does it act?', *British Journal of Dental Science*, 1868, 11, pp. 318–20.
12 Duncum, *The Development*, p. 294.
13 Davies M.L., 'Nitrous oxide as an anæsthetic', *Medical Press and Circular*, 1869, 8 NS, p. 505.
14 'Nitrous oxide gas', *Medical Press and Circular*, 1870, 9 NS, p. 358.

Chapter 7

Ether's Return

Declan Warde

The author of an editorial in the *British Medical Journal* (*BMJ*) of 6 May 1871 wrote:

> It might be well that the less lethal influence of other anæsthetics than chloroform should be more extensively employed. If it be true, as there seems good reason to believe, that ether is by far less dangerous, and that nitrous oxide gas be almost absolutely safe, the sooner our almost absolute preference for chloroform is reconsidered the better. Speaking for ourselves, we should be glad to see chloroform absolutely interdicted in dental practice: we should be glad to see nitrous oxide introduced into every operating-theatre in the limited range (but large number) of rapid procedures for which it is fitted. And we are disposed to ask for a renewed consideration of ether as an anæsthetic, too largely and too rapidly superseded by chloroform for reason of the greater rapidity and convenience of action of the more dangerous agent.[1]

This was the first shot in what was to become an extended campaign by the journal for the reintroduction of ether, but the moment was not right, and few gave it any consideration.[2]

In October of the same year, Dr J. Warrington Haward, surgical registrar and chloroformist to St George's Hospital, London read a paper on 'Ether and chloroform as anæsthetics' at a meeting of the Royal Medical and Chirurgical Society. He had investigated ether as an anaesthetic over the previous year and had concluded that it was to be preferred to chloroform for several reasons. These were that ether was not so marked a cardiac depressant, that it was 'antagonistic to the effects of the shock of an operation', and that it was less likely to induce postoperative sickness.

Haward's conclusions found little support. The president regretted that no notice had been taken of the Society's Chloroform Committee's previous recommendation to use the A.C.E. mixture; Spencer Wells had tried ether but found it very troublesome, while Charles Kidd, who had also tried it, found its use tedious. Nevertheless, he advocated inducing the patient with chloroform and continuing the anaesthesia with ether. Joseph Clover stated that he had been in the habit of giving nitrous oxide first and then ether, as the great difficulty was to get patients to inhale it freely.[3]

Benjamin Joy Jeffries, an ophthalmic surgeon of Boston, Massachusetts travelled to London in August 1872 to attend an ophthalmology conference but also with the intention of spreading information about American methods of etherisation among British chloroformists.

After successful demonstrations by him in a number of London hospitals, some of his English counterparts were persuaded to give ether a trial. A few decided to use the agent for induction of anaesthesia, but then continued with chloroform. Others began by having the patient take a few breaths of chloroform, and then continued with ether. However, as a body, chloroformists were not easily to be transformed into etherists.[4]

On 16 November 1872, however, the British Medical Association, through the *BMJ*, stated that:

> In the face of the great mortality from chloroform, and the almost deathless record of ether, it has become our duty to interpose, to call the urgent attention of professional men throughout the country to the claims which ether has upon their confidence, and to urge that the anæsthetic which was thrust out of repute by the ready and convenient fluid introduced by Simpson, shall have an extended and a fair trial.[5]

The results were immediate. One week later, the journal observed, 'Three weeks ago, the administration of ether was a rare exception; we have reason to believe that it is already becoming the rule ... Thus far only the most favourable reports reach us'.[6] *The Lancet* was sceptical, claiming that Jeffries had said nothing that older doctors had not heard many many times before and had mainly converted the young, to whom 'it was to some extent a novelty, and so attracted'.[7]

Some practitioners wondered why there had been such a sudden and virtually

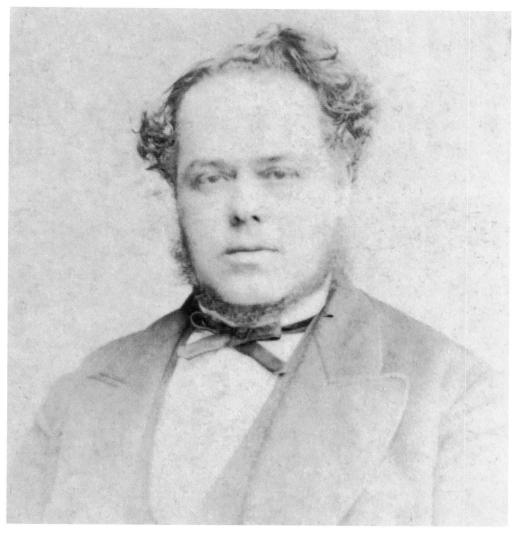

Photograph of Professor John Morgan 1829 – 76. Courtesy of the Royal College of Surgeons in Ireland.

complete replacement of ether by chloroform 25 years earlier, while it was not to be too long before others began to downplay what had always been considered to be the major advance made by James Young Simpson with his introduction of the latter agent: 'It is by no means certain that the vulgarisation of chloroform by the energy of Simpson was not a disadvantage rather than an advantage to humanity; ether being probably the safer and not less efficient anæsthetic'.[8]

John Morgan was born in Dublin in 1829 and became a Licentiate of the Royal College of Surgeons in Ireland (LRCSI) in 1850. He was elected professor of surgical and descriptive anatomy to the college in 1861, having become a fellow four years earlier. He subsequently served on its council and worked as a surgeon in Mercer's and the Westmoreland Lock Hospitals in Dublin.[9]

On 31 July 1872, shortly *before* Jeffries' visit to London, the *Medical Press and Circular* had published the first of four parts of a lengthy paper by Morgan on the theme of 'ether versus chloroform'. The Dublin surgeon began by pointing out that following the introduction of anaesthesia into surgical practice, the great object of producing a temporary state of insensibility had been successfully achieved through the use of ether, chloroform, a mixture of both or nitrous oxide. In Britain and Ireland, chloroform, had 'carried the palm', and had the most extensive use. However, the danger associated with this agent was recognised by the profession and anxiously questioned by the public.

He went on to refer to the Chloroform Committee's report of 1864 and the conclusion formed that 'it would be advantageous to have available an agent which produced the desired insensibility yet was not as dangerous as chloroform.' Ether, to a certain extent, fulfilled these conditions, but its odour was disagreeable, it was slow in operation, and gave rise to greater excitement. Morgan wrote that he had etherised and operated on 30 patients over the previous 10 days with the most satisfactory results, and the most comfortable sense of security. He believed that the triple argument against ether (odour, tediousness and liability to excitement) was insignificant when compared with chloroform's danger to life. He described a limited number of comparative investigations carried out by him with the two agents in rabbits; these had led him to the conclusion that ether was safer, and as efficacious, as chloroform.[10] One week later, Morgan wrote concerning a number of ether anaesthetics in patients in whom he had previously employed chloroform and stated, 'Ether produced incomparably superior results in every way accompanied by a much greater sense of security'. He quoted a number of authorities as to the safety of ether over chloroform and provided statistics from various large hospitals, stating that ether continued to be far more widely used in America. He believed that the arguments in the agent's favour were unanswerable where the great question of danger to life was concerned and that the convenience of chloroform was not a valid excuse for using it. By combining American statistics collected by Dr Edmund Andrews of Chicago, and others from England by Dr Benjamin Ward Richardson of London, it had been calculated that the anaesthetic mortality from chloroform was 1 in 2,873, whereas that from ether was as low as 1 in 23,204. He asked:

Will chloroform maintain its present popularity as an anæsthetic in surgery? We do not believe it will; unless some method other than we have at present, is devised to lessen the risk dependent on its use, we cannot but think its popularity must decline ...

and concluded:

The surgeon who makes use of chloroform will employ an agent not only eight times more dangerous than ether but is actually the most dangerous of the other agents in use. Should he not have put these issues before the patient and should any casualty occur, his responsibility may be indeed brought seriously into question.[11]

In the third part, Morgan commented that the report of the Royal Medical and Surgical and Chirurgical Society had stated:

The essential difference between the action of ether and chloroform is to be found in the effect produced upon the heart. The first operation of both agents is to stimulate the heart and augment the force of its contractions; but after this, chloroform depresses the heart's action, whereas ether appears to exert but little influence upon the muscular movements of that organ.[12]

The committee had investigated the effect of the two agents on the heart using a hemadynamometer, an instrument by which the pressure of the blood in the arteries was measured by the height to which it raised a column of mercury. Morgan wrote that readouts of pulse volume which he had produced using another device, the sphygmograph, which used a system of levers to amplify the radial pulse,

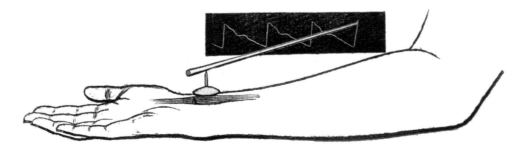

Sphygmograph, as used by John Morgan for observation of pulse writing during ether anaesthesia. Medical Press and Circular, 21 August 1872.

77

confirmed its finding in respect of ether. He stated, 'It is therefore established that while chloroform exerts a depressing influence on the heart, ether exerts a stimulating one; and that chloroform is the most dangerous, while ether is immeasurably the safest of all anæsthetics' while 'the only argument in favour of the use of chloroform is that of its being convenient'. He accepted that one of the objections to the use of ether was its disagreeable odour, but observed, quoting a paper of Henry Napier Draper's published in the previous year that 'this was not sufficient to prevent many from imbibing it for its exhilarating effects'.[13]

Morgan began the final section by stating that he did not believe that there was any real difference in induction time between ether and chloroform, but that even if an extra few minutes were consumed, the safety of etherisation amply counterbalanced the inconvenience. He outlined the diversity of opinion on how inhalational induction of anaesthesia with ether should be conducted, with regard to both the apparatus used and the admission or exclusion of air during the process – he was among those who believed that air should be excluded. He went on to provide brief details but no illustration of the inhaler used by him which, he remarked:

> is constructed so as to collect the ether vapour rapidly and have it inhaled through the flexible tubing which, with the mouthpiece, suits any position of the patient. The respiration is allowed to carry on freely by means of an india-rubber diaphragm at the top of the instrument, which by corresponding with each respiration, is self-accomodating. The internal arrangement is such that ample provision is made for the collection of the ether vapour.[14]

In response to Morgan's paper, Dr Francis Trenar of Omagh, County Tyrone wrote shortly afterwards in the *Medical Press and Circular*:

> I am for more than twenty years apothecary to the Tyrone Infirmary ... and during that time I have had charge of the administration of chloroform to the patient about to be operated on, and I have never had an untoward event or a case to create the slightest alarm while the patients were under its influence.[15]

In late November 1872, the author of an editorial comment in the same publication wrote that the revulsion, as he termed it, that was taking place in

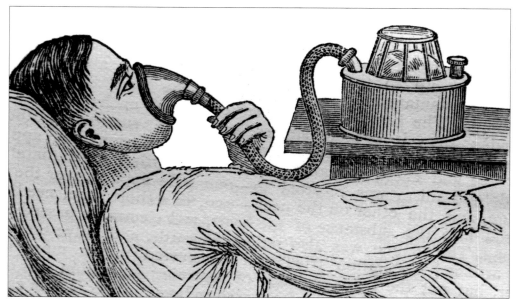

John Morgan's ether inhaler. British Medical Journal, *23 November 1872.*

favour of ether or, at all events, in favour of a safer anaesthetic than chloroform, was remarkable. Believing that the former agent should be in more general use, he urged his professional brethren to closely examine its value by practical experience.[16]

Morgan addressed a meeting of the Surgical Society of Ireland on 29 November 1872. He referred to Morton's 1846 ether demonstration and the fact that the agent had held its ground in America since that year and then remarked that since November 1847, when Simpson introduced chloroform, it was the anaesthetic used by most practitioners in the United Kingdom. He went on to speak of sudden death in the early stages of chloroform anaesthesia and to quote the mortality figures referred to in his paper in the *Medical Press and Circular*. He mentioned the various ways in which he had tried to improve the mode of administering ether and exhibited his inhaler, the principles of which were very simple, namely the exclusion of air and causing the patient to breathe the same vapour over and over again; a patient could be etherised in three minutes. Morgan had used it in a large number of patients, fit and unfit, for a wide range of operations, with few if any ill-effects. He left it to the gentlemen around him to say whether chloroform deserved their confidence, whether ether was not a safer anaesthetic, and whether its difficulties might not be overcome by a simple arrangement such as he had described. He contended that when these conditions were complied with, there would be no excitement, no sickness of stomach, and the patient would come quickly under the influence of the anaesthetic.[17]

Before the end of the year, papers written by Morgan outlining his experience with ether anaesthesia and the advantages of his inhaler had also been published in both the *Dublin Journal of Medical Science* and the *British Medical Journal*. In the former, he wrote:

> In this country, apprehension more or less accompanies the process of chloroformisation; in the smaller operations in surgery it is almost given up; in dentistry, where a safe anæsthetic would be invaluable, it is also almost abandoned ... The struggling or spasm is due to the imperfect modes hitherto pursued in the administration, where a sponge is used, or a cone of paper, or a towel, or, in fact, where air is freely admitted; this, I believe, is a mistake. Air should be more or less perfectly excluded, and the patient be allowed to breathe the ether vapour repeatedly.

He made brief reference to nitrous oxide, commenting that it had gained some support as an anaesthetic and that, like ether, it acted most efficiently when breathed without the admixture of air. He was of the view that the main reason ether fell out of favour in the first place was down to imperfect equipment and technique, rather than being the fault of the agent itself. His *BMJ* paper was written in similar vein and concluded:

> I have used ether in hundreds of cases, and have had no ill effects. The day I etherised six patients in periods varying from three to five minutes, the anæsthesia was in all cases perfect and most satisfactory; the patients sometimes becoming insensible while applying the mouthpiece themselves, while the inhaler gets rid of all the inconveniences that have been found in the rougher and more wasteful method of applying by the sponge or towel.[18,19]

Joseph Clover of London was among those to try Morgan's inhaler; he found it to be effective and economical but felt that those patients who used it complained more of headache afterwards.[20]

On 1 January 1873, the *Medical Press and Circular* reported that Morgan's address at the 29 November meeting of the Surgical Society of Ireland had attracted unusual interest and that a special committee of the society had, as a result, been appointed to investigate the relative merits of both ether and chloroform and to scrutinise the results of their administration in Dublin.[21]

The first few months of the year also saw the appearance of Charles Kidd's final submissions, of which there had been a very great number over the years, to this and other publications. His opinion regarding the safety of nitrous oxide had changed again in that he now considered it to be not quite as safe as he had previously believed, especially when administered by unskilled practitioners such as dentists' assistants.[22]

What was clearly intended to be a preliminary report of the Ether and Chloroform Committee of the Surgical Society of Ireland was published at the end of May. Details of 226 anaesthetics (217 ether, 9 chloroform) administered in either one of eight Dublin hospitals or 'in private' were included. In those patients in whom ether was used, patient age ranged from 3 to 74 years, anaesthesia induction time from 2 to 14 minutes and duration of anaesthesia from 2 to 80 minutes. Vomiting occurred in 11 of 210 patients in whom Morgan's inhaler was employed, and in 3 of 7 where an India-rubber bag over the face was used. In no case was there any report of apprehension or danger to life. Three of the nine patients to whom chloroform was administered vomited while a fourth became very weak and caused great concern to those present.[23] The Medical Press and Circular commented that the results to date seemed greatly in favour of ether.[24] No final report of the committee has been located at the time of writing.

John Morgan died of peritonitis, probably secondary to typhoid fever, in March 1876. An obituarist wrote:

> His labours in the investigation of anæsthetics are well known, and he is entitled to the credit of having reintroduced the use of ether to Irish surgery. By the inhaler which bears his name he placed at the disposal of the profession the only satisfactory means of administering that anæsthetic, and by the influence of his writings and example he succeeded in great measure in banishing chloroform from a place in Irish surgery.[25]

He hadn't, however, been the only Dublin doctor to invent an ether inhaler in the early 1870s. Surgeon to the Adelaide Hospital, **Benjamin Wills Richardson (1819–1883)**, who was also an early Dublin microscopist and who should not be

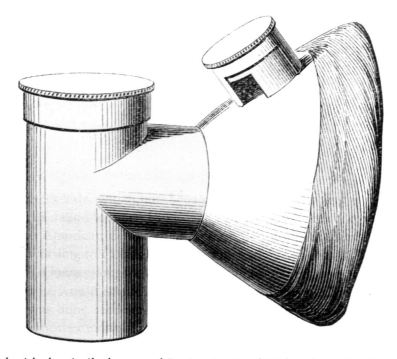

confused with the similarly named Benjamin Ward Richardson, London physician, thought it advisable 'to have constructed a simple and moderate-priced inhaler for etherisation in hospital practice' and also proposed what would have been a prospective, matched study of ether and chloroform anaesthesia. His inhaler incorporated a sliding or rotating cap in order to regulate the admission of air, which Richardson, unlike Morgan, favoured during induction of anaesthesia. He commented in passing reference to a recent case in which a solicitor acting for the family of a patient who had died in a Dublin hospital 'under the administration of chloroform' had made application to the police-court for a summons against the doctor for the incautious use of the anaesthetic agent: 'in the present medico-legal aspect of the relative safety of ether over chloroform for the production of anæsthesia, it would not, perhaps, be injudicious, upon the part of the administrator, to permit the patient to select the anæsthetic'.[26]

The only inquiry of the time designed to compare and contrast the usage of different anaesthetic agents in Britain and Ireland was carried out by **Henry MacNaughton-Jones (1844–1918)**. Born in Cork city, he received his medical education at Queen's College Cork (now University College Cork), graduating in 1864. He was to become a major figure in the development of medicine in

Cork, not least because of his role in the foundation of various hospitals in the city. He founded the Cork Eye, Ear and Throat Hospital in 1868 and four years later, was co-founder of the Cork Maternity Hospital on Nile Street which was established to provide free care to pregnant women in their homes and to educate nurses. He later became professor of midwifery in Queen's College, and in 1881, examiner in the same subject at the Royal University of Ireland. For 11 years, he acted as physician to the Cork Fever Hospital, and for a good period, he was surgeon to the South Infirmary. He was also co-founder of the County and City of Cork Hospital for the Diseases of Women and

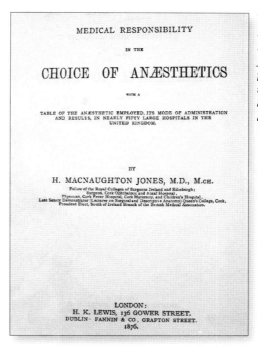

MEDICAL RESPONSIBILITY

IN THE

CHOICE OF ANÆSTHETICS

WITH A

TABLE OF THE ANÆSTHETIC EMPLOYED, ITS MODE OF ADMINISTRATION AND RESULTS, IN NEARLY FIFTY LARGE HOSPITALS IN THE UNITED KINGDOM.

BY

H. MACNAUGHTON JONES, M.D., M.CH.

Fellow of the Royal Colleges of Surgeons Ireland and Edinburgh;
Surgeon, Cork Ophthalmic and Aural Hospital;
Physician, Cork Fever Hospital, Cork Maternity, and Children's Hospital,
Late Senior Demonstrator (Lecturer on Surgical and Descriptive Anatomy) Queen's College, Cork,
President Elect, South of Ireland Branch of the British Medical Association.

LONDON:
H. K. LEWIS, 136 GOWER STREET.
DUBLIN · FANNIN & CO., GRAFTON STREET.
1876.

Title page of Dr Henry MacNaughton-Jones' 1876 pamphlet on the use of various anaesthetic agents in the United Kingdom.

Children on Union Quay, which was renamed the Victoria Hospital in 1901.[27,28]

MacNaughton-Jones addressed a meeting of the County and City of Cork Medico-Chirurgical Society held on 22 December 1876. In his paper, which was later published as a pamphlet, he indicated that cognisant of the ongoing debate concerning the relative safety of the two most commonly used anaesthetic agents, he had contacted many of the larger hospitals in the United Kingdom regarding the usage of such drugs therein. He had received 42 replies, 14 from Irish hospitals (all but one of which were in Dublin, the exception being Belfast Royal Hospital, now the Royal Victoria Hospital), and 28 from Great Britain.[29] The responses revealed that there was no great difference between hospitals on the two sides of the Irish Sea in terms of the anaesthetic agents generally employed – despite the upsurge of interest in ether, chloroform was still slightly more popular overall although anaesthetists in many hospitals were using both (Table 1). From some centres, the respondents, usually either surgeons or house surgeons, indicated that ether had just recently been introduced in their institutions. There was some regional variation in agent usage in Great Britain; replies were received from four Scottish hospitals and, perhaps not surprisingly, chloroform continued to be used exclusively in all. It is clear from the brief 'remarks' received from Dublin practitioners (Table 2) that chloroform was considered easier to use than ether and also that a variety of modes of administration were employed. Of interest, the respondent from the Royal Belfast Hospital indicated that chloroform, administered on a sponge, had been given there on more than 5,000 occasions with 'not one death'. MacNaughton-Jones commented that he was aware that, up to that time, chloroform was the agent that had generally been employed in Cork. He stated, however, that he had decided, quite recently, to use ether exclusively henceforth, whenever it 'could be availed of'.[29]

Table 1. Anaesthetic agents used in certain United Kingdom hospitals, 1876 (MacNaughton-Jones)

Agent(s) Used	Ireland	Great Britain
Ether	3	7
Chloroform	5	9
Both ether and chloroform	5	8
Nitrous oxide/ether sequence	0	2
Chloroform, also a mixture of ether, chloroform and rectified spirit	0	1
Mixture of ether, chloroform and rectified spirit	1	0
Bichloride of methylene	0	1
Hospitals	14	28

Joseph Clover had introduced his apparatus for administering chloroform, the 'chloroform bag', in 1862. It was too clumsy to be adopted for general use and the mere sight of it was known to appal nervous patients.[30] He devised an ether inhaler some 11 years later; this was followed in 1874 by the first of a series for use in a nitrous oxide-ether sequence, claiming the advantages of rapid response, regulated control of anaesthetic concentration and greater economic value. His portable regulating ether inhaler was first described by him in January 1877.[31–33]

Lambert Hepenstal Ormsby (1849–1923) was born to Irish parents in Auckland, New Zealand; the family returned to Ireland shortly afterwards. He was apprenticed to George Porter, surgeon to the Meath Hospital, Dublin at a young age and qualified as a licentiate of the Royal College of Surgeons in Ireland

Table 2. Anaesthetic agents used and remarks from Dublin hospitals and Belfast Royal Hospital 1876 (MacNaughton-Jones)

Hospital	Agent(s) Used	Remarks
Adelaide	Ether by Richardson's apparatus, also chloroform administered on lint	Both satisfactory
Belfast Royal	Chloroform	Given over 5000 times, not one death; administered on a sponge
City of Dublin	Anhydrous ether	Partially satisfactory, objection to slowness of action and sick stomach which ensues; Richardson's apparatus used
Dr Steevens'	(a) Chloroform; (b) ether principally used; (c) mixture of chloroform and rectified spirit	(a) Most satisfactory, especially with children; (b) generally satisfactory, but the patients troublesome; (c) data not sufficient to give opinion
Dublin Eye and Ear Infirmary	Chloroform	Perfect satisfaction if properly administered; air must be altogether excluded if possible, Morgan's inhaler alone effects this purpose; the ether must be the best and the patient's stomach empty
Jervis Street	Chloroform	Perfect in its results, administered with a plain wire framed inhaler with free admission of air
Mater Misericordiae	Ether	Satisfactory, several inhalers, sub-judice
Meath	Chloroform, sometimes ether	Both satisfactory
Mercer's	Chloroform	Satisfactory
National Eye and Ear Infirmary	Ether generally, chloroform sometimes	Satisfactory, except for the length of time in putting the patient under its influence, and sick stomach ensuing; Richardson's apparatus used, requires too much ether and does not sufficiently exclude the air; anæsthetics not much used; no anæsthetic for cataract or iridectomy; only used for such operations as enucleation, plastic, or painful or protracted ones
Richmond	Chloroform; ether lately introduced	Not capable as yet of forming an opinion on ether
St Mark's Ophthalmic	Chloroform	Satisfactory
St Vincent's	Ether; chloroform administered only in exceptional cases	Properly administered, quick, and satisfactory, if not so, tedious and may fail altogether; a large quantity of the vapour given at once
Sir Patrick Dun's	Chloroform	Most satisfactory; Skinner's inhaler and a dropping bottle used

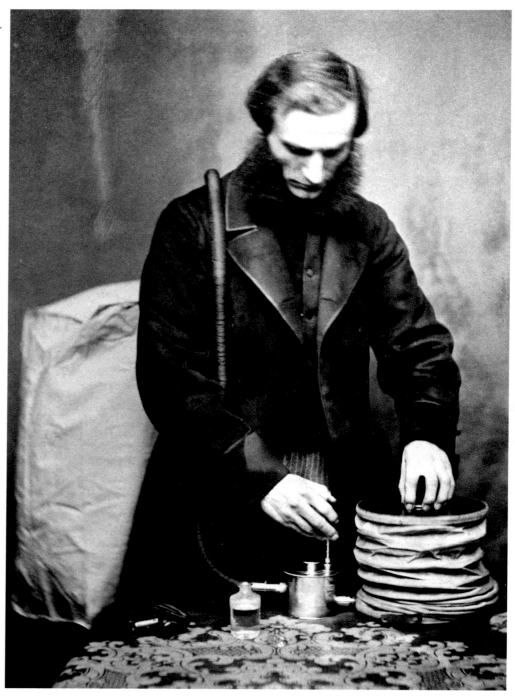

Photograph of Dr Joseph Clover and his chloroform apparatus, which could also be used for nitrous oxide administration. Courtesy of the Anaesthesia Heritage Centre.

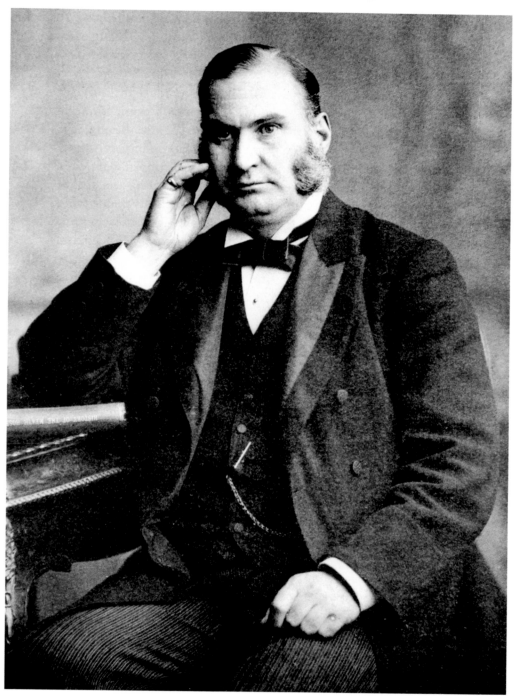

Photograph of Sir Lambert Hepenstal Ormsby, surgeon to the Meath Hospital, Dublin and inventor of Ormsby's ether inhaler. Reproduced from Ormsby L.H. Medical History of the Meath Hospital and County Dublin Infirmary, Fannin, 1888.

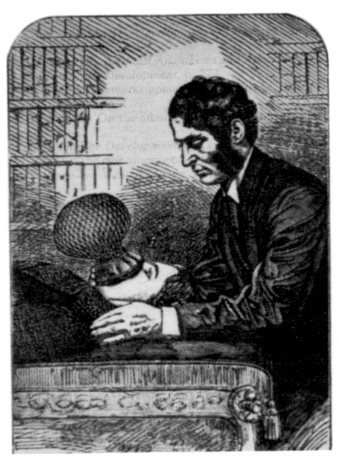

Ormsby's portable ether inhaler, 1877, the bag covered with netting to prevent over-expansion during expiration. Wellcome Collection.

(RCSI) and of the King and Queen's College of Physicians in Ireland (KQCPI) in 1869. He was elected to the post of surgeon in the Meath three years later and subsequently gained degrees in arts and medicine from Trinity College Dublin and also the RCSI fellowship in surgery (FRCSI).[34,35] His MD award from Trinity in 1879 was for a thesis on the subject of anaesthesia.

Just three weeks after the initial description of Clover's portable ether inhaler was published, a letter from Ormsby recounting details of a new portable inhaler of his own appeared in *The Lancet*. He wrote, 'For the last nine months I have been using an ether inhaler which I am now desirous of introducing to the profession'. His device consisted of (i) an india-rubber bag, covered with netting in order to prevent undue expansion during expiration, (ii) a soft metallic face-piece lined with rubber so that it would fit more closely and (iii) a valve, to either admit air or allow it to escape if necessary. In the body of the inhaler there was a cone-shaped wire cage, into which fitted a similarly shaped hollow sponge into which the ether was poured, the inhaler then being ready for use. Further ether could be added if required without raising the face-piece from the face. The advantages claimed by Ormsby for his new apparatus included that it was simple in construction and application, inexpensive and portable, prevented undue loss or evaporation of ether vapour, and provided great safety for the patient during ether administration. He stated that he had used it in patients of all ages and both sexes, in nearly all the usual operations in surgery, and had received testimonials in its favour from many of Dublin's leading surgeons.[36]

Ormsby's inhaler achieved more immediate popularity than Clover's, possibly because Clover was not himself particularly enamoured of his own model, preferring his gas-ether apparatus. Nevertheless, it is by the portable regulating ether inhaler that he is chiefly remembered.[37,38] Writing in June 1877, Ormsby was able to say, 'I have been informed by Messrs. Coxeter & Son ... that many of the leading hospitals in London, Dublin, and the provincial towns of England, including those of Manchester, Birmingham, Leeds and Liverpool, are using the ether inhaler suggested by me'.[39]

Sixteen years later, Frederic Hewitt, probably the leading London anaesthetist of the day, compared the two:

> For inducing anæsthesia by means of ether there is no apparatus which can compare with that invented by Clover, for the anæsthetic vapour may be admitted so gradually that the initial discomforts are reduced to a minimum. But for maintaining ether anæsthesia, Ormsby's inhaler is equal, and in many cases superior to Clover's. I have on several occasions changed from Clover's to an Ormsby's inhaler with marked improvement in the symptoms of the patient. For example, I have often known cyanosis to quickly vanish and the breathing to become less hampered by effecting this change of inhalers during deep ether anæsthesia.[40]

Hewitt actually used his own modification of Ormsby's inhaler. It was designed to prevent the temperature of the sponge becoming too low during administration – this had always been an objection to the device.[41]

In 1876, Ormsby had established the National Orthopaedic and Children's Hospital, a forerunner of the National Children's Hospital, Harcourt Street, Dublin where he was senior surgeon. He was particularly interested in advancing the nursing profession and was involved in various charitable and other publicly-spirited activities. However, he was also arrogant, outspoken on a number of issues and completely oblivious to any offence caused. Notwithstanding his undoubted unpopularity in some quarters, he became president of RCSI serving from 1902–4.[34]

The metallic inhaler introduced by Benjamin Wills Richardson in 1873 had never become popular. The inventor himself admitted that it was rather expensive and he later devised one made of rubber which he wrote 'works efficiently, economises ether, and may be purchased for a few shillings' and which, at the time of writing (1880), had been used for several months in almost every operative case in the Adelaide Hospital. He stated that he had, by then, ceased using chloroform and that it was a matter of surprise to him that its use was not more limited.[42]

References

1   'Editorial. Deaths from anæsthetics', *British Medical Journal*, 1871, 1, p. 480.
2   Stratmann L., *Chloroform: The Quest for Oblivion*, Stroud: Sutton Publishing 2003, p. 145.
3   'Report of the Royal Medical and Chirurgical Society meeting of October 24th 1871', *Medical Times and Gazette*, 1871, 2, pp. 603–4.
4   Duncum B.M., *The Development of Inhalation Anaesthesia*, London: Oxford University Press, 1947, pp. 311–5.
5   'Editorial. The administration of ether as an anæsthetic in Great Britain', *British Medical Journal*, 1872, 2, pp. 554–6.
6   'Anonymous, 'Ether as an anæsthetic', *British Medical Journal*, 1872, 2, p. 583.
7   'Special report on anæsthetics and anæsthesia', *The Lancet*, 1872, 2, pp. 722–4.
8   'Anonymous, 'The discovery of the anæsthetic powers of chloroform', *British Medical Journal*, 1879, 1, p. 880.
9   Cameron C.A., *History of the Royal College of Surgeons in Ireland, and of the Irish Schools of Medicine: Including a Medical Bibliography and a Medical Biography*, 2nd Edition, Dublin: Fannin, 1916, pp. 629–30.
10 Morgan J., 'Ether versus chloroform. On the use of ether as an anæsthetic in surgical operations; as a safer and more efficacious agent than chloroform in producing the avoidance of pain, with a description of an inhaler, and the mode of administration', *Medical Press and Circular*, 1872, 14 NS, pp. 81–4.
11 *Ibid.*, pp. 104–6.
12 *Ibid.*, pp. 145–7.
13 Draper H.N., 'On the use of ether as an intoxicant in the north of Ireland', *Medical Press and Circular*, 1870, 9 NS, pp. 117–8.
14 Morgan, 'Ether versus chloroform', pp. 165–7.
15 Trenar F., 'Chloroform and its waning popularity', *Medical Press and Circular*, 1872, 14 NS, p. 380.
16 'Editorial. The ether question and the anæsthetic controversy', *Medical Press and Circular*, 1872, 14 NS, pp. 463–4.
17 'Surgical Society of Ireland', *Medical Press and Circular* 1872, 14 NS, pp. 549–52.
18 Morgan J., 'The dangers of chloroform and the safety of ether as a means of producing insensibility to pain', *Dublin Journal of Medical Science*, 1872, 54, pp. 360–8.
19 Morgan J., 'The administration of ether, and its superiority to chloroform as an anæsthetic agent', *British Medical Journal*, 1872, 2, p. 575.
20 Clover J.T., 'Remarks on the production of sleep during surgical operations', *British Medical Journal*, 1874, 1, pp. 200–3.

21 'Ether', *Medical Press and Circular*, 1873, 15 NS, p. 10.
22 Kidd C., 'Nitrous oxide deaths', *Medical Press and Circular*, 1873, 15 NS, p. 218.
23 'The Dublin Ether and Chloroform Report', *Medical Press and Circular* 1873, 15 NS, p. 469.
24 'The anæsthetic controversy', *Medical Press and Circular*, 1873, 15 NS, p. 497.
25 'Obituary. John Morgan FRCSI', *Medical Press and Circular*, 1876, 21 NS, p. 209.
26 Richardson B.W., 'Description and illustration of an ether inhaler for the inhalation of ether as an anæsthetic, with a few observations upon a mixture of chloroform and spirit of wine for producing anæsthesia', *Dublin Journal of Medical Science*, 1873, 55, pp. 227–9.
27 McCarthy K., 'One of Cork's medical pioneers', *Cork Independent*, available at www.corkindependent.com/weekly/ourcityyourtown/articles/2018/05/02/ 4155530-one-of-corks-medical-pioneers/ (accessed 1 November 2020).
28 'Obituary. Henry MacNaughton-Jones, M.D., M.Ch., M.A.O., F.R.C.S.I. and Edin.', *British Medical Journal*, 1918, 1, pp. 521–2.
29 MacNaughton-Jones H., *Medical Responsibility in the Choice of Anæsthetics with a Table of the Anæsthetic Employed, its Mode of Administration and Results, in nearly Fifty Large Hospitals in the United Kingdom*, London: Lewis, 1876.
30 Duncum, *The Development*, p. 244.
31 *Ibid.*, p. 323.
32 Maltby J.R., 'Joseph Clover Lecture: Joseph Thomas Clover 1825–1882' in J.R. Maltby (ed.), *Notable Names in Anaesthesia*, London: Royal Society of Medicine, 2002, pp. 39–42.
33 Clover J.T., 'Portable regulating ether inhaler', *British Medical Journal*, 1877, 1, pp. 69–70.
34 O'Donnell B., 'Ormsby, Sir Lambert Hepenstal PRCSI 1902–1904' in B. O'Donnell (ed.), *Irish Surgery and Surgeons in the Twentieth Century*, Dublin: Gill & MacMillan, 2008, p. 293.
35 'Sir Lambert Hepenstal Ormsby (1849–1923)' in *Dictionary of Ulster Biography*, available at newulsterbiography.co.uk/index.php/home/viewPerson/2149 (accessed 31 October 2020).
36 Ormsby L.H., 'A new ether inhaler', *The Lancet*, 1877, 1, p. 218.
37 Bryn Thomas K., *The Development of Anaesthetic Apparatus*, London: Blackwell, 1975, p. 8.
38 Duncum, *The Development*, p. 350.
39 Ormsby L.H., 'Ether inhalation', *The Lancet*, 1877, 1, p. 863.
40 Hewitt F.W., *Anæsthetics and their administration*, London: Griffin, 1893, pp. 150–1.
41 Duncum, *The Development*, p. 352.
42 Richardson B.W., 'Description of an india-rubber inhaler for ether anæsthesia', *Medical Press and Circular*, 1880, 30 NS, p. 6.

Chapter 8

From Cork to Hyderabad

Declan Warde

From 1847, when anaesthesia in Ireland and elsewhere was in its infancy, the country's obstetricians had written regularly on the subject. Little had changed as the penultimate decade of the nineteenth century dawned. The *Dublin Journal of Medical Science* issues of February, March and April 1881 contained a lengthy paper divided into three parts and pertaining to anaesthesia, written by Henry MacNaughton-Jones, who was now professor of midwifery at Queen's College Cork.

Over the series as a whole, MacNaughton-Jones provided both a comprehensive history of the early attempts at anaesthesia up to the time of Morton's 1846 demonstration in Boston and a detailed review of the anaesthesia literature from both sides of the Atlantic at the time of writing. He recounted his own extensive experience and offered his personal opinion on various anaesthetic agents and techniques. Apart from historical aspects, the first part dealt in detail with nitrous oxide and its use, and concluded with advice on the management of what he termed asphyxia during anaesthesia, laying particular emphasis on elevation of the lower jaw and drawing the tongue forwards with forceps.[1]

He began the second part by impressing upon readers the desirability of using anaesthesia for even what might be regarded as trivial operations, many of which can be exceedingly painful. However, he also commented that some patients bear pain much better than others, suffer less shock, and under such circumstances, especially when they did not wish for anaesthesia, it was better not to press its use. On the other hand, he believed that anaesthesia was indicated when muscle relaxation was required, and in delicate manipulations and critical operations, even when not very painful.

MacNaughton-Jones continued by addressing in detail the opinions of several authors on the question of sudden death under chloroform, and concluded that in the majority of cases, the cause of death was syncope – stoppage of the heart, sudden and often impossible to foresee. He stated that the first fatality in Cork had been in one of his own patients and wrote a lengthy account of the event:

It might appear strange that the first death from chloroform that occurred in this city should have been in a patient of our own ... In February 1880 a patient, aged fifty, was admitted to the South Infirmary with a luxation of the femur into the sciatic notch. The accident had occurred some weeks previously and attempts had been made thrice under chloroform to reduce the dislocation unsuccessfully. We determined to attempt reduction by manipulation under an anæsthetic. We had not given chloroform for a few years in any case, save to children and in some operative obstetric cases. We somehow had the idea that we should have a better chance of reduction under chloroform than with ether ... Some fresh chloroform (Duncan & Flockhart's) was obtained. The man's heart was examined previous to administration, and nothing detected abnormal. A few of the ribs were injured – one broken – by the injury, but the lung was not affected; otherwise he appeared a strong healthy man. The resident-surgeon proceeded to give the chloroform ... on a folded piece of lint ... The pulse was felt at either side by two medical friends present. A little over a drachm was given, when he appeared to pass rapidly under the chloroform, having addressed some remarks a minute before to the resident. We turned aside to take off our cuffs, up to this point watching the countenance of the patient, and we then went to the limb – Dr Sandiford, who was administering the chloroform, saying that he was now ready. Just as we took the limb in our hands, Dr Atkins, who had his hand on the pulse, noticed it fail, and the chloroform was withdrawn. On glancing at the man's face we saw that a death-like pallor overspread it, and that his appearance was most alarming. We at once went to his chin, drawing it well up, and had the body inverted. The pupils were greatly contracted. After a short time he gave a few gasps, Sylvester's method of respiration being practised at the same time. In the meantime a strong battery was brought. The pupils changed and we hoped that he was coming

SAFETY AS WE WATCH

to. Warmth was applied to the body and mustard to the heart, but again he relapsed; and, despite of reinversion, faradisation in the course of the pneumogastric and over the heart, with continued artificial respiration, he sank. The coroner unfortunately had no post mortem. This, after a constant administration of anæsthetics for fourteen years, was the only fatal accident we have seen … From that day to the present we have not given chloroform to an adult, though we have chloramyle and bichloride of methylene; we invariably employ ether. From henceforth we intend to use the combined method of Clover.[1]

In the third part, MacNaughton-Jones wrote on methods that had been used up to that time to produce local anaesthesia including cold, ice and electricity. While mentioning Samuel Little Hardy's work, he regarded Benjamin Ward Richardson as being the modern scientist to whom humanity was most indebted for his experiments with ether and the production of a freezing jet six degrees below zero; he stated that the latter's spray was widely used in cases of abscess, fistula and haemorrhoids. He believed that local anaesthesia should be more frequently resorted to than was generally the case, particularly in cases not suitable for general anaesthesia. Dealing with the medicolegal aspects of anaesthesia he was, like John Snow a number of years before, unequivocal in his view that valuable lives should not be placed in the hands of uninformed individuals: 'skill, judgement, discretion, experience – all are required in the administration of anæsthetics'. He concluded with a discussion of various inhalers in use at the time, including those of Morgan: 'We have administered ether several hundreds of times with Morgan's inhaler. We must say that it gave us every satisfaction' and Ormsby: 'It has given satisfaction but we prefer the others described', and also those of Snow and Joseph Clover.[1]

MacNaughton-Jones' failure to gain the chair of either Materia Medica (1875) or of Surgery (1880) at Queen's College may have precipitated the Cork doctor's move in 1883 to Harley Street, London.[2] He maintained a deep interest in his native city, founding the Old Corkonians Graduate Club (1905) in London. He made clear his own objections and those of the club to the change of name from Queen's College Cork to University College Cork in 1908. He was thrice president of the Irish Medical Schools Graduates Association, twice president of the British Gynaecological Society, and also president of the Obstetrics and

Gynaecology Section of the Royal Society of Medicine. In addition to his publications on anaesthesia and those on midwifery, a subject on which he was an acknowledged expert, he was the author of a number of medical books and scientific papers on a variety of other subjects including ophthalmology, surgery and, in particular, otology. He died in London on 26 April 1918.[1] Two years prior to his death, he endowed a prize to provide a gold medal in Obstetrics and Gynaecology, awarded to this day to the student who obtains the highest mark in the subject in the final-year RCSI examinations.

MacNaughton-Jones' Dublin colleague Lambert Ormsby had retained his interest in anaesthesia and in 1885, wrote:

> all anæsthetics are dangerous, and will induce death if pushed too far; but of all anæsthetics I believe ether, properly and judiciously administered, to be the safest of all, for ether will neither produce syncope nor failure of the heart's action, no matter how much is given; but it will produce asphyxia or a failure of respiratory action; but as this is a very slow process compared to the former, time and warning is given to the anæsthetist to anticipate and prevent any untoward result, whereas syncope comes on and ends so rapidly that no time whatever is given'.

He suggested:

> That all anæsthetists should understand the properties and dangerous effects of each anæsthetic administered,
> That all administrators should be qualified physicians or surgeons and that they should carefully understand the process and degrees of anæsthesia before undertaking the very solemn duty of placing a human being into the mysterious sleep of insensibility,
> That previous to any anæsthetic being administered, a careful and thorough examination of the thoracic cavity be made, so as to detect before it is too late any bronchitis or other pulmonary affection, and
> That the administration of ether or any other anæsthetic should not be prolonged beyond the actual time required for the performance of any surgical operation …[3]

However, apothecaries and others who were not medically qualified continued to provide anaesthesia, as evidenced by an extract from the minutes of a November 1886 meeting of the Medical Board of the Mater Misericordiae Hospital in Dublin:

> The following resolution was proposed by Mr Chance, seconded by Mr Lentaigne and passed:
> That patients about to be operated on should, if it is thought desirable, be anæsthetised before being carried into the operating theatre, and that in order to carry out this arrangement a room close to the theatre should be provided with a second operating table where the apothecary with assistants could administer ether.[4]

Change was on the way and before the end of the year, **Dr Paul Piel (*c.* 1851–1924)** (see Chapter 24) was appointed to administer anaesthetics on two mornings per week in the Adelaide Hospital, Dublin, thereby becoming the first doctor to be employed in a designated anaesthetic post in Ireland.[5] He appears to have mainly used ether given by Clover's inhaler, but he occasionally commenced anaesthesia with chloroform or nitrous oxide in order to provide a more pleasant and smoother induction.[6] While the latter agent had by then been used successfully by the country's dentists for over 20 years, it seems that its employment in hospital practice remained quite limited.

Three years after Henry MacNaughton-Jones suggested that local techniques should be used more widely, **Carl Koller (1857–1944)** of Vienna discovered the local anaesthetic properties of cocaine on the eye. Unable to afford the train fare to attend the gathering himself, his findings were first presented by one of his colleagues at a meeting of the German Ophthalmological Society in Heidelberg on 15 September 1884; it was not long before the drug's use in surgery was widely adopted.[7,8] Upon learning of the paper presented in Germany, **Arthur Benson (1852–1912)**, a surgeon at St Mark's Hospital in Dublin, ordered some hydrochlorate of cocaine and carried out experiments with it on a patient, a medical colleague and himself. The initial results were disappointing. However, it transpired that the cocaine he had used had been contaminated with the parasympathomimetic alkaloid eserine and subsequent experiments with a new supply were far more satisfactory – he found that repeated applications of a 2 per cent solution produced almost total corneal and conjunctival anaesthesia in two to three minutes. He successfully used the technique for removal of corneal

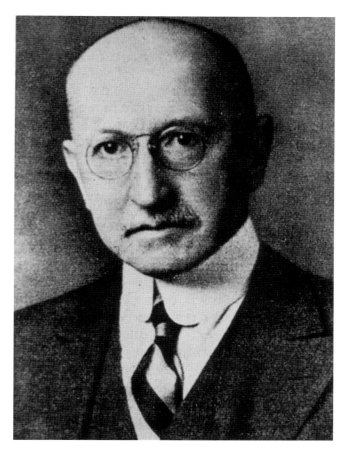

Photograph of Dr Carl Koller, Austrian ophthalmologist who was first to use cocaine as a local anaesthetic for eye surgery. Wellcome Collection.

foreign bodies, iridectomy, cataract extraction and also in removing a large polyp growing from the middle ear. Benson presented his findings on 11 December 1884 at a meeting of the Ophthalmological Society of the United Kingdom, expressing the view that cocaine would ultimately prove to be one of the most valuable drugs ever discovered.[9]

The first report from Ireland of surgery following the injection of a local anaesthetic agent was written by the Dublin surgeon **George Mahood Foy (1843–1934)** (see Chapter 24). The patient, a man aged 30 years, underwent excision of a tumour situated below the angle of the left scapula and fixed deeply. He did not feel the incision, but experienced pain when fibrous bands attaching it to the thoracic parietes were divided, and also while the wound was being sutured. The injections of cocaine were given by **Dr Ephraim MacDowel Cosgrave (1853–1925)**, future president of the Royal College of Physicians of Ireland (1914–16).

Foy wrote, 'Except for superficial incisions, the drug will probably not be much used in general surgery. Its depressing action on the heart and its tendency to render respiration irregular and shallow prohibit its use in any but minor operations'.[10]

While John Snow, James Young Simpson and others had written books on anaesthesia and anaesthetic agents as far back as the 1840s and 1850s, it was not until 1888 that what might reasonably regarded as the first textbook on the subject was published in the United Kingdom.[11] Its author was **Dudley Wilmot Buxton (1855–1931)**, a London anaesthetist who believed that every doctor entering practice should have a competent knowledge of anaesthetics. Buxton's book, extending to 164 well-illustrated and indexed pages, was reviewed for the *Irish Journal of Medical Science* by Henry MacNaughton-Jones who was, by that time, working in London himself.

Buxton, in the preface to his book, described it as having been written 'purely from the standpoint of every-day practice'. MacNaughton-Jones was of the view that it would be well if the same principle were adopted by: 'many more of our modern medical writers'. He wrote:

> For it can hardly be gainsaid that much of the padding of medical textbooks, so far as the requirements of the practitioner are concerned, might well be cut out. The difficulty, amidst the legion of authors, is to find one who is satisfied with giving the necessary information required for 'every-day' practice, avoiding abstruse disquisitions on disputed theories and modes of treatment which the average practitioner has neither the time nor the inclination to trouble itself about.

He believed that Buxton, having conceived that there was a want of a handy manual, had provided in condensed but sufficiently clear language all the necessary knowledge of anaesthetics demanded in ordinary hospital or general practice, had executed his plan well, and as a result, had produced a thoroughly useful and valuable little work on a most important subject.

Departing from discussion of the book itself, the Irish reviewer also recommended that a short course in anaesthetics be part of the training of every medical student. He stated:

> It is a fact that the majority of students finish their hospital course

98

without having had the opportunity of administering an anæsthetic under the supervision of a skilled and experienced anæsthetist. Nor have they been taught the necessary precautions to be taken before, during and after the administration. Those who have occasionally to entrust the administration of ether or chloroform to some assistant who has had no special instruction or experience in their use, must acknowledge how his anxieties and responsibilities are increased, and his attention diverted by the dangerous and often reckless acts of the administrator. It is a matter of surprise how readily men undertake to administer chloroform or ether who are quite ignorant of the proper mode of administration, the true signs of danger, and the immediate management of the patient when alarming signs are observed.

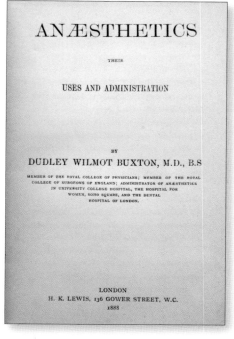

ANÆSTHETICS

THEIR

USES AND ADMINISTRATION

BY

DUDLEY WILMOT BUXTON, M.D., B.S

MEMBER OF THE ROYAL COLLEGE OF PHYSICIANS; MEMBER OF THE ROYAL
COLLEGE OF SURGEONS OF ENGLAND; ADMINISTRATOR OF ANÆSTHETICS
IN UNIVERSITY COLLEGE HOSPITAL, THE HOSPITAL FOR
WOMEN, SOHO SQUARE, AND THE DENTAL
HOSPITAL OF LONDON.

LONDON
H. K. LEWIS, 136 GOWER STREET, W.C.
1888

Title page of Dr Dudley Wilmot Buxton's Anæsthetics: Their Uses and Administration, *1888.*

Returning to Buxton's book, MacNaughton-Jones concluded:

Altogether, the little work to which we have drawn attention is just the class of book likely to meet the wants of the hospital assistant surgeon, or house surgeon, and the practitioner. It is clear, concise and a pleasure to read.[12]

Though Paul Piel had been appointed as anaesthetist to the Adelaide Hospital two years previously, it is evident that, in the reviewer's opinion, it would be some time before the practice in many hospitals of delegating the administration of anaesthetics to junior staff would cease.

At a meeting on 6 April 1888 of the Section of State Medicine of what had become the Royal Academy of Medicine in Ireland during the previous year, George Foy presented a paper on hypnotism and specifically the use in surgery of mesmerism, named after the German physician **Franz Anton Mesmer (1734–1815)** who first described his theory of 'animal magnetism' in the late eighteenth century. The practice attained some popularity in Britain in the 1830s but its use declined dramatically after the introduction of ether and chloroform. Foy reported that there had recently been renewed interest in mesmerism's usefulness in France, Italy and some other countries, although he was not himself an enthusiast. He contended that it was 'a remedy which threatens reason, is liable to gross abuse, and is uncertain in its action stands self-condemned, and cannot, in our present insufficiency of knowledge of psychology look for support from scientific medicine'.[13]

In spite of the various reports that had been published over the years, disagreement persisted between medical practitioners, both in Ireland and abroad, regarding the relative safety of ether and chloroform as anaesthetic agents and also as to whether the primary factor in chloroform deaths, when they did occur, was the drug's effect on respiration or that on the heart. **Edward Lawrie (1846–1915)** of the Indian Medical Service had, in 1885, been appointed residency surgeon to the State of Hyderabad in India where he also had charge of the medical school. Lawrie, a disciple of James Young Simpson and the Scottish surgeon James Syme, had used chloroform safely for many years and read with disbelief the frequent reports of chloroform deaths in Europe, and particularly in England.[14] He believed that the drug was not being administered correctly and that deaths, when they did occur, were due to the fact that inadequate attention had been paid to the patient's respiration. He refused to accept that chloroform could kill because of a direct effect on the heart.

With financial support from the Nizam of Hyderabad, Lawrie organised an investigation into the safety of the agent through experiments on dogs. This concluded in late 1888 and the findings of what later became known as the First Hyderabad Chloroform Commission were entirely in support of his views. They were first revealed by him in January 1889 during a speech at a prize presentation of the Hyderabad Medical School. One month later, *The Lancet* published an account of what Lawrie had said at the prize-giving.[15] In June of the same year, George Foy, a chloroform 'supporter', referred to the work of the Hyderabad Commission in the last of his series of eight 'Anæsthetics' papers in the *Dublin Journal of Medical Science*, although he mistakenly stated that *The Lancet* account had appeared in the *British Medical Journal*.[16] Also in 1889, the death occurred coincidentally of the Irish-born **Sir William Brooke O'Shaughnessy (1809–1889)** (see Chapter 24) who, in March 1847, had overseen the

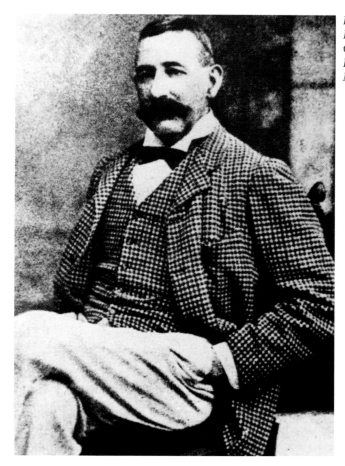

Photograph of Lieutenant-Colonel Edward Lawrie, Indian Medical Service.

administration of the first anaesthetic in India.

The Lancet was not impressed by the experiments organised by Lawrie, whereupon the latter approached the Nizam, who agreed to provide 1,000 pounds for the journal to send an independent representative to India to repeat the study. **Dr (later Sir) Thomas Lauder Brunton (1844–1916)** was chosen – he had an international reputation in pharmacology and appeared, at first sight, to be admirably suited to the work. Moreover, he had hitherto believed that chloroform killed by stopping the heart. However, he lacked recent experience in anaesthesia and was also an old friend of Lawrie.[17] Brunton sailed for India in October 1889. Within weeks of arriving, he had been completely out-manoeuvred by Lawrie and had changed his views about chloroform completely. He informed The Lancet that chloroform could not possibly kill by a direct action on the heart and that its only danger was from respiratory depression.[14,18] This opinion was repeated in the eagerly awaited report of the Second Hyderabad Chloroform Commission which was published, in parts, over the first few months of 1890: 'The administrator should be guided as to the effect entirely by the respiration ... Chloroform may be given in any case requiring an operation with perfect ease and absolute safety so as to do good without the risk of evil'.[19]

The *Dublin Journal of Medical Science* soon printed a lengthy editorial comment which was firmly supportive of the findings of the Commission.[20] The *Medical Press and Circular*'s writer, probably Foy, commented that if the rules drawn up by the Commission for its administration were implicitly followed, the percentage of deaths would be lessened, but that the conclusion that chloroform could ever be used 'with perfect ease and absolute safety' was too sanguine. He remarked, however, that it would tend to be rehabilitated in the eyes of many who had come to look on it as a convenient but dangerous agent.[21] This prediction proved to be correct and although *The Lancet* and many leading United Kingdom anaesthetists remained sceptical, in particular those who were working in London and firmly in the ether 'camp', the Commission's two reports emboldened others to continue using chloroform for many more years.

At the end of the decade, the 1890 *Medical Directory* entry for **John George Cronyn (c. 1857–1935)** indicated that he was anæsthetist to the (Incorporated) Dental Hospital of Ireland, now the Dublin Dental University Hospital. It seems likely that rather than being directly employed, he would have attended by arrangement with dentist colleagues to provide anaesthetic services to patients as required. Cronyn, a native of Kilkenny, attended Trinity College and qualified LRCSI 1880, LRCPI 1881. He described himself in his 1901 Census of Ireland return as 'Physician and Anæsthetist'; he was living at the time with his wife and children in Clare Street, Dublin.[22] His home was within a few yards of the Dental Hospital which had relocated from near St Stephen's Green to Lincoln Place two years earlier. Although approximately 57 years of age at the outbreak of World War One, by which time he was living and practising in England, he volunteered and served as physician and anaesthetist, attaining the rank of temporary captain and working in the Royal Herbert Hospital, Woolwich, London which treated wounded soldiers.[23]

The Cronyn name is of significance where the history of Irish rugby is concerned. Abraham Cronyn, a brother of John, played for Ireland against England in the first international between the two countries in February 1875 and later became a Church of Ireland clergyman. John himself represented

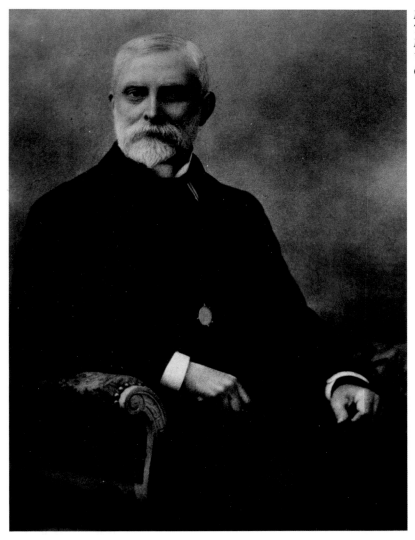

Photograph of Sir Thomas Lauder Brunton. Wellcome Collection.

Munster against Leinster in the first (unofficial) match between the two provinces which took place in Dublin two years later. He also had a prominent role in the 1879 discussions between the Irish Football Union and the Northern Football Union, held in Trinity College, which resulted in the three provinces of Ulster, Leinster and Munster agreeing to join together and form the Irish Rugby Football Union (IRFU). He later described the meeting thus: 'Goulding, Neville and myself did most of the talking and eventually we wore out the North!'[24]

103

References

1   MacNaughton-Jones H., 'Report on Anæsthetics', *Dublin Journal of Medical Science*, 1881, 71, pp. 150–70, 225–39, 336–49.

2   McCarthy K., 'One of Cork's medical pioneers', available at www.corkindependent.com/weekly/ourcityyourtown/articles/2018/05/02/4155530-one-of-corks-medical-pioneers/ (accessed 1 November 2020)

3   Ormsby L.H., 'The administration of anæsthetics', *Medical Press and Circular* 1885, 39 NS, pp. 268–9.

4   Mater Misericordiae Hospital, Minutes of the Medical Board Meeting of 3 November 1886.

5   Mitchell D., A *'Peculiar' Place: The Adelaide Hospital, Dublin 1839–1989*, Dublin: Blackwater Press, 1989, p. 124.

6   Clarke R., 'Anaesthesia', in B. O'Donnell (ed.), *Irish Surgery and Surgeons in the Twentieth Century*, Dublin: Gill & MacMillan, 2008, p. 590.

7   Keys T.E., *The History of Surgical Anesthesia*. New York, Schuman's, 1945, p. 40.

8   Maltby J.R., 'Carl Koller Medal, Carl Koller Research Fund', in J.R. Maltby (ed.), *Notable Names in Anaesthesia*, London: Royal Society of Medicine Press, 2002, pp. 105–7.

9   Benson A.H., 'Observations on the action of hydrochlorate of cocaine in the eye', *Transactions of the Ophthalmological Society of the United Kingdom*, 1884–5, 5, pp. 211–6.

10 Foy G., 'Operation under cocaine anæsthesia', *Medical Press and Circular* 1888, 46 NS, p. 363.

11 Buxton D.W., *Anæsthetics: Their Uses and Administration*, London: Lewis, 1888.

12 MacNaughton-Jones H., 'Book review, Anæsthetics: Their Uses and Administration by Dudley Wilmot Buxton', *Dublin Journal of Medical Science*, 1888, 86, pp. 329–38.

13 Foy G.M., 'Hypnotism, in Royal Academy of Medicine in Ireland, Section of State Medicine, Meeting of April 6th 1888', *Dublin Journal of Medical Science*, 1888, 85, pp. 450–1.

14 Ellis R.H., 'The Scottish Tradition', in A. Marshall Barr, T.B. Boulton and D.J. Wilkinson (eds), *Essays on the History of Anaesthesia.*, London: Royal Society of Medicine Press, 1996, pp. 49–58.

15 'Hyderabad Medical School: Chloroform Inhalation', *The Lancet*, 1889, 1, p. 394.

16 Foy G., 'Anæsthetics', *Dublin Journal of Medical Science*, 1889, 87, pp. 486–99.

17 Stratmann L., *Chloroform: The Quest for Oblivion*, Stroud: Sutton Publishing 2003, pp. 194–5.

18 'Annotation. The Lancet and the Hyderabad Chloroform Commission', *The Lancet*, 1889, 2, p. 1183.

19 Lawrie E., Brunton T.L., Bomford G. and Hakim R.D., 'Report of the Second Hyderabad Chloroform Commission', *Indian Medical Gazette*, 1890, 25, pp. 33–40, 65–8, 100–5.

20 'The Hyderabad Chloroform Commission', *Dublin Journal of Medical Science*, 1890, 89, pp. 189–92.

21 'The Hyderabad Chloroform Commission', *Medical Press and Circular* 1890, 50 NS, p. 96.

22 Census of Ireland, 1901. John Cronyn's household return, available at census.nationalarchives.ie/reels/nai/003731129/ (accessed 25 January 2021).

23 Casey P.J., Cullen K.T. and Duignan J.P., *Irish Doctors in the First World War*, Dublin: Merrion Press, 2015, p. 260.
24 'The History of Dublin University Football Club', available at dufc.ie/club-history/ (accessed 25 January 2021).

Chapter 9

Another Committee
and Successors to Piel

Declan Warde

The Second Hyderabad Chloroform Commission's continued focus on the respiratory system rather than the heart led to the introduction of yet another chloroform inhaler designed by an Irish doctor. **Alexander Duke (1845–1915)** graduated LRCP & SI in 1874 and was awarded membership of the King and Queen's College of Physicians of Ireland (MKQCPI) seven years later. He became obstetric physician to Dr Steevens' Hospital, Dublin and in 1891 published details of his 'Safety Inhaler for Chloroform'. The main advantage claimed for it was that every inspiration and expiration, no matter how faint, caused a set of valves through which the air had passed to produce a sound audible to the administrator thereby giving immediate notice of danger. Duke believed that his inhaler, if given a fair trial, would be a great saver of anxiety.[1] It never achieved great popularity.

At a meeting of the British Medical Association (BMA) held in Bournemouth, England in July of that year, Thomas Lauder Brunton read a paper with the title 'Remarks on death during chloroform anæsthesia' which stated the case from the Hyderabad Commission's point of view. The members also heard a contrary opinion expressed by L.E. Shore, demonstrator in physiology at the University of Cambridge in his paper 'Remarks on the effects of chloroform on the respiratory centre, the vasomotor centre and the heart'; it was based on work carried out by him in association with W.H. Gaskell, lecturer in physiology at the same institution.[2] At the end of the discussion that followed, Dr Christopher Childs of Weymouth moved 'that a committee be formed to investigate the clinical evidence with regard to anæsthetics, especially the relative safety of the various anæsthetics, and the best methods of administering them'. His motion was passed, a committee was formed, and so as to obtain evidence, it requested all anaesthetists throughout the United Kingdom to record their cases during 1892. In order that the observations might be as uniform as possible, record

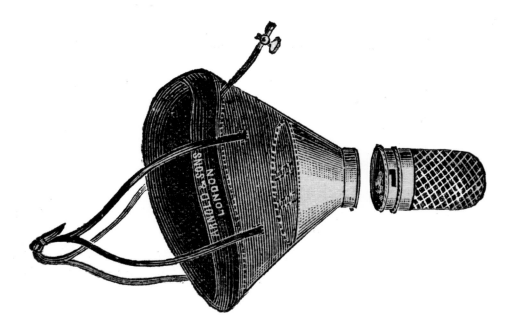

Dr Alexander Duke's 'Safety Inhaler for Chloroform', Medical Press and Circular, 28 October 1891.

books were drawn up containing columns for noting the consecutive number, date, hour, sex, age, general state of the patient, nature of the operation, anaesthetic employed, method, duration, quantity used, source where the anaesthetic had been obtained, and after effects in each case.[3]

Dudley Wilmot Buxton spoke on the matter at a meeting of the Section of Obstetrics, Royal Academy of Medicine in Ireland held in Dublin on 8 January 1892 and attended by many of the leading practitioners in the city. He stated that although anaesthetics had been applied in surgery for nearly 50 years, imperfect attempts, with very few exceptions, had been made to treat the subject from a clinical standpoint. He pointed out that the various commissions and investigations in the past had conflicted in their findings, so that no definite conclusions could be rationally accepted. He urged that the time had come for the profession itself to take up the matter, and to collect reliable records of the action of anaesthetics on human beings. He told the meeting of the committee that had been formed by the BMA in order to initiate an exhaustive inquiry into the action of anaesthetics and pointed out that evidence might be collected from (i) post-mortem reports following death under anaesthetic, (ii) from symptoms in cases where difficulties had arisen during the course of an anaesthetic and (iii) for cases in which anaesthesia had proceeded normally, and that the inquiry was

107

Photograph of Dr Dudley Wilmot Buxton. Wellcome Collection.

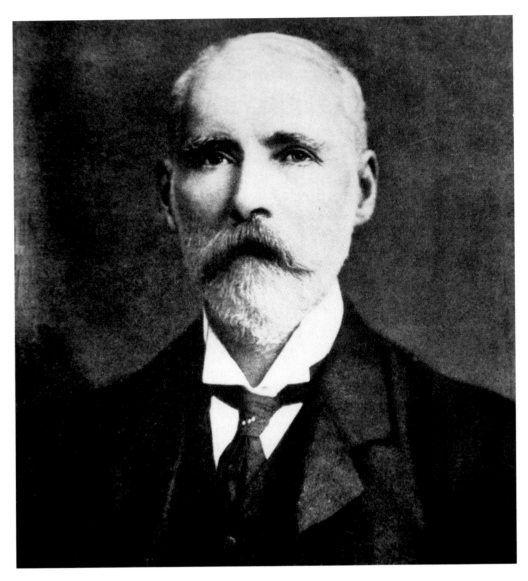

also seeking information on matters such as the age, sex, race of patients, the purity of the anaesthetic used etc. He believed that a thorough investigation could not fail to result in a vast increase in knowledge concerning the actions, dangers and complications of anaesthetics.[4,5]

During what was clearly a lively discussion that followed, Henry Gray Croly, President of the Royal College of Surgeons in Ireland, said that he had been asked to form a subcommittee in Ireland in connection with the Anæsthetic Committee, and he hoped to do so as soon as possible. He pointed out that the anaesthetic question was one of vital importance to every member of the medical profession, and also to each individual who takes an anaesthetic. While he had never been present at a death from an anaesthetic, he had seen several 'touch and go' cases. He confessed that he was always more afraid of the anaesthetic than the operation. Lambert Ormsby stated that he hoped something definite would come from the commission but that this would only happen if an experienced committee, whose members really took trouble in the matter, was appointed.

Dr Robert Harley of Dublin believed that there had been a panic about anaesthetics displayed at the meeting which was quite uncalled for. He had been practising for 20 years and had never heard of more than two or three deaths in all that time from an anaesthetic, and had never even had a case of what Mr Croly called 'touch and go'. Thomas Myles, surgeon to the Richmond Hospital, was dismissive of the methodology to be employed, pointing out that the experimental method was the only one from which reliable results could be drawn while William Stokes, professor of surgery at RCSI, was disappointed that a definite line of investigation was not indicated by Dr Buxton. He feared that if the results of the labours of the committee were to be nothing but a record of cases to which anaesthetics had been administered, the statistics would be unsatisfactory. George Foy made a brief contribution in which he pointed out that outside London and the New England States of America, chloroform remained the favoured anaesthetic. He did not approve of the advocacy of certification where anaesthesia was concerned; in his opinion, there were already too many certificates.[4,5]

The initiation of the BMA's inquiry did not prevent those who had already made up their own minds from continuing to promulgate their views. Over one year after its initial publication, a review, over 40 pages in length, of the full report of the second Hyderabad commission was published in two parts in the *Dublin Journal of Medical Science*. Although anonymous, the tenor and phrasing were typical of those usually employed in his writings by Foy. He wrote:

> Acting on the doctrine of possibilities there are no good grounds for thinking other than favourably of chloroform after its successful issue from all the tests supplied. No anæsthetic has been submitted to so many and such various tests as chloroform. The second Hyderabad Commission has performed its work with

a fullness and completeness hitherto unknown; and the fact that the decision of the commission coincides with that of the great majority of the medical profession, both at home and abroad, is eminently satisfactory, and well calculated to allay the public anxiety as to the value of the drug which enthusiastic etherists created.[6]

Buxton responded to a report in the *Medical Press and Circular* of what had transpired at the Dublin meeting by letter. He expressed his gratitude for the consideration with which he had been received but considered that the report did not represent either the tone or the sense of the discussion as it took place, and went on to write:

It was in answer to an express invitation that I visited Dublin and sought to enlist the sympathies of its surgeons in a line of research which commends itself to the profession, and I trust that any inadequacy on my part will not prejudice a cause the claims of which rest upon a foundation far firmer than the mere success or failure of a half-hour's speech.[7]

In January 1893, 156 report books with details of 25,920 anaesthetics in hospital and private practice were returned to the BMA. Each book and case was reviewed by the Analysis Subcommittee which consisted of four persons, and included both Buxton and Frederic Hewitt. The final report, extending to almost 150 pages, was not ready for publication for a number of years. It included a list of the individual institutions and practitioners throughout the United Kingdom by whom reports had been submitted. The number received from Ireland must surely have been a source of some disappointment to the organisers and in particular to Buxton – it seems that his Dublin 'appeal' had fallen on deaf ears. Just four Irish hospitals, the County Infirmaries in Armagh, Wexford, Lisburn in County Antrim and Maryborough in Queen's County (now Portlaoise in County Laois), none of which were in major population centres, had responded. Two individual doctors, working in Armagh and Maryborough, had also submitted information pertaining to their 'off-site' private practices.[8]

Overall, the anaesthetics that had been most frequently used in the United Kingdom were chloroform (52 per cent), ether (18 per cent), nitrous oxide (11 per cent) and 'gas and ether' (8 per cent) followed by the A.C.E. mixture and various combinations of the agents already named. On the 'clinical evidence regarding anaesthetics generally' the subcommittee concluded that: (i) anaesthetic complications and danger were more likely in males, (ii) excluding infancy, complications and dangers of anaesthesia increased with advancing age, (iii) danger to life was especially likely to be incurred in early periods of administration of anaesthetics, (iv) the tendency for complications increased with the gravity of the operation, (v) the most important factor in the safe administration of anaesthetics was the experience of the administrator, (vi) in many instances, the anaesthetic completely transcended the operation in gravity and importance and in those cases, it was essential that the anaesthetist had large experience and (vii) practitioners everywhere must, in emergencies, be prepared to administer anaesthetics and that, therefore, no one should be allowed to qualify until he or she had shown proficiency in that very important branch of medical work.[9]

The subcommittee found that chloroform, alone or in combination, caused a danger-rate six-fold higher than that caused by ether in the reported cases. Contrasting chloroform alone with ether alone, chloroform had a danger-rate more than eight times that of ether.[10]

Also in 1893, the first edition of Frederic Hewitt's classic *Anæsthetics and their Administration* was published.[11] It was described by a *Dublin Journal of Medical Science* reviewer as 'the best treatise on the subject we have yet read' and would become the standard anaesthesia textbook in Britain and Ireland for some decades to come.

It seems that it was eight years after Paul Piel commenced work in the Adelaide Hospital before another doctor was formally appointed to an anaesthetic post in Ireland. At a meeting of the Medical Board of the Mater Misericordiae Hospital held on 12 November 1894, the secretary reported that he 'was requested by Sr Mary Berchmans to report to the board that she had appointed **Mr** [*sic*] **Michael O'Sullivan** as anæsthetist to the hospital for one year from 1st October 1894'.[12]

O'Sullivan had attended the Catholic University School of Medicine in Temple Bar, Dublin and graduated from the Royal University of Ireland in 1892. His *Medical Directory* entry of the time indicates that he worked as both anaesthetist and pathologist in The Children's Hospital, Temple Street for a short period prior to commencing in the Mater; this may not have been in an official salaried capacity. A somewhat similar appointment was that of Dr Richard Shaw, who in 1895, became both anaesthetist and pharmaceutist to St Vincent's

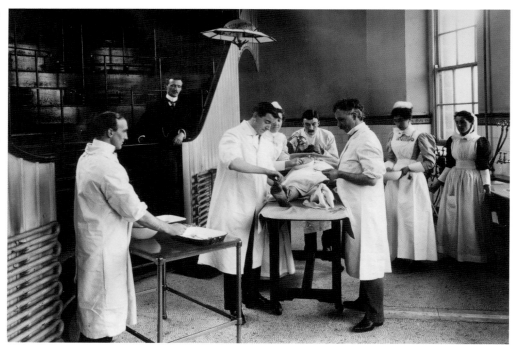

Photograph of an operation in progress at the Mater Misericordiae Hospital, Dublin c.1898. Dr Michael O'Sullivan is administering the anaesthetic. Reproduced by kind permission of the Royal College of Physicians of Ireland (RE/2/9).

Hospital in Dublin. Shaw has been described as 'a gentleman of the old school'; although he also had a flourishing general practice, he attended the hospital every day, dressed in a frock coat, tie and tall hat.[12]

While O'Sullivan's original appointment was for a period of one year, it was renewed on a regular basis over the following decade or so. His salary from November 1896 was 30 pounds per annum – this was significantly less than that of the assistant surgeon, assistant physician or medical registrar, each of whom were being paid 50 pounds per year. This was in spite of the fact that he was taking on additional duties; a Medical Board meeting of the same month agreed, regarding recently-installed x-ray equipment, 'That the care and working of the expensive photographic and electrical installation be entrusted to Dr O'Sullivan subject to the supervision of the committee'.[13] The position of anaesthetist was perceived as needing no training, and the administration of an anaesthetic was seen as a 'procedure' rather than a 'specialty'.[14] His salary was, however, increased by ten pounds per year from 1898 onwards. By 1901, he was working as both anaesthetist and surgical registrar and his annual income had risen to approximately 120 pounds. Michael O'Sullivan died of multiple sclerosis, aged 37 years, in November 1906.

Charles O'Neill (1861–1924) was born in Crossnacreevy, County Down. He studied medicine at Queen's College Belfast and graduated from the Royal University of Ireland in 1886. He worked as a general practitioner and anaesthetist in Belfast and was superintendent medical officer of Health for Castlereagh Rural District. He does not appear to have had a formal hospital anaesthetic appointment but wrote in 1897 concerning a personal series of 600 cases without a fatality under various headings including patient age, quantity of anaesthetic used, the average time taken to produce anaesthesia and postoperative problems. He provided a comprehensive overview of the methods used by him, including preoperative preparation of the patient and methods of administration of anaesthetic agents. He also addressed the relative merits of methylene and chloroform, the two agents used by him on a regular basis, and resuscitation of the collapsed patient.[15, 16]

Over the final four years of the nineteenth century, the number of doctors working as 'official' anaesthetists in Ireland finally began to increase, with at least eight positions being filled during that period. Those appointed included Drs James Lynass (assistant surgeon and chloroformist, Belfast Hospital for Sick Children, 1897), Richard Kennan (anaesthetist, Sir Patrick Dun's Hospital, Dublin, 1898), Victor Fielden (anaesthetist, Ulster Hospital, Belfast, 1898), Thomas Percy Claude 'Percy' Kirkpatrick (anaesthetist, Dr Steevens' Hospital, Dublin, 1899; see Chapter 24), Edward Fannin and S. Wesley Wilson (anaesthetists, Drumcondra Hospital, Dublin, c. 1899), Nathaniel Henry Hobart (anaesthetist, Eye, Ear and Throat Hospital, Cork, 1900 – he had previously worked for some years as assistant anaesthetist at St Bartholomew's Hospital in London) and Robert Johnstone (anaesthetist, Royal Victoria Hospital, Belfast, 1900).

The general pattern of the time was to employ young doctors, often budding surgeons, to serve as anaesthetists for a short time before they moved on as their careers progressed. The choice of anaesthetic agent and technique very often remained in the hands of the surgeon.[17] Among those appointed before 1901, James Lynass became surgeon to the Belfast Hospital for Sick Children in 1900, a year in which he performed '51 chloroform induced surgeries'.[18] Richard Kennan also became a surgeon and joined the Colonial Medical Service, while Robert Johnston was a future professor of gynaecology at Queen's University Belfast. Nathaniel Hobart succeeded his father as surgeon to the North Infirmary in Cork and Edward Fannin who was a member of the Fannin family, well-known retailers of medical books and equipment, later worked as a general practitioner in Dublin. Irish surgeons continued to write on anaesthetic topics, with one noteworthy 1907 example, on death following chloroform anaesthesia due to acute fatty degeneration of the liver, coming from Robert Campbell (1866–1920) who, at the time, was assistant surgeon at the Royal Victoria Hospital, Belfast.[19]

Victor George Leopold Fielden (1867–1946) was one of the few anaesthetists of the time who remained in the developing specialty for more than a year or two. He was born near Plymouth, Devon and after his family moved to Belfast in 1881, he completed his school education at the Royal Belfast Academical Institution and then studied at Queen's College in the city. He graduated in pharmacy in 1890 and in medicine, from the Royal University of Ireland, two years later. After working as anaesthetist at the Ulster Hospital for two years, he was appointed, in addition, to the Royal Victoria Hospital (RVH), Belfast in 1900, where he was to be the pillar of anaesthesia for the rest of his working life. His MD was awarded with gold medal by Queen's University in 1912 for a thesis on the pharmacology of ethyl chloride; he had read a paper on his use of the agent at a meeting of the Ulster Medical Society as early as 1904.[20] His work on it was supported by many experiments on laboratory animals, dogs, cats, rabbits and frogs. In his preface he stated, 'It is an attempt to add to the limited knowledge of the action of an anæsthetic which is now largely used but whose pharmacological effects have not received much attention.'

Fielden was probably the first doctor in Ireland to practise anaesthesia exclusively and in addition to authoring many papers on chloroform administration techniques, he was an early advocate of the combined administration of oxygen with nitrous oxide in anaesthesia for general surgery, summarising his thoughts on the matter in the following way:

> (i) A mixture of nitrous oxide and oxygen constitutes an excellent anæsthetic for short, painful examinations, dressings and operations, (ii) The dangers are practically nil, (iii) After-effects, if any, are very slight, (iv) Anæsthesia is rapidly induced, and the recovery to perfect consciousness is even more rapid and (v) The patient is able to move about almost immediately, so that it is the best anæsthetic to administer when one is desired in the surgeon's consulting room.[21]

Victor Fielden served with the Queen's University Officer Training Division of the Royal Army Medical Corps during World War One. Within the Royal Victoria Hospital, no other anaesthetist achieved similar status for many years,

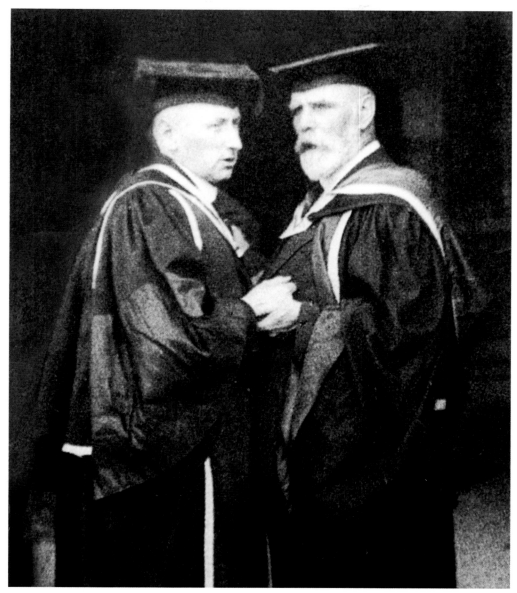

Photograph of Dr Victor Fielden (on right) with Dr John Morrow at a 1933 Queen's University graduation ceremony. By kind permission of Belfast Health and Social Care Trust.

and following his retirement it was to be some time before he was replaced on the attending staff. Away from medicine, he was a keen cyclist and bell-ringer and rang peals in St Thomas's Church, Lisburn Road, Belfast after the deaths of both Queen Victoria and King Edward VII.[22,23]

References

1   Duke A., 'New safety chloroform inhaler', *Medical Press and Circular*, 1891, 52 NS, pp. 440–1.

2   Duncum B.M., *The Development of Inhalation Anaesthesia*, London: Oxford University Press, 1947, p. 458.

3   *Ibid.*, pp. 460–1.

4   Buxton D.W., 'Anæsthetics: A clinical study. Section of Obstetrics, Royal Academy of Medicine in Ireland, Meeting of January 8th 1892', *Medical Press and Circular*, 1892, 53 NS, pp. 83–4.

5   Buxton D.W., 'Anæsthetics: A clinical study. Section of Obstetrics, Royal Academy of Medicine in Ireland, Meeting of January 8th 1892', *Dublin Journal of Medical Science*, 1892, 93, pp. 155–9.

6   'Report of the Hyderabad Chloroform Commission', *Dublin Journal of Medical Science*, 1892, 93, pp. 301–21, 490–511.

7   Buxton D.W., 'Anæsthetics', *Medical Press and Circular*, 1892, 53 NS, pp. 147–8.

8   'British Medical Association: Report of the Anæsthetics Committee (appointed 1891)', London, 1900.

9   Duncum, *The Development*, p. 464.

10 *Ibid.*, p. 463.

11 Hewitt F.W., *Anæsthetics and Their Administration*, London: Charles Griffin, 1893.

12 Meenan F.O.C., *St Vincent's Hospital 1834–1994*, Dublin: Gill & MacMillan, 1995, p. 12.

13 Mater Misericordiae Hospital, Minutes of the Meetings of the Medical Board 1861–899. Meetings of 12 November 1894, 3 November and 1896, 28 June 1898.

14 Nolan E., *Caring for the Nation: A History of the Mater Misericordiae University Hospital*, Dublin: Gill and MacMillan, 2013, p. 53.

15 Clarke R.S.J., *A Directory of Ulster Doctors (who qualified before 1901)*, Belfast: Ulster Historical Foundation, 1913, pp. 889–90.

16 O'Neill C., 'The safe administration of anaesthetics: With special reference to chloroform and methylene', *British Medical Journal*, 1897, 1, pp. 1465–6.

17 'Clarke R.', in B. O'Donnell (ed.), *Irish Surgery and Surgeons in the Twentieth Century*, Dublin: Gill & MacMillan, 2008, pp. 586–7.

18 Robinson D., 'Ulster's Fulton Physicians', *Ulster Medical Journal*, 2016, 85, pp. 29–32.

19 Campbell R., 'Acid intoxication following general anæsthesia', *Medical Press and Circular*, 1907, 84 NS, pp. 198–201.

20 'The Ulster Medical Society. Meeting held in the Medical Institute, Belfast; April 22nd 1904', *Medical Press and Circular*, 1904, 78 NS, pp. 473–4.

21 Fielden V.G.L., 'Nitrous oxide and oxygen as an anaesthetic in general surgery', *Dublin Journal of Medical Science*, 1902, 114, pp. 189–94.

22 Clarke R.S.J., *A Directory*, p. 344.

23 Clarke R., *The Royal Victoria Hospital Belfast: A History 1797–1997*, Belfast: Blackstaff Press, 1997, pp. 123–4.

Chapter 10

The Early Twentieth Century

Declan Warde

Not all Irish doctors who contributed to the advancement of the developing specialty ever practised as anaesthetists. **Nathaniel Henry Alcock (1871–1913)**, born near Letterkenny, County Donegal to a naval surgeon and his wife, obtained both his MB and MD from Trinity College Dublin in 1896 with honours and prizes in various subjects. He subsequently taught physiology at Trinity and anatomy at the Victoria University of Manchester. After working in a research capacity in the University of Marlburg, Germany, he was appointed demonstrator in physiology at the University of London in 1903, and lecturer in the same subject to St Mary's Hospital Medical School, Paddington during the following year, becoming the school's vice dean in 1906.[1]

At the University of London, Alcock had worked under Augustus Desire Waller who was interested in the morbidity and mortality associated with chloroform, and was very aware of the importance of knowing the dosage being administered. In 1903, he (Waller) reported on a series of animal experiments in which the effects of known inhaled concentrations of chloroform were observed. Five years later, undoubtedly influenced by the work of his former superior, Alcock published a description of his chloroform apparatus, which was probably the first accurately calibrated, temperature compensated, plenum vaporizer.[2] In some respects, it was many decades ahead of its time – it was not until the late 1950s that such vaporizers became a common feature of anaesthetic machines. However, despite being endorsed by noted figures such as Joseph Blumfeld and Alfred Goodman Levy, it never achieved great popularity among practising anaesthetists. There were a number of reasons for this: (i) the BMA Chloroform Committee Report of 1910 recommended an alternative design by Vernon Harcourt, (ii) it was complex and not very portable, important considerations for the 'itinerant' anaesthetists of the day and (iii) many practitioners felt that there was, in any event, no need for a dosimetric method of chloroform administration.[3]

Photograph of prototype Alcock vaporizer – this example is incomplete, with no provision for temperature compensation. Courtesy of the Science Museum / Science & Society Picture Library.

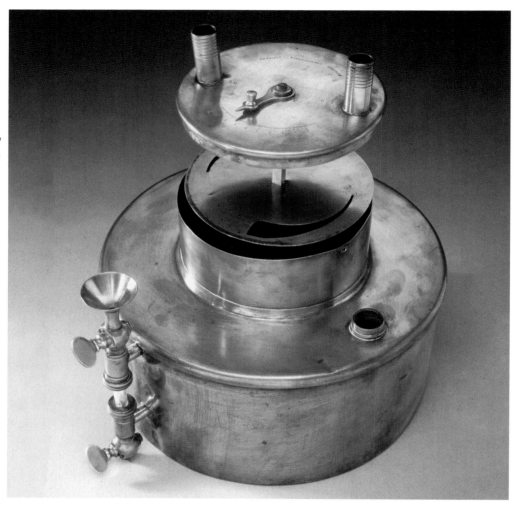

Alcock was awarded a doctorate in science (DSc) for his physiological researches by the University of London in 1909. He retained links with his native country by examining at both the Royal College of Physicians of Ireland and the National University of Ireland. He became professor of physiology at McGill University, Montreal, Canada in 1911 but unfortunately, held the post only briefly as he died aged 42 years in 1913. Sir William Osler wrote, 'The death of Dr Alcock is a great loss to the Faculty of Medicine … The energy and enthusiasm he displayed, though suffering for nearly three years from medullary leukaemia, were remarkable'. His widow and young children returned to the United Kingdom, and in recognition of her late husband's contribution to medical education, Prime

Minister Herbert Asquith granted Mrs Alcock the unusual distinction of a pension from the Civil Service Fund.[1]

While practitioners such as Fielden in Belfast and Kirkpatrick in Dublin worked hard to advance the status of anaesthesia in Ireland, the reality was that the methods and agents used by most of those anaesthetising patients had not changed greatly when compared with 50 years earlier. Either open ether or chloroform was generally used, sometimes with ethyl chloride for induction and for short procedures. The anaesthetic was still not thought to be important by many, and was often given by the least experienced doctor or a medical student.[4] Moreover, the limited number of skilled anaesthetists was almost invariably engaged in both general and anaesthetic practice and therefore available for only a minority of cases. The further development of the specialty was not helped by the fact that until 1946, the only academic meetings in Dublin at which discussion of subjects of interest to anaesthetists took place were those of the Dublin Clinical Club (which had a limited membership) and gatherings of specialists in other disciplines, e.g. the Sections of Surgery, Obstetrics or State Medicine of the Royal Academy of Medicine in Ireland. Outside the largest city, the Ulster Medical Society, founded in 1862 through the amalgamation of three other medical groups, and the Cork Medical and Surgical Society, the successor to the City and County of Cork Medico-Chirurgical Society, provided occasional fora for debate. For many years to come, medical journals would continue to provide the only source of ongoing education on the subject for those working elsewhere on the island.

The number of doctors either employed as anaesthetists or attached to the larger hospitals as 'visiting' anaesthetists continued to grow. It is hoped, over the following pages, to provide some insight into the contributions made either to anaesthesia, other areas of medical practice or society in general by some of these individuals.

James (Jim) Beckett, son of William Beckett, a successful building contractor, and his wife Frances, was born in Dublin in 1884. He entered Trinity College in 1902, graduating in medicine nine years later. Mercer's Hospital advertised for 'an Anaesthetist unpaid' in 1913 and Beckett, who had been working in England, returned to his native city to take up the position.[5] He became honorary anaesthetist to the Royal Victoria Eye and Ear Hospital, Adelaide Road some months later but in October 1914, applied for leave of absence, which was granted, in order that he might work with the Royal Army Medical Corps during World War One.[6] He served from July 1915 until the end of the war, attaining the rank of Temporary Honorary Major,[7] working primarily at the St John Ambulance Brigade Hospital

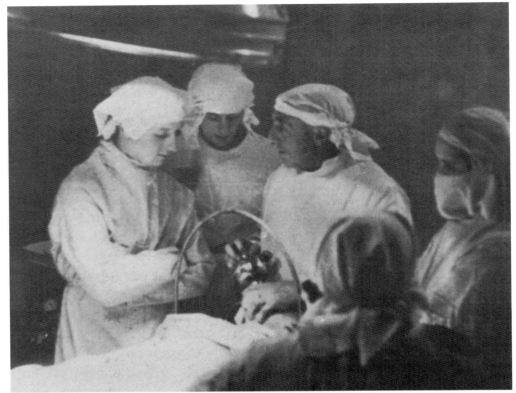

Photograph of Dr James Beckett at work in the operating theatre of the Adelaide Hospital, Dublin. Reproduced from Mitchell D. A 'Peculiar' Place: The Adelaide Hospital, Dublin 1839–1989, Blackwater, 1989.

in Étaples, near Boulogne, France. The hospital provided 520 beds for soldiers wounded in nearby fighting and was regarded as one of the finest and best-equipped in the country. Following his return to Dublin, he resumed his previous positions and also worked for a time as honorary radiologist to Monkstown Hospital.

At a meeting of the Adelaide Hospital Managing Committee held on 29 March 1927, it was noted, 'The Medical Board reported that Dr Ella Webb having resigned her position as Anaesthetist to the hospital, they had appointed Dr J. Beckett to fill the vacant post. The appointment was approved'.[8] It was to the Adelaide and its patients that Jim Beckett was to devote most of the remainder of his working life, serving the hospital with distinction for over 20 years. He was active in the Association of Anaesthetists of Great Britain and Ireland from shortly after its inception as District Representative for Ireland; he later became the first Irish member to be elected to council, serving from 1936–44. Two years prior to his retirement in 1948, he wrote on the subject of 'Anaesthetic fatalities'. At that time, chloroform was still being used in some centres. He stated unequivocally that the agent's dangers were so widely appreciated that there was no argument in favour of its continuance as an anaesthetic.[9]

While Beckett undoubtedly had a distinguished anaesthetic career, it was for his remarkably wide-ranging sporting achievements, as both a participant and an administrator, that he was best known to the Irish public. Apart from being involved in athletics and hockey while in Trinity College and twice becoming university heavyweight boxing champion, he was also an accomplished rugby player. He played for Old Wesley for many years and captained the club to a Leinster Cup victory in 1905. He was capped by Leinster on three occasions and was also captain of the Dublin Hospitals team at least twice when they played against their London counterparts.

However, watersports were Beckett's real strength. A member of Pembroke Swimming Club, he set numerous Irish swimming records at different distances, with his 100 yards freestyle record not being bettered for over 30 years. He first played water polo for Ireland aged just 16, and continued to play at international level for almost a quarter of a century. He had the distinction of captaining the team at the 1924 Olympic Games in Paris, a particularly significant sporting occasion for the country as it was the first Games at which Ireland competed as an independent nation. While still involved as a competitor, he fulfilled a number of sporting administrative roles – he was secretary of the Leinster Rugby Football Union in 1905–6, president of the Leinster Swimming Union on five occasions and president of the

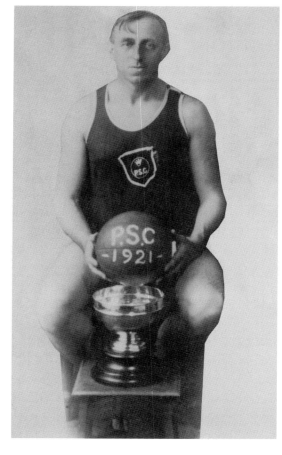

Photograph of Dr James (Jim) Beckett, Captain of Pembroke Swimming Club's water polo team, winners of the Irish Senior Cup in 1921.
Courtesy of his daughter, Margo Magan.

121

Irish Amateur Swimming Association in 1923. He was president of the Association of Referees, Leinster Branch in 1929–30 having become a top-level referee after he ceased to play rugby. Beckett's daughter, Margo Magan, was also an Irish swimming champion and won the inaugural Irish Senior Women's Golf Championship.[10–12]

An uncle of Samuel Beckett, the 1969 Nobel Prize winner for Literature, Jim Beckett suffered from major complications associated with diabetes mellitus and other illnesses in later life. It was a sad ending for a man who had a medical career of note and had once cut such an impressive figure, brimming over with athleticism, confidence and good humour.[13] He died at his Dublin home on 19 March 1971.

Jim Beckett and John Cronyn were just two of approximately 3,300 Irish doctors and medical students who served with the British forces during World War One; over 260 of these died in the war.[14] Approximately 40 served prior to, during or after anaesthetic careers; some of them are introduced below.

Charles Molyneux Benson (c. 1878–1919) graduated from Trinity College Dublin in 1904. He was anaesthetist to Dr Steevens' Hospital from 1904–6, leaving to work in a similar post for some years in Sir Patrick Dun's Hospital, to which he was appointed as a surgeon in 1916. He served as surgeon to the 83rd (Dublin) General Hospital in Boulogne during 1917–18, and died some months after his return to Ireland.[15]

Alfred Ernest Boyd (1872–1949) was another Trinity College medical graduate, qualifying in 1896. After undertaking postgraduate study in Vienna and working in Public Health, he was appointed, along with Dr John Meyler, as anaesthetist to the Richmond Hospital in 1905. He was senior anaesthetist to the hospital for two decades and consulting anaesthetist for a further 24 years. Boyd served at the rank of captain in the Royal Army Medical Corps, spending most of the final year of World War One at the 83rd (Dublin) General Hospital in Boulogne.[16]

As early as 1847, rectal, or more properly, colonic etherisation had been practiced by Nikolai Ivanovich Pirogoff in Petrograd, Russia. Liquid ether, sometimes mixed with water, was first used but this was subsequently abandoned in favour of ether vapour. The method fell into disuse but was revived to some extent in the late nineteenth century. However, the reported complications and fatalities precluded the technique from entering into general application. James Tayloe Gwathmey of New York introduced oil-ether colonic anaesthesia in 1913 and wrote in detail of his experience two years later.[17] Boyd had experience with Gwathmey's approach, beginning in 1918, while he was serving in France. He wrote in 1920 that the technique, although simple, subjected the patient to a deal of disturbance in terms of preparation and preliminary medication, while it also called for an extreme degree of watchfulness on the part of the anaesthetist in view of the instances reported in which deep and dangerous anaesthesia supervened with great rapidity. He went on to describe a number of cases in which he had used a combined 'rectal and inhalation' method which he found to be more satisfactory.[18] Aside from medicine, Alfred Boyd was a member of the Royal Irish Yacht Club and was well known as an authority on the history of Old Dublin.[19]

Isaac Alexander Davidson (1869–1942) graduated from Queen's College Belfast in 1892 and became anaesthetist to the Belfast Hospital for Sick Children in 1901; the unsuccessful candidate was a woman, Dr Eleanor Sproull, who obtained her degree from the Edinburgh Medical College for Women in 1900. His designation was 'Honorary Anaesthetist to the Staff' which implies that he was not an 'Honorary Attending'.[20] Davidson was also anaesthetist to the Benn Ulster Eye, Ear and Throat Hospital 1902–9, and to the Royal Victoria Hospital. He subsequently became a surgeon who served in the Royal Army Medical Corps during World War One, as an ophthalmic specialist with the rank of captain, and was ophthalmic surgeon to the Ulster Hospital for Women and Children 1914–34.[21]

Victor Ormsby McCormick (1897–1970) was one of the most prominent anaesthetists in Ireland for over 40 years. Born in Dublin, he received his school education in his native city and Cambridge. He joined the British Army at 18 years of age and was commissioned as Second Lieutenant in the Leinster Regiment. During World War One he saw active service in Macedonia where he was wounded and invalided home in 1917. Having obtained a Bachelor of Arts degree from Trinity College in 1919, he graduated in medicine four years later. After qualifying, McCormick worked initially in general practice. He was appointed as anaesthetist to Sir Patrick Dun's Hospital in 1926 and remained on the staff until his retirement over 40 years later. He held additional appointments in the Rotunda and Monkstown Hospitals. At a time when there were no postgraduate anaesthetic qualifications, he took the MRCPI examination in 1928 and became FRCPI two years later. In 1942, when the Diploma in Anaesthetics (DA) was instituted by the Conjoint Board of the Royal Colleges of Physicians and Surgeons in Ireland, McCormick was chosen as first examiner.[22] He succeeded Percy Kirkpatrick as lecturer in anaesthetics to his alma mater, Trinity College, in 1948 and was a foundation fellow of the Faculties of Anaesthetists of the Royal Colleges of Surgeons in both England (1948) and Ireland (1960).[23] He became president of the

Photograph of Dr Victor Ormsby McCormick. Reproduced by kind permission of the Royal College of Physicians of Ireland (PDH/6/5/2).

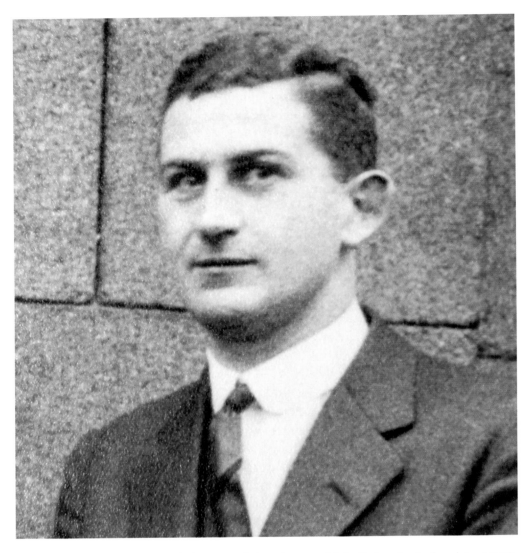

Section of Anaesthetics of the Royal Academy of Medicine in Ireland in 1949, served as the first vice dean of the Irish faculty (1959–64) and was vice president of the Association of Anaesthetists of Great Britain and Ireland (1961–4). He also found time to write extensively, publishing on such subjects as trichloroethylene, curare and the future of the growing specialty and its practitioners.

Victor McCormick died at his Dublin home on 6 March 1970. He had been known for many years as 'The Boss'; one of his many obituarists remarked that he was, however: 'A boss who never cracked a whip and who had the character to lead others by kindliness and encouragement' and also that 'The status of the anaesthetist was his constant concern. No man did more ... to earn respect for the science and art of anaesthesia'.[24]

George Pugin Meldon (1875–1950) was born in Dublin to Dr Austin Meldon, reputed to have been the first man in Ireland to ride a bicycle, and his second wife Katherine Pugin. She was a daughter of the renowned English architect and designer Augustus Pugin whose work included designing the interior of the Palace of Westminster and its iconic clock tower, which houses the bell known as Big Ben. Meldon was educated at Clongowes Wood College and Trinity College Dublin's medical school. He graduated MB BCh BAO in 1897, was awarded a doctorate in medicine (MD) during the following year and became FRCSI in 1901. He obtained the DA in 1937; it had been established in London two years earlier.

Following graduation, he had commenced his working life at the Charitable Infirmary in Jervis Street, Dublin and was appointed to the Westmoreland Lock Hospital shortly afterwards, remaining on its staff for over 40 years. He became anaesthetist to the Royal City of Dublin Hospital, Baggot Street in 1909 and worked there until his retirement in 1948. He was a regular attender at and contributor to meetings of various sections of the Royal Academy of Medicine in Ireland and was a member for some years of the RCSI Council. In the mid-1920s, the use of carbon dioxide as a respiratory stimulant during induction, maintenance and recovery from anaesthesia had become popular in some centres. The concentrations used, up to 25 per cent on occasion, seem remarkably high today. George Pugin Meldon reviewed a number of papers on using the gas to 'dominate' or 'control' respiration for the *Irish Journal of Medical Science* and suggested that its application in such a manner was also relevant to the management of asphyxia of the newborn, alcoholic intoxication, carbon monoxide poisoning and other related conditions.[25]

He took a prominent part in the St John Ambulance Brigade during the 1916 Rising and is said to have acted with great gallantry in bringing in wounded under fire; he also served as temporary captain in the Royal Army Medical Corps at the Dublin Hospital in Boulogne during the latter part of 1917.[26–29]

References

1 Zuck D., 'The Alcock chloroform vaporizer', *Anaesthesia*, 1988, 43, pp. 972–80.
2 Alcock N.H., 'A new apparatus for chloroform anaesthesia', *British Medical Journal*, 1908, 2, pp. 372–3.
3 Zuck D., 'A forgotten chloroform vaporizer in its historical context (N.H. Alcock)', in *Proceedings of the History of Anaesthesia Society*, 1988, 3, pp. 59–64.

4   Hewitt J.C. and Dundee J.W., 'Development of anaesthesia in Northern Ireland', *Ulster Medical Journal*, 1970, 39, pp. 97–107.

5   Lyons J.B., *The Quality of Mercer's: Story of Mercer's Hospital 1734–1991*, Dublin: Glendale, 1991, p. 131.

6   Crookes G., *Dublin's Eye and Ear, the Making of a Monument*, Dublin: TownHouse, 1993, p. 103.

7   J. Beckett, available at www.forces-war-records.co.uk/records/4917415/temporary-honorary-major-j-beckett-british-army-royal-army-medical-corps/ (accessed 7 December 2020).

8   Minute Book of the Adelaide Hospital Managing Committee, Meeting of 29 March 1927, MARLOC 11270/2/1/1/2/8, Trinity College Dublin.

9   Beckett J., 'Anaesthetic fatalities', *Irish Journal of Medical Science*, 1946, 21, pp. 656–61.

10 Shanahan J. .Beckett, James C[rothers?] ('Jim')', in *Dictionary of Irish Biography*, vol. 1, A–Burchill, Cambridge: Royal Irish Academy and Cambridge University Press, 2009, pp. 400–1.

11 Knowlson J., *Damned to Fame: Life of Samuel Beckett*, London: Bloomsbury, 1997, pp. 8–9.

12 'The History of the Association of Referees, Leinster Branch I.R.F.U. 1902–1977', National Library of Ireland, Pamphlet volume A28148.

13 Knowlson, *Damned to Fame*, p. 581.

14 Casey P.J., Cullen K.T. and Duignan J.P., *Irish Doctors in the First World War*, Dublin: Merrion Press, 2015, p. 5.

15 'J.W.M. In Memoriam: Charles Molyneux Benson, MD, MA Univ. Dubl., FRCSI; Surgeon to Sir Patrick Dun's Hospital, Dublin', *Dublin Journal of Medical Science*, 1919, 147, pp. 195–6.

16 Casey, Cullen, Duignan, *Irish Doctors*, p. 230.

17 Gwathmey J.T., 'Ether-oil colonic anesthesia', in *American Year-Book of Anesthesia and Analgesia*, New York: Surgery Publishing, 1915, pp. 182–212.

18 Boyd A.E., 'Oil ether colonic anæsthesia', *Dublin Journal of Medical Science*, 1920, 1, pp. 121–33.

19 'Obituary. Dr A.E. Boyd', *Irish Times*, 29 December 1949, p. 5.

20 Calwell H.G., *The Life and Times of a Voluntary Hospital: The History of the Royal Belfast Hospital for Sick Children, 1873 to 1948*, Belfast: Brown, Cox and Dunn, 1973, pp. 65, 84.

21 Clarke R.S.J., *A Directory of Ulster Doctors (who qualified before 1901)*, Belfast: Ulster Historical Foundation, 1913, pp. 248–9.

22 'T.J.G. Obituary. V.O. McCormick', *British Medical Journal*, 1970, 2, p. 486.

23 Warde D. 'Dr Victor Ormsby McCormick' available at rcoa.ac.uk/dr-victor-ormsby-mccormick (accessed 8 December 2020).

24 Whyte F. de B., 'Victor Ormsby McCormick', *Irish Times*, 17 March 1970, p. 8.

25 Meldon G.P., 'Carbon dioxide in anæsthesia', *Irish Journal of Medical Science*, 1927, 2, pp. 85–6.

26 Kirkpatrick T.P.C., 'Irish Medical Obituary; Meldon, George Pugin', *Irish Journal of Medical Science*, 1950, 25, p. 430.

27 Casey, Cullen and Duignan, *Irish Doctors*, p. 393.

28 'Obituary. Dr G.P. Meldon', *Irish Times*, 3 July 1950, p. 5.

Chapter 11

The First Ladies

Declan Warde

In 1885, the Royal College of Surgeons in Ireland (RCSI) on St Stephen's Green in Dublin became the first third-level institution in the country to admit a female student to its medical school. The lady concerned, Agnes Shannon, did not complete her studies. She was followed into RCSI in November 1886 by Mary Josephine Hannan, the daughter of Dublin banker Benjamin Hannan and his wife Grace. She qualified in 1890, thus becoming the first woman to both study medicine and graduate in Ireland. Dr Hannan subsequently practised in Dublin, India, Wales and South Africa, which is believed to have been the country of her mother's birth. Her particular interests were in paediatrics and dermatology.[1] In marked contrast to the present day, when over half of those studying medicine are female, male medical students remained overwhelmingly in the majority for many years (over 99 per cent of the total in 1898).

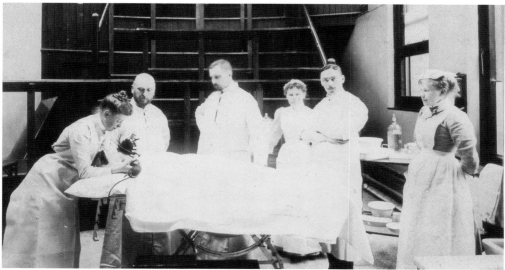

Photograph of Dr Sara McElderry anaesthetising a patient in the Mater Infirmorum Hospital, Belfast c.1901. Reproduced by kind permission of Dr Mark Gormley, Honorary Archivist, Mater Infirmorum Hospital.

The first female doctor to administer anaesthetics in Ireland may have been Sara Kyle McElderry, born in Ballymoney, County Antrim in 1877, who graduated in 1900 from the Medical College for Women in Edinburgh. She worked as a junior resident doctor in the Mater Infirmorum Hospital, Belfast prior to relocating in 1903 or so to a mission hospital in Bombay (now Mumbai), India where she spent the next 30 years. The initial official appointment of a female anaesthetist (**Ella Webb (1877–1946)**, see Chapter 24) to an Irish hospital did not take place until 1918. Webb was followed by **Ruth Mary Slade**, who was appointed as anaesthetist to the Belfast Hospital for Sick Children in 1921; she also worked in the Samaritan Hospital for Women, Belfast Maternity Hospital and a Salvation Army home but died of bronchopneumonia in January 1923. The author of her obituary in the *British Medical Journal* expressed the view that her illness had been caused by excess work.[2,3]

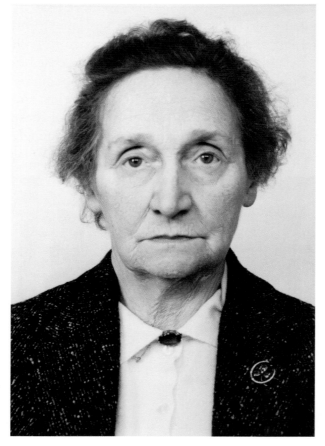

Photograph of Dr Mary Hearn. Reproduced by kind permission of the Royal College of Physicians of Ireland (VM/1/2/H/22).

Mary Hearn (*née* **Cummins, 1891–1969**), daughter of William Cummins, professor of medicine at Queen's College/University College Cork (UCC), and his wife Jane was born in Cork city in 1891. She began to study medicine in UCC but interrupted her studies in 1911 to marry Robert Thomas Hearn, vicar of Shandon, who later became Church of Ireland bishop of Cork, Cloyne and Ross. Their two children Ellice and Robert were born in 1912 and 1913. Hearn later returned to medical school and graduated in 1919 with first class honours. She worked in the North Infirmary until

1922, when she was appointed honorary anaesthetist to the Victoria Hospital. After a year or two, she was promoted to the position of assistant physician and she continued to serve the hospital up to her retirement, working primarily as a gynaecologist. Also in 1922, she attained membership of the Royal College of Physicians of Ireland (MRCPI) and two years later was elected as the college's first female fellow (FRCPI). A study and research room in its Kildare Street, Dublin building is named the Hearn Room in her memory.

An Irish hockey international herself from 1908 to 1912, three of Mary Hearn's sisters also played for Ireland. Following her death in the Victoria Hospital in 1969, a library for the hospital's nurses was created as a memorial to her. Dr Mary Hearn Park which is located beside St Ann's Church, home to Cork's famed Bells of Shandon, was officially opened in 2011.[4-7]

Olive Margery Anderson (1894–1986) was born in Belfast and educated at Coleraine High School and Queen's University, qualifying MB BCh BAO in 1917. Following graduation she served as a medical officer in the Women's Army Medical Corps, working in military hospitals in Britain from 1917–19 before returning to Belfast where she combined anaesthesia with general practice. She was sufficiently progressive and enthusiastic in the early 1920s to spend several weeks at the Westminster Hospital, London learning from Ivan Magill.

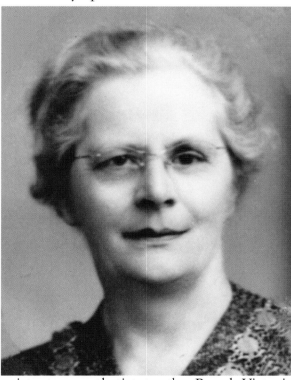

Photograph of Dr Olive Margery Anderson OBE. Courtesy of the Ulster Medical Society.

Anderson was appointed assistant anaesthetist to the Royal Victoria Hospital, Belfast in 1923 where she remained (with short breaks) until 1944. She provided anaesthetic services principally to patients in the Department of Obstetrics and Gynaecology where she was well-known for her calmness and composure with even the most turbulent of surgeons. She had become interested in the provision of contraceptive services early in her career from 1940 and worked voluntarily as medical officer to the new family planning clinic at the Royal Maternity Hospital, Belfast; she pioneered this work in Northern Ireland with Dr Elizabeth Robb. Olive Anderson obtained an MD in 1932 and the Diploma in Anaesthetics four years later. In 1957, after it had been in existence for almost 100 years, she became the first female president of the Ulster Medical Society. The main subject of her presidential address was her namesake Elizabeth Garrett Anderson who had been the first woman to qualify as a physician and surgeon in Britain. She was awarded the OBE in the 1967 New Year's Honours List for services to medicine.[8-11]

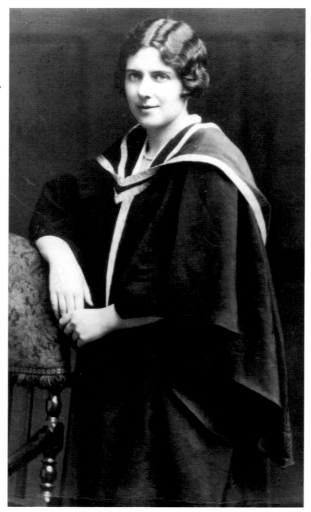

Photograph of Dr Clare McGuckin. Courtesy of her grandson, Andrew Kennedy.

Clare Mary McGuckin (later McSparran), born on 4 November 1901 to Belfast publican Hugh McGuckin and his wife Marion (*née* McMahon), was another early female Belfast anaesthetist. She qualified as a medical doctor from Queen's University in 1923 and moved to London shortly afterwards. While there, she spent some months as resident anaesthetist in the West Middlesex Hospital and learned to use Boyle's and Shipway's apparatus, Clover's and ethyl chloride inhalers, and also Magill's technique of endotracheal anaestheia, which she introduced to Northern Ireland. Upon her return to her native city, she was appointed on 3 November 1923 as the first paid anaesthetist at the Mater Infirmorum Hospital, located within 200 yards or so of the house in which she was born, and worked as anaesthetist there for the next three and a half years. She may have been the first full-time anaesthetist in Ireland. She relinquished her post shortly after marrying James McSparran, barrister-at-law and prominent nationalist politician, in University Church, Dublin in 1927. Her husband, an avid Glasgow Celtic supporter, collapsed and died on 15 April 1970 in the Director's box at the European Cup semi-final between Celtic and Leeds United in Hampden Park, Glasgow.[9,12–14]

Nannette Norris (later Quin) (1899–1989) was born at Ederney, near Irvinestown, County Fermanagh to Thomas Duke Norris, a district inspector in the Royal Irish Constabulary and his wife Helena. A 1921 medical graduate of Trinity College Dublin, she was anaesthetist to Dr Steevens' Hospital in 1926. In February of that year, she had married James Sinclair Quin, a Dublin physician and gynaecologist and interestingly, while he was noted in the Register of Marriages as a 'Medical Doctor, MD TCD, MRCPI', her post or profession was stated to be 'Lady' although she had qualified some five years previously. She continued to work in anaesthetic practice for some time and by 1933, was assistant anaesthetist to Silver Deane-Oliver in the Meath Hospital, where she was referred to as 'Mrs Quin'.

Nannette Quin and her husband were invited to the inaugural meeting, held in a Dublin hotel on 31 January 1931, of what later became the National Council for the Blind of Ireland (NCBI); the couple worked ceaselessly to assist blind people for the rest of their lives with James being a long-serving NCBI treasurer and Nannette (Nancy) acting as chairman of the Ladies Committee for many years. She was an indefatigable fundraiser for the organisation and started the concept of 'The Little Shop' which was the first charity shop in Ireland. Apart from running shops from NCBI premises, she regularly persuaded business people to provide vacant premises rent-free, often in the weeks leading up to Christmas, thus enabling her to open a series of what would now be termed 'pop-up' shops.[15] They were stocked, in part, through her own cajoling of friends and acquaintances into donating gowns, furs and even jewellery, thus raising significant funds for the charity.[16] Her efforts were to lead in time to NCBI's countrywide chain of over 100 outlets which were named Mrs Quin's Charity Shops in her memory in 1996; they were rebranded as NCBI Retail in 2012/13.

Sarah (Sal) Joyce O'Malley (1896–1959), born in Connemara, County Galway to a sheep farmer and his wife, graduated MB, BCh BAO from University College Galway in 1923. After working for a year in her native county, she moved

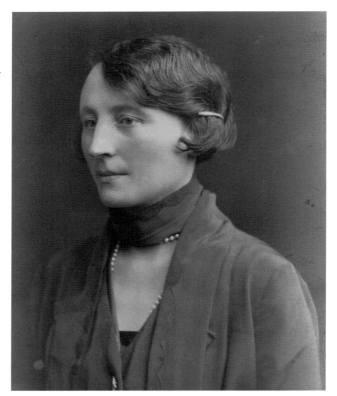

to London and obtained anaesthetic experience in a number of hospitals including University College Hospital, Charing Cross Hospital and the Chelsea Hospital for Women. Having been working as anaesthetist to the Central Hospital, Galway on an honorary basis for some years beforehand, she was appointed by the Local Appointments Commission as part-time visiting anaesthetist in 1929. She was the sole trained anaesthesia provider in the hospital for over 20 years, often working with her husband Conor O'Malley, who was professor of ophthalmology in University College Galway and also practised ear, nose and throat surgery. For over 15 years, her starting salary of £100 per annum remained unchanged, while that of her surgical colleagues rose significantly. She wrote to the hospital authorities seeking an increase; in support of her claim, she pointed out that in many thousands of anaesthetics administered by her, including over 4,500 for tonsillectomy alone, there had not been a single fatality. This was a remarkable record when one considers that, at the time, chloroform was still used extensively, skilled assistance was rarely if ever available, artificial airway support was uncommon and intraoperative monitoring consisted merely of close observation and clinical examination.

After protracted correspondence over many years, her remuneration was increased in the mid-1950s to just over £800 per annum, signifying some belated recognition for the excellent service she had provided for so long. The gender pay gap in Ireland during the 1940s was over 40 per cent; by 2017, it had fallen to a little over one-third of that figure. Sarah Joyce O'Malley's personal campaign surely played its own small part in causing the great inequity to be addressed. She never had the opportunity to enjoy retirement as she was still working as an anaesthetist when she died in 1959 aged just 62 years.[17–20]

Other women engaged in anaesthesia practice in Ireland during the 1920s included **Mary O'Leary** who graduated from the National University of Ireland in 1915. She was appointed to Dr Steevens' Hospital, Dublin in 1923 and also worked in child welfare as a schools medical officer but was lost overboard in unexplained circumstances while on a Mediterranean cruise in late 1934.[21]

Margaret Adelaide Esther Silver Deane-Oliver (1899–1988), generally known as Silver Deane-Oliver, worked as a Voluntary Aid Detachment (VAD) nurse from 1917–19 at the Irish Counties War Hospital in Glasnevin, Dublin and also at Burcote House Hospital near Abingdon, Oxfordshire.[22] She commenced her medical studies in Trinity College Dublin in 1921 and qualified five years later. Following house officer posts, she worked for many years as anaesthetist to the Meath Hospital, Dublin and also at the Royal Victoria Eye and Ear and National Children's Hospital, Harcourt Street. In 1960, she became a foundation fellow of the Faculty of Anaesthetists, RCSI.

Maude Warren McKnight (later Henry), the daughter of a publican, was born in Belfast in 1898. A 1922 Queen's University graduate, she was honorary anaesthetist to the Royal Victoria Hospital for about five years from 1927. She later worked in both Nigeria and South Africa.

Dorothea Alexandra McEntire (later Bennett), a 1925 Trinity College medical graduate, worked in a number of Dublin hospitals most notably the National Children's Hospital in Harcourt Street where she acted for a number of years from around 1930 as both anaesthetist (along with Silver Deane-Oliver) and radiologist.

Ita Dympna Brady, born in 1895, qualified from University College Dublin in 1923 and was appointed as anaesthetist to Temple Street Children's Hospital in about 1931. She was promoted to the position of assistant physician some years later and also served as assistant medical officer of health for County Dublin for over 20 years.

One of the longer serving female anaesthetists of the time was **Emily Quin** who graduated from Queen's University in 1916 and worked in the County Antrim Infirmary, Lisburn for about 15 years from 1932.

Two years later **Sheila Kenny (1909–1990)**, perhaps the premier female Irish anaesthetist of the twentieth century, was appointed to the Adelaide Hospital (see Chapter 24).

Of the 13 female anaesthetists referred to above, it appears that all but Mary Hearn and Clare McGuckin practised anaesthesia for five years or more. At least eight of the women married. Of these, seven continued to work afterwards; this was unusual in that over 90 per cent of married women in Ireland described themselves in 1926 as being engaged in home duties.[23] Male doctors who took up anaesthetic posts at the time often did so as a prelude to obtaining employment in other medical disciplines. Where early Irish female practitioners were concerned it seems that, for most, anaesthesia was their chosen specialty from the outset. At a time when opportunities for women doctors were limited, particularly in hospital medicine, their work undoubtedly helped to enhance the career prospects of all their female colleagues.

References

1 'Dr Mary Josephine Hannan (1859–1936)', available at women.rcsi.com/women/dr-mary-josephine-hannan (accessed 3 January 2021).
2 Calwell H.G., *The Life and Times of a Voluntary Hospital: The History of the Royal Belfast Hospital for Sick Children, 1873 to 1948*, Belfast: Brown, Cox and Dunn, 1973, p. 133.
3 'Obituary, Mrs Ruth Mary Slade M.B.', *British Medical Journal*, 1923, 1, p. 355.
4 Barry J.M., *The Victoria Hospital Cork – A History*, Midleton: Litho Press, 1922, p. 280.
5 Cummins N.M., *Some Chapters of Cork Medical History*, Cork: Cork University Press, 1957, p. 55.
6 Hayes C. 'Hearn, Mary Ellice Thorn' in *Dictionary of Irish Biography*', vol. 4, G–J, Cambridge: Royal Irish Academy and Cambridge University Press, 2009, pp. 580–1.
7 'Dr. Mary Hearn', *Cork Examiner*, 6 June 1969, p. 11.
8 'Clarke R.', in B. O'Donnell (ed.), *Irish Surgery and Surgeons in the Twentieth Century*, Dublin: Gill & MacMillan, 2008, p. 593.
9 Hewitt J.C. and Dundee J.W., 'Development of anaesthesia in Northern Ireland', *Ulster Medical Journal*, 1970, 39, pp. 97–107.
10 Clarke R., *The Royal Victoria Hospital Belfast: A History 1797–1997*, Belfast: Blackstaff Press, 1997, pp. 124–5.
11 Anderson O.M., 'Elizabeth Garrett Anderson and her contemporaries', *Ulster Medical Journal*, 1957, 26, pp. 97–106.
12 Kelly L., *Irish Women in Medicine, c. 1880s–1920s*, Manchester and New York: Manchester University Press, 2012, p. 222.
13 'Clarke R.', in *Irish Surgery and Surgeons*, p. 597.
14 Lynn B., 'McSparran, James' in *Dictionary of Irish Biography*, vol. 6, McGuire–Nutt, Cambridge: Royal Irish Academy and Cambridge University Press, 2009, pp. 187–8.
15 '80th 1931–2011', National Council for the Blind of Ireland, available at yumpu.com/en/ncbi.ie (accessed 11 January 2021).
16 'Who is Mrs Quin?', available at mrsquincharityroscrea.weebly.com/mrs-quin-foundation.html (accessed 11 January 2021).
17 Murray J.P., *Galway: A Medico Social History*, Galway: Kenny's, n.d., pp. 161–2, 242.

18 O'Malley Kelly A., 'Sal O'Malley, pioneering anaesthetist – a memoire', *Journal of the Galway Archaeological and Historical Society*, 2015, 67, pp. 202–8.

19 O'Brien K. and O'Brien B., 'Sarah Joyce O'Malley, Irish anaesthetist (1896–1959)', *British Journal of Anaesthesia*, 2020, 124, E187–E189.

20 Ibec, 'Measures to Address the Gender Pay Gap in Ireland', available at cdn.the journal.ie/media/2017/10/ibecs-observations-on-the-measures-to-address-the-gender-pay-gap-in-ireland.pdf (accessed 9 January 2021).

21 'Dr Mary M.A. O'Leary', *Irish Times*, 1 January 1935, p. 7.

22 'Miss Margaret Adelaide Esther Silver Deane-Oliver', available at vad.redcross.org.uk/en/Card?fname=&sname=OLIVER&id=163541 (accessed 10 January 2021).

23 Kiely E and Leane M., '"What would I be doing at home all day?": Oral narratives of Irish women's working lives 1936–1960', *Women's History Review*, 2004, 13, pp. 427–45.

Chapter 12

Developments, 1920s to early 1940s

Declan Warde

espite the various innovations introduced over the decades, it would be reasonable to state that by the beginning of the 1920s, the methods and agents used by anaesthetists had not changed greatly since Morton's first public demonstration in Boston almost 75 years earlier. Open ether and chloroform were still widely employed, while ethyl chloride and nitrous oxide were generally reserved for induction of anaesthesia or dental surgery. The use of local or regional techniques remained limited while, apart from clinical observation, intraoperative monitoring was still virtually non-existent. The following two decades were to bring a number of advances, some of which would change the developing specialty forever.

In 1920, **Ivan Magill (1888–1986)** (see Chapter 24) described the forceps which to this day bear his name and also recorded his first use of a wide-bore tube inserted through the nostril and passed down into the trachea, through which anaesthetic agents could be delivered to the patient. It took a few more years for him to find suitable tubing to cut to different lengths, bevel and smooth in order to prepare what later became known as the Magill endotracheal tube. As a consequence, he did not write and publish a full paper on the details of his technique until 1928. Magill's success with what was soon to become known as blind nasal intubation excited the curiosity of other anaesthetists to whom he taught his principles at meetings of the Section of Anaesthetics of the Royal Society of Medicine in London.[1-3] The introduction of endotracheal intubation not only ensured that the anaesthetist no longer needed to be in almost continuous contact with the patient's face but also that he or she could provide positive pressure ventilation at will.[4]

Alfred Boyd's use of oil-ether anaesthesia was discussed in Chapter 9. In 1926, tribromoethanol (Avertin), another agent that could be administered rectally, was first clinically employed by Butzengeiger in Germany.[5] In early 1928,

APPLIANCES AND PREPARATIONS.

Forceps for Intratracheal Anaesthesia.

DR. IVAN W. MAGILL (Anaesthetist, Queen's Hospital, Sidcup) writes: Following on Dr. Rowbotham's article in the JOURNAL of October 16th on intratracheal anaesthesia by the nasal route, the accompanying illustration of a forceps, made for me by Messrs. Meyer and Phelps for a similar purpose, may be of interest. The forceps are constructed with a bend to clear the field of vision, as in Heath's nasal forceps, the ends which grasp the catheter representing a cylinder split longitudinally and

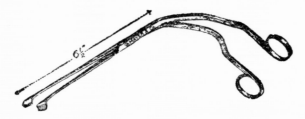

serrated on the inner surface. Introduction of the catheter into the trachea is carried out with the aid of an electrically illuminated speculum, as in Dr. Rowbotham's method, but I find in the forceps the following advantages over Dr. Rowbotham's guiding rod:

1. There is no injury to the end of the catheter, and therefore no liability of small pieces of the friable material being left in the trachea.
2. The catheter is more easily picked up in the oral pharynx, and once grasped the hold is secure, without the necessity of holding the free end which protrudes from the nose, as is the case with the guiding rod.
3. The forceps can be used at the side of, as well as inside, the speculum.
4. The field of vision is always clear.

I need hardly add that in operations involving bleeding into the pharynx the fixation of a suitable suction pump to the expiratory nasal tube provides even a clearer field for the surgeon by removing blood without continual swabbing.

Dr (later Sir) Ivan Magill's 1920 letter to the British Medical Journal describing his 'forceps for intratracheal anaesthesia'. British Medical Journal, 30 October 1920.

prior to its general release in Britain and Ireland, a consignment for research purposes was sent to an anaesthetics committee set up by the Medical Research Council (UK) and the Section of Anaesthetics of the Royal Society of Medicine.[6] This was redistributed, in turn, to three prominent London anaesthetists but also, for reasons that are unclear, to a surgeon in Bradford, England and to **Francis 'Pops' Morrin (1893–1967)**, also a surgeon, who worked in St Vincent's Hospital, Dublin. Morrin's impressions of tribromoethanol were published in June of the following year.[7] He described the anaesthesia produced as resembling normal

137

Photograph of Dr August Karl Gustav Bier, who in 1898 was first to administer a spinal anaesthetic. Courtesy of NIH Digital Collections.

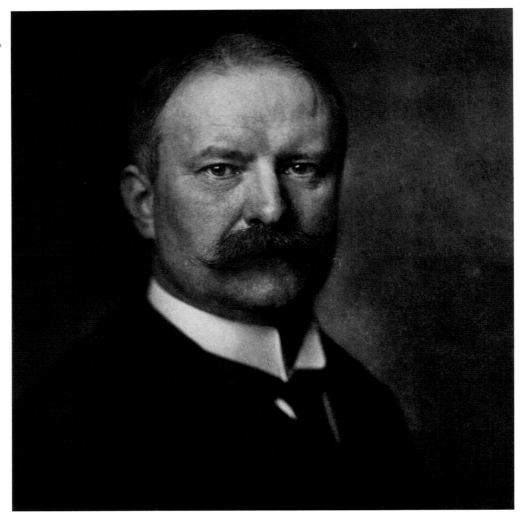

sleep and wrote that problems only developed when high doses were used. The average systolic blood pressure fall in his patients was 27 mm Hg., while the average duration of anaesthesia was sufficient for all major operative work. Analgesia that lasted for some hours after the end of surgery was a feature of the recovery period. He noted, as some previous investigators had found, that failure to obtain full anaesthesia was occasionally encountered. He had used tribromoethanol in 54 cases altogether, many of them patients with advanced head and neck cancer, and found it to be very satisfactory overall. He was particularly impressed with its value in cases for which the use of diathermy was necessary. The agent was widely used for five years or so, but was ultimately abandoned because of a high incidence of complications, including death.

On 16 August 1898 in Kiel, Germany, **August Bier (1861–1949)** had performed the first operation under spinal anaesthesia when he administered intrathecal cocaine to a man aged 34 years who had suffered severe adverse effects from a previous general anaesthetic and was about to undergo resection of a tuberculous ankle joint. The technique was soon used extensively in a number of European countries but acceptance was slower elsewhere. Its popularity waxed and waned until the 1930s when usage became widespread, but there was a sharp decline again in the 1950s due to adverse publicity concerning neurological sequelae.[8–10] **Richard Atkinson Stoney (1877–1966)**, visiting surgeon to the Royal City of Dublin Hospital in Baggot Street, may have been the first in Ireland to employ spinal anaesthesia; in 1911, he described its successful use for prostatectomy in a patient considered unfit for general anaesthesia.[11]

By 1928, **Andrew Hope Davidson (1895–1967)**, who later became professor of midwifery at the Royal College of Surgeons in Ireland and was master of the Rotunda Hospital from 1933 to 1940, had used spinal anaesthesia in some 30 to 40 patients undergoing either gynaecological surgery or Caesarean section and wished to provoke discussion on and provide some impetus to a procedure which he considered deserved a definite place in the provision of anaesthesia for both general surgical and obstetrical operations. He wrote that novocain and stovain were the two drugs in general use at the time, with the latter probably being the more satisfactory. He described the sitting technique used by him, the patient having been premedicated with morphine and scopolamine beforehand, and considered the definite indications for the technique to be heart disease, lung disease, oral sepsis, renal disease and, in fact, any condition which made the patient a bad subject for a general anaesthetic. Davidson referred to the fact that the chief disadvantage of spinal anaesthesia was depression of the general circulation, that nausea and vomiting could develop during the operation or after the patient's return to bed, and that very severe headache sometimes followed. He had found that the way to relieve such headache was by the intravenous injection of 20 ccs of a 20 per cent solution of sodium chloride but made no reference to pre-loading with intravenous fluid prior to the procedure. Writing that respiratory failure, when it occurred, was due to faulty technique, he stated that although very terrifying, it could be overcome by artificial respiration and the giving of cardiac stimulants. In rare cases, the injection of a caffeine-strychnine preparation into the spinal canal might be required.

Davidson also considered that there was a well-marked place for local anaesthesia in obstetrics and gynaecology using novocain with adrenaline, for example in the removal of cysts and other operations on the vulva, perineum or anus. In addition, he wrote that there existed another regional technique called caudal, extradural or epidural analgesia, which he considered to be a very valuable method and described his technique for carrying out a caudal epidural injection, again using novocain with adrenaline. He cautioned against injecting the solution too rapidly and stated that, with care, any after-effects observed tended to be of little moment. He did not reveal the extent of his experience with the procedure but opined that extradural injection provided splendid anaesthesia of the entire pelvic floor and viscera. He believed, quite presciently, that its main usefulness would prove to be during labour.

Overall, Davidson considered that regional anaesthesia, especially in obstetric and gynaecological practice, was worthy of much more attention than had been given to it previously. He concluded by expressing the view that it should not yet be allowed to become routine, but that if the correct patient was chosen, her cooperation obtained and she was made comfortable, the operator will have made a friend for life.[12]

A more wide-ranging account of pain relief in labour was provided by another Irish-born obstetrician, **Dame Anne Louise McIlroy (1874–1968)**. A native of Loughguile, a few miles from Ballycastle, County Antrim, she enrolled as a medical student at the University of Glasgow in 1894 and graduated four years later. She also studied in London, Dublin, Vienna and Berlin. During World War One she worked at the Scottish Women's Hospital in Troyes (France), and also served in Serbia (where she established a nurse training school), Greece and finally with the Royal Army Medical Corps in Constantinople (Istanbul). In 1921, she became professor of obstetrics and gynaecology at the London School of Medicine for Women and the Royal Free Hospital, thus becoming the first female medical professor in the United Kingdom.[13]

McIlroy wrote, in 1930, that in every case of labour, pain should be alleviated as far as possible within the limits of safety for the mother and infant and provided a comprehensive account of the use of various analgesic regimens during the first stage, including opioids alone and the combination of an opioid with scopolamine in order to produce 'twilight sleep'. She believed that the pain of the second stage could be relieved in almost every case if proper methods were applied and was of the view that more satisfactory results could be obtained by the use of intermittent anaesthetic inhalations than from morphine. Wary of

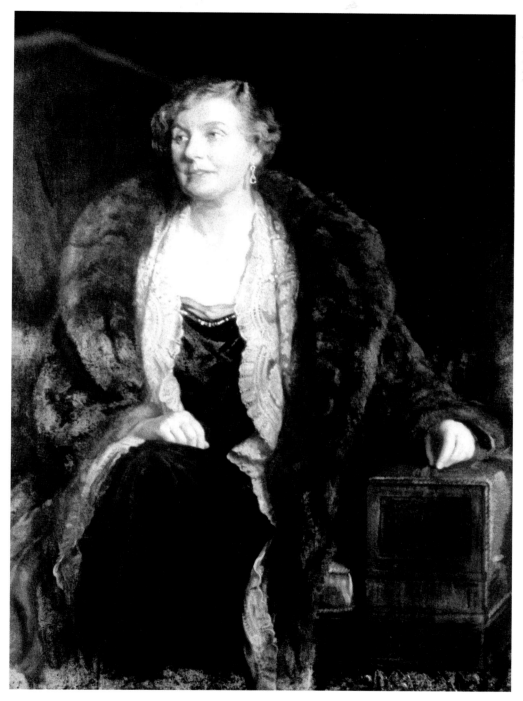

Portrait of Dame Anne Louise McIlroy. Courtesy of History Ireland.

chloroform but not dismissing it entirely, she wrote that in London at least, ether was the most widely used anaesthetic during labour. In her opinion, a mixture of nitrous oxide (80 per cent) and oxygen (20 per cent), administered by a competent anaesthetist, was by far the safest and most satisfactory anaesthetic for the second stage – she considered it to be the anaesthetic of the future in obstetric practice. She commented, although she had little personal experience, that the injection of novocain into the sacral canal rendered the latter part of labour and delivery almost painless, and at the same time gave good relaxation of the tissues. Finally, McIlroy believed that the use of anaesthetics during the third stage of labour was undesirable, except for manual removal of the placenta or when repair of the cervix or perineum proved necessary.[14]

The first issue of the *British Journal of Anaesthesia*, the earliest United Kingdom anaesthetic journal, was published in 1923. Eight years elapsed before the appearance of a paper written by a practitioner based in Ireland.[15] Dr Oswald Murphy, anaesthetist to St Vincent's Hospital in Dublin, wrote that ether remained the most satisfactory and reliable agent for routine work. He went on to discuss the relative advantages of the open and closed methods of administration, coming down firmly in favour of the latter.

As far back as 1874, Pierre-Cyprien Oré of Bordeaux, France had reported to the French Academy of Sciences what is believed to have been the first use of intravenous anaesthesia in man. He had employed chloral hydrate but, despite his enthusiasm for both the drug and technique, and reports in the contemporary literature by other Frenchmen, a significantly high mortality rate prevented further development until after the turn of the century. Nicholas Krockow (1865–1925) used hedonal (methylpropylcarbinol urethane) in St Petersburg, Russia from 1909; it was the first anaesthetic for intravenous use that produced fairly adequate surgical anaesthesia with a moderate degree of safety.[16,17] Three years later, **Herbert de Lisle Crawford** (a 1910 Trinity College graduate) who was honorary assistant surgeon to Dublin's Richmond Hospital, described his experience in using the drug by continuous infusion in 30 patients, and stated that he obtained full surgical anaesthesia in all. While his overall impressions of hedonal were positive, he considered the intravenous technique to be unnecessarily complicated for minor operations and commented that both induction of and recovery from anaesthesia were slow.[18] These were precisely the reasons why hedonal's use effectively came to an end following the later introduction of intravenous barbiturates. While Crawford worked primarily as a surgeon, he had a significant interest in anaesthesia; in 1913, he described an apparatus he had developed for the intratracheal insufflation of ether, while, in 1920, he was awarded a doctorate for his thesis on the choice of anaesthetic in dangerous cases.[19,20]

Although both alcohol and tribromoethanol had been tried previously, 'Pernoston', a barbiturate, was the first drug to attain anything approaching widespread use as an intravenous anaesthetic after it was introduced by the German obstetrician Bumm in 1927.[21] Two years later, John Lundy of the Mayo Clinic drew attention to the intermittent administration of amylobarbitone as a method of increasing the quality and safety of anaesthesia.[22] It was subsequently used for a short period by both Ronald Jarman in London and Henry Featherstone in Birmingham. In 1931, pentobarbitone was employed as both an intravenous anaesthetic and oral premedicant by, among others, Ivan Magill.[23] However, it should be pointed out that at the time, the barbiturates used, all of which had a relatively slow onset time, were simply regarded as being basal narcotics that bridged the gap between consciousness and unconsciousness – inhalational agents remained synonymous with general anaesthesia. The first rapidly acting intravenous anaesthetic was hexobarbitone. Its use for induction of anaesthesia was first reported in the German literature in 1932 and two years later, John Cameron Crawford, honorary dental anaesthetist to the Belfast Hospital for Sick Children, employed it by intermittent injection for 50 dental anaesthetics in children aged between 6 and 12 years.[24] The drug was an immediate success and it was estimated that it had been administered to ten million patients in the first 10 years after its introduction.

On 8 March 1934, **Ralph Waters (1883–1979)**, in Madison, Wisconsin, was the first to use thiopental sodium (thiopentone) in man.[25] It was to become, until the introduction of propofol over 50 years later, the intravenous induction agent of choice for most purposes. The first account from Britain was published in February 1936. In December of the same year, **Edward Solomons**, who was to become professor of obstetrics and gynaecology at the State University of New York in 1954, described its use in 43 patients, most of whom were on the labour ward of the Rotunda Hospital, Dublin where he was assistant master.[26,27] It had been employed as a sole agent for a variety of indications, the majority of which were evacuation of the retained products of conception, forceps delivery or perineal suturing. In a number of instances, the operator gave the injection and carried out the procedure. Solomons wrote that, at the time, thiopentone was not yet on the market in Ireland but that he had been provided with a supply by the manufacturer. From the perspective of year 2021, it seems remarkable that as recently as the mid-1930s, what appears to have been the earliest paper from Ireland on a drug that was soon to become such an important part of the anaesthetist's armamentarium was written by an obstetrician, who was also the person who had investigated its effects on patients.

Ralph Waters and his colleagues were also the first to use cyclopropane in clinical anaesthetic practice. Having commenced animal experiments in 1930, their initial paper on their experience with the gas in almost 450 patients was published in spring 1934.[28] Meanwhile, the agent had been introduced to Britain in December of the previous year by Royden Muir, a South African anaesthetist, who had brought a cylinder with him from America and administered it to several patients in the Royal Cancer Hospital in London.[29] In late 1934, Stanley Sykes of Leeds reported on its use in a small personal series of just 13 cases.[30] John Boyd (see below) was definitely using it in Belfast from 1938 but it seems likely that it was employed at an earlier date both in that city and in other Irish centres.

Just one year after the first cyclopropane communication, Striker and colleagues in Cincinnati, Ohio wrote of their initial experience with another new inhaled anaesthetic agent, trichloroethylene.[31] Principally because of safety concerns, it did not come into widespread clinical use for a further six years, after the publication of a 1941 paper by Christopher Langton Hewer of St Bartholomew's Hospital ('Barts') in London.[32,33]

As early as the 1930s, a few Irish anaesthetists were working primarily in 'niche' areas that were of particular interest to them; examples included anaesthesia for children or for patients undergoing specific types of surgical operations. Nowadays there are almost as many 'special interests' for anaesthetists as there are surgical specialties with many spending much if not all of their time outside the operating theatre working in areas such as chronic pain management or critical care.

A number of similar appointments to that of Isaac Davidson had been made during the first two decades of the twentieth century at the Belfast Hospital for Sick Children. The arrangement cannot have been entirely satisfactory, for in 1923, the staff requested the appointment of a second house surgeon, part of whose duties would be to administer anaesthetics. They brought to the notice of the hospital board that Miss Annie Knox, the matron, had been giving most of the anaesthetics for a great number of years, and they wished to relieve her of this duty because she had too much to do.[34] Within five years, a major change occurred. Although he combined working as an anaesthetist and as a general practitioner for much of his professional life, **John Boyd (1902–1981)** might be

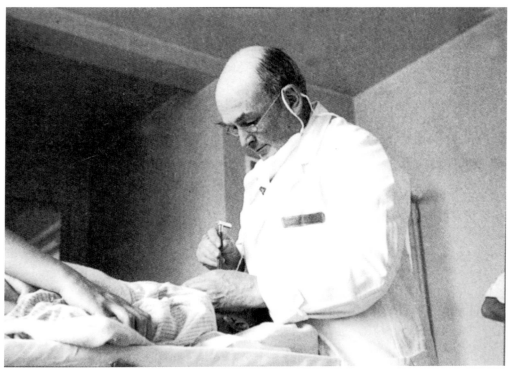

considered to have been the first Irish anaesthetist with a definite subspecialty interest. The son of a Belfast baker, he paid his own way through the Royal Belfast Academical Institution and Queen's University medical school by dint of hard work and business enterprise – selling Ulster soda bread. After graduating MB, BCh BAO in 1926 and working as a house surgeon in the Royal Victoria Hospital and Queen Street Hospital for Children, he was appointed honorary anaesthetist to the latter in 1928 by his medical colleagues, apparently without any reference to hospital management. One of his first requests was for permission to order a nitrous oxide and oxygen apparatus. He became assistant anaesthetist to the Royal Victoria Hospital in 1937; eight years later, the Board of Management at the Belfast Hospital for Sick Children (later designated Royal), which had relocated to Falls Road in the interim, created the post of honorary visiting anaesthetist on condition that the appointee be engaged exclusively in the practice of anaesthesia. Boyd's candidature was unanimously approved and he gave up general practice. He was appointed consultant anaesthetist at the Royal Victoria Hospital in 1948.

145

Boyd's MD, awarded in 1933, was for his thesis was on the role of rectal tribromoethanol. He published extensively on its use as a complete anaesthetic in paediatric practice, and also on cyclopropane anaesthesia. He was especially well-known for his technique of blind nasal intubation in children, a procedure at which his skill was said to be unparalleled. He obtained his DA (RCP&SI) in 1943 and was later elected a foundation fellow of both the English and Irish Faculties of Anaesthetists. He was a dedicated Bible student whose expert opinion was regularly sought regarding the interpretation of various passages and who, in his spare time, was happiest teaching holy writ in a small gospel hall in Crossgar, County Down.[35-37]

Paul Finbarre Murray (1905–1981), son of Hugh Murray, chief transfer clerk of the Great Northern Railway, and his wife Josephine, was born in Sandycove, County Dublin. Educated at Blackrock College and the Royal College of Surgeons in Ireland, he graduated LRCP & SI in 1929. He worked initially in house surgeon and physician posts at the Richmond Hospital and later as assistant physician to the Children's Hospital, Temple Street and anaesthetist to the City of Dublin Skin and Cancer Hospital. He became anaesthetist to the Richmond Hospital, Dublin in 1936.[38] He obtained his DA (London) in 1941, was a foundation fellow of the Faculty of Anaesthetists, RCSI and served on its first board.

The surgeon **Adams Andrew McConnell (1884–1972)** began developing a neurosurgical service in the Richmond in 1913 and by the time of Murray's appointment, the specialty was well-established in the hospital. Although he continued to work part-time in general practice for a few years, Murray soon developed a particular interest and expertise in anaesthesia for neurosurgery. A special October 1946 issue of the *Irish Journal of Medical Science*, commemorating the centenary of Morton's first public demonstration in Boston, included a comprehensive paper by him on the subject. He believed that the ideal anaesthetic for intracranial exploration consisted of premedication with papaveretum and scopolamine, followed by local infiltration of the scalp using novocain with adrenaline. For those cases in which general anaesthesia was required, he stressed the importance of endotracheal intubation and care with positioning in order to ensure an unobstructed airway; he pointed out that this was of particular importance in patients undergoing posterior cranial fossa surgery which was carried out with the patient in the prone position. He considered a combination of nitrous oxide and oxygen with tribromoethanol to be the general anaesthetic of choice. His paper included a copy of his anaesthetic

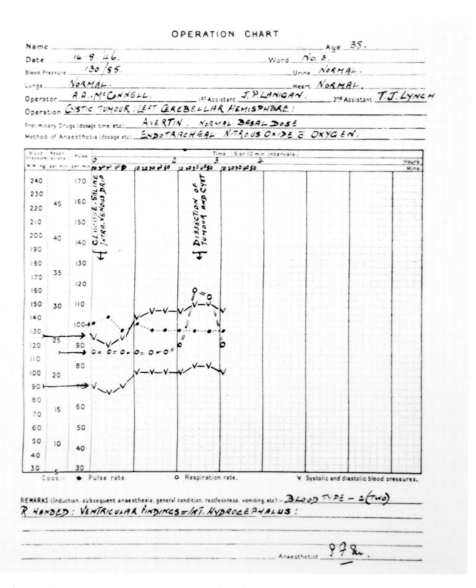

OPERATION CHART

Name _____ Age 35.
Date 16-8-46.   Ward No. 3.
Blood Pressure 130/85.   Urine NORMAL.
Lungs NORMAL.   Heart NORMAL.
Operator A.R. McCONNELL.   1st Assistant J.P LANIGAN.   2nd Assistant T.J. LYNCH
Operation CYSTIC TUMOUR : LEFT CEREBELLAR HEMISPHERE :
Preliminary Drugs (dosage time etc.) AVERTIN. NORMAL BASAL DOSE
Method of Anaesthesia (dosage etc) ENDOTRACHEAL NITROUS OXIDE & OXYGEN.

REMARKS (Induction, subsequent anaesthesia, general condition, restlessness, vomiting, etc) – BLOOD TYPE – 2 (TWO)
R. HANDED : VENTRICULAR FINDINGS = INT. HYDROCEPHALUS :

Anaesthetist _____

Anaesthetic chart of a patient anaesthetised by Dr Paul Murray in 1946 for excision of a tumour of the left cerebellar hemisphere. Courtesy of Springer Nature.

record relating to a recent operation for the removal of a cerebellar tumour.[39] Ten years later, he was co-author of a significant article on the importance of correct positioning of patients undergoing spinal surgery in preventing venous congestion.[40]

The results of the first clinical trials of what, at the time, was a revolutionary new inhalational anaesthetic agent, halothane, were published in September and

147

October 1956.[41,42] By November, Paul Murray was using it in his neuroanaesthesia practice. Two years later, he reported that he had employed halothane in all types of neurosurgical cases, some 500 in all, the patients' ages having ranged from three weeks to 75 years. The overall results were very satisfactory; he considered the agent's hypotensive effect, easily reversed, to be a particular advantage in anaesthesia for neurosurgery.[43] While there had been at least one earlier publication on the use of the new drug in neurosurgical patients,[44] the Richmond Hospital series, when it appeared in print, seems to have been by far the largest published up to that time.

Murray's skills extended far beyond the operating theatre. Mary Hearn (hockey) and Jim Beckett (watersports) had already represented Ireland in international sport, but he could be said to have gone one step further. A member of Wanderers Rugby Club, he was capped for Ireland at senior international level on 19 occasions between 1927 and 1933, scoring 33 points. In 1930, he was selected for the British Lions squad (as it was known at the time) that toured New Zealand and Australia. He played in three of the four Tests against New Zealand, missing the third because of injury. The Lions won the first but lost the other three. He played in 17 matches altogether on the tour, including the one Test against Australia, which the Lions lost 6-5. Murray became president of the Leinster Branch of the Irish Rugby Football Union (IRFU) in 1935, an Irish international selector (1935–7) and IRFU president (1965–6). Also an accomplished amateur golfer, he won the South of Ireland championship in 1940.[45–47] Fifty-five years later, his grandson Jody Fanagan partnered Padraig Harrington to defeat Tiger Woods and John Harris of the USA in the 1995 Walker Cup played at Royal Porthcawl Golf Club in Wales.

Born in Scotland in 1914, **Dr Jay Fleming** (*née* Fairweather) was a 1938 graduate of the University of Glasgow. In 1939, Andrew Hope Davidson suggested to Dr Fleming, whose husband had recently been assistant master in the Rotunda Hospital, that she should go to London and train as an anaesthetic specialist. This she did and worked under Ronald Jarman who, along with Lawrence Abel, had introduced the use of both hexobarbitone (1934) and thiopentone (1935) into British anaesthesia practice. Following her return to Dublin, she was appointed to the Rotunda and was perhaps the first specialist obstetric anaesthetist in Dublin. She obtained the Diploma in Anaesthetics in 1943 and was elected FFARCSI in 1962. Fleming was considered an expert in the administration of spinal anaesthesia; this was of great importance in the 1940s as there were times when inhalation anaesthesia was unavailable for

148

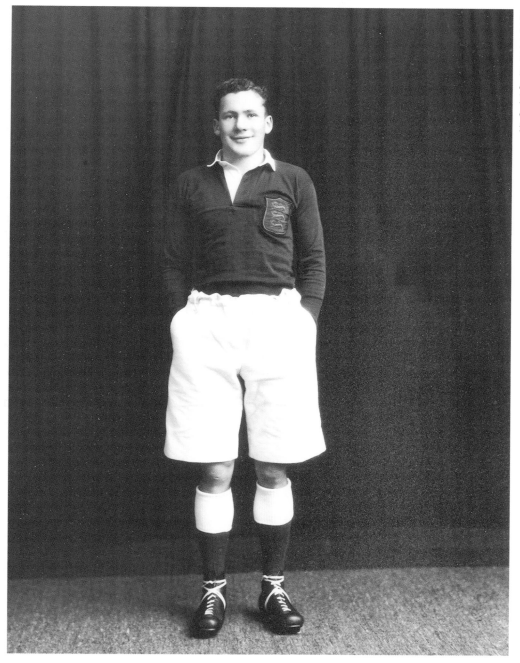

Photograph of Dr Paul Murray, 1930 British Lions tour of New Zealand and Australia. By kind permission of the Murray family.

operations such as Caesarean section due to a shortage of oxygen and nitrous oxide. In addition to her contribution to anaesthesia, she also designed an inexpensive portable infant resuscitation kit for use in developing countries; she introduced the kit personally in Addis Ababa, Ethiopia.[48-50]

References

1   Magill I.W., 'Forceps for intratracheal anaesthesia', *British Medical Journal*, 1920, 2, p. 670.

2   Calverley R.K., 'Intubation in Anaesthesia', in R.S. Atkinson and T.B. Boulton (eds), *The History of Anaesthesia: Proceedings of the Second International Symposium on the History of Anaesthesia held in London 20–23 July 1987*, London and New York: Royal Society of Medicine, 1989, pp. 333–41.

3   Magill I.W., 'Endotracheal anæsthesia', *Proceedings of the Royal Society of Medicine*, 1928, 22, pp. 83–8.

4   Dundee J.W., 'Anaesthetics, with special reference to Ivan Magill', *Ulster Medical Journal*, 1987, 56, pp. 587–90.

5   Keys T.E., *The History of Surgical Anesthesia*, New York: Schuman's, 1945, p. 48.

6   Edwards G., 'The introduction of Avertin', *British Journal of Anaesthesia*, 1938, 15, pp. 154–7.

7   Morrin F.J., 'Rectal narcosis with Avertin', *Irish Journal of Medical Science*, 1929, 4, pp. 256–61.

8   Wulf H.F.W., 'The centennial of spinal anesthesia', *Anesthesiology*, 1998, 89, pp. 500–6.

9   Brown T.C.K., 'History of pediatric regional anesthesia', *Pediatric Anesthesia*, 2012, 22, pp. 3–9.

10 Maltby J.R., Hutter C.D.D. and Clayton K.C., 'The Woolley and Roe case', *British Journal of Anaesthesia*, 2000, 84, pp. 121–6.

11 Stoney R.A., 'The use of spinal anæsthesia in prostatectomy', *Medical Press and Circular*, 1911, 92 NS, pp. 575–7.

12 Davidson A.H., 'Regional and spinal anæsthesia in obstetrics and gynæcology', *Irish Journal of Medical Science*, 1928, 3, pp. 268–72.

13 'Surgeon Anne Louise McIlroy', available at universitystory@gla.ac.uk/ww1-biography/?id=4481 (accessed 7 June 2021).

14 McIlroy L., 'Analgesia and anæsthesia in labour', *Medical Press and Circular*, 1930, 129 NS, pp. 302–6.

15 Murphy O.J., 'Ether – open or closed?', *British Journal of Anaesthesia*, 1930, 8, pp. 11–14.

16 Keys, *The History*, p. 56.

17 Kissin I. and Wright A.J., 'The introduction of hedonal: A Russian contribution to intravenous anesthesia', *Anesthesiology*, 1988, 69, pp. 242–5.

18 Crawford, H. de Lisle., 'Hedonal as an anæsthetic', *Medical Press and Circular*, 1912, 94 NS, pp. 515–7.

19 'Transactions of the Royal Academy of Medicine in Ireland, Section of Surgery Meeting of March 28th 1913. Intratracheal insufflation of ether – report of cases and demonstration of apparatus', *Medical Press and Circular*, 1913, 95 NS, p. 423.

20 'Crawford, Herbert de Lisle' in *1929 Medical Directory*, London: Churchill, 1929, p. 585.

21 Dundee J.W. and McIlroy P.D.A., 'The history of the barbiturates', *Anaesthesia*, 1982, 37, pp. 726–34.

22 Lundy J.S., 'Intravenous anesthesia: Particularly hypnotic, anesthesia and toxic effects of certain new derivatives of barbituric acid', *Current Researches in Anesthesia and Analgesia*, 1930, 9, pp. 210–7.

23 Magill I.W., 'Nembutal as a basal hypnotic in general anaesthesia', *The Lancet*, 1931, 1, pp. 74–5.

24 Crawford J.C.C., 'Intravenous anaesthesia with evipan sodium in children', *Ulster Medical Journal*, 1934, 3, pp. 191–3.

25 Dundee J., 'Editorial. Fifty years of thiopentone', *British Journal of Anaesthesia*, 1984, 56, pp. 211–12.

26 Jarman R., Abel A.L., 'Intravenous anaesthesia with pentothal sodium', *The Lancet*, 1936, 1, pp. 422–3.

27 Solomons E., 'Pentothal sodium in obstetrics', *Irish Journal of Medical Science*, 1936, 11, pp. 746–51.

28 Stiles J.A., Neff W.B., Rovenstine E.A. and Waters R.M., 'Cyclopropane as an anesthetic agent: A preliminary clinical report', *Current Researches in Anesthesia and Analgesia*, 1934, 13, pp. 56–60.

29 Rowbotham S., Chester A., Phillips G.R., Jarman R. and Vaile T.B., 'Cyclopropane anaesthesia: A report on 200 cases', *The Lancet*, 1935, 2, pp. 1110–3.

30 Sykes W.S., 'Cyclopropane anaesthesia', *British Medical Journal*, 1934, ii, pp. 901–2.

31 Striker C., Goldblatt S., Warm I.S., Jackson D.E., 'Clinical experiences with the use of trichloroethylene in the production of over 300 anesthesias and analgesias', *Current Researches in Anesthesia and Analgesia*, 1935, 14, pp. 68–71.

32 Hewer C.L., 'Trichloroethylene as an inhalation anaesthetic', *British Medical Journal*, 1941, 1, pp. 924–7.

33 Parkhouse J., 'Trichloroethylene', *British Journal of Anaesthesia*, 1965, 37, pp. 681–7.

34 Calwell H.G., *The Life and Times of a Voluntary Hospital: The History of the Royal Belfast Hospital for Sick Children, 1873 to 1948*, Belfast: Brown, Cox and Dunn, 1973, p. 84.

35 Boyd J., 'Avertin as a complete anaesthetic in children. A study of 700 cases', *British Medical Journal*, 1935, 1, pp. 1120–2.

36 Boyd J., 'Cyclopropane anaesthesia', *Ulster Medical Journal*, 1946, 15, pp. 58–77.

37 Love H., *The Royal Belfast Hospital for Sick Children – A History, 1948–1998*, Belfast: Blackstaff, 1998, pp. 91–2.

38 'Clarke R.', in B. O'Donnell (ed.), *Irish Surgery and Surgeons in the Twentieth Century*, Dublin: Gill & MacMillan, 2008, p. 589.

39 Murray P.F., 'Anaesthesia in neurosurgery', *Irish Journal of Medical Science*, 1946, 21, pp. 680–3.

40 Taylor A.R., Gleadhill C.A., Bilsland W.L. and Murray P.F., 'Posture and anaesthesia for spinal surgery with particular reference to intervertebral disc surgery', *British Journal of Anaesthesia*, 1956, 28, pp. 213–9.

41 Johnstone M., 'The human cardiovascular response to cardiovascular anaesthesia', *British Journal of Anaesthesia*, 1956, 28, pp. 392–410.

42 Bryce-Smith R. and O'Brien H.D., 'Fluothane: A non-explosive volatile agent', *British Medical Journal*, 1956, 2, p. 969.

43 Murray P.F., 'Fluothane in neurosurgery', *Irish Journal of Medical Science*, 1958, 33, pp. 433–8.

44 Brindle G.F., Little D.M. and Tovell R.M., 'The use of fluothane for neurosurgery: A preliminary report', *Canadian Anaesthetists Society Journal*, 1957, 4, pp. 265–81.

45 Coleman M., 'Murray, Paul Finbarre', in *Dictionary of Irish Biography*, vol. 6, McGuire–Nutt, Cambridge: Royal Irish Academy and Cambridge University Press, 2009, pp. 834–5.
46 'Paul Murray', available at lionsrugby.com/history/ (accessed 5 February 2020).
47 'Paul Murray', available at en.espn.co.uk./scrum/rugby/player/3388.html (accessed 5 February 2020).
48 Gardiner J., 'Anaesthesia and Analgesia in the Rotunda' in A. Browne (ed.), *Masters, Midwives and Ladies-in-Waiting: The Rotunda Hospital 1745–1995*, Dublin: A & A Farmar, pp. 180–5.
49 Organe G., 'Obituary. Ronald Jarman DSC, FRCS, FFARCS, FFARCSI (Hon)', *Anaesthesia*, 1973, 28, p. 197.
50 'Report of the Rotunda Hospital (1st November 1940–31st October 1941)', *Irish Journal of Medical Science*, 1942, 200, pp. 273–397.

PART II

Chapter 13

Organisations and Academic Developments in the Twentieth Century: An Overview

Joseph Tracey

In 1893, Dr Frederick Silk founded the Society of Anaesthetists in London, the first body to bring practitioners of the specialty together. Its objectives were to encourage the study of anaesthetics and to foster friendly relations between its members through debates, discussions and scientific papers.[1] In 1908, this society then joined the newly formed Royal Society of Medicine (RSM) to become the 'Section of Anaesthetics'. As the specialty developed, it was realised that the group needed a forum to organise working conditions, terms of employment and remuneration. However, the RSM was confined to purely scientific activities, so members of the section decided to form a body to deal with contractual and other matters. Thus, the Association of Anaesthetists of Great Britain and Ireland was founded in 1932 by Dr Henry Featherstone who had just retired as president of the Section of Anaesthetics of the RSM.

1932: The Association of Anaesthetists of Great Britain and Ireland
(see Chapter 14)
The practice of anaesthesia took its first steps towards specialty recognition in 1932 with the formation of the Association of Anaesthetists of Great Britain and Ireland. A number of Irish anaesthetists were involved in the foundation of this body, notably Dr (later Sir) Ivan Magill from Larne, County Antrim. The Association wanted to improve the safety of anaesthesia by developing proper training and Magill, in particular, was insistent about the need for a suitable postgraduate qualification. After discussions between the Royal Colleges of Physicians and Surgeons in the UK, the Conjoint Diploma in Anaesthetics (DA) was introduced there in 1935. As this was the only formal examination in the specialty in the British Isles, a number of Irish anaesthetists took the exam (e.g. Drs Olive Anderson, Stafford Geddes and Patrick Nagle in 1936; Dr Tommy

Gilmartin in 1937; Dr John Dorman in 1941; Dr Maurice Brown in 1945; Dr Edmund Delaney in 1955 and Dr Joe Galvin in 1959).[2]

1942: Conjoint Diploma in Anaesthetics

In Ireland, the first discussions on developing a similar diploma took place at a council meeting of the Royal College of Surgeons in Ireland on 10 July 1941, when the question of the award of a diploma in anaesthetics was raised.[3] This was then referred to the Examinations Committee to draw up a scheme and report back to the council. The committee duly responded in October recommending that the council should award a diploma. Regulations for an examination were discussed and the registrar of the college was instructed to obtain further information from the English Conjoint Board regarding their DA exam. Subsequently, a letter was received from the English board in December 1941 stating that their candidates were required to submit a list of 1,000 operations for which they had administered anaesthetics. The candidates had also to set out, in each case, the nature of the operation and the type of anaesthetic used. This list had to be submitted to the committee of management who would then decide whether or not it included 500 major operations. The Dublin committee decided to adopt a similar principle with the total number of cases being reduced to 600 of which 300 should be major. In January 1942, the council received a request from the Royal College of Physicians of Ireland that the diploma be a conjoint one. At the next council meeting, Mr William 'Bill' Doolin (a surgeon at St Vincent's Hospital) suggested that it might be appropriate to award the DA *honoris causa* to certain anaesthetists of long standing, and this was duly accepted.

The first examination for the Conjoint Diploma in Anaesthetics of the Royal College of Physicians of Ireland and the Royal College of Surgeons in Ireland (RCP & SI) was held in December 1942 (just seven years after the introduction of the DA in the UK). There were eight candidates in total, of whom four passed. The successful candidates were Drs Leo Darley Keegan, Patrick W.M. Kiernan (Richmond Hospital, Dublin), Ethel Sheila Kenny (Adelaide Hospital, Dublin) and William Robert Murphy. In February 1943, the DA was granted to four doctors without examination but on payment of a fee of ten guineas: Drs Silver Margaret Deane-Oliver (Meath Hospital), Thomas James Gilmartin (Mercer's Hospital), Oswald Joseph Murphy (St Vincent's Hospital) and Richard William Shaw (Dr Steevens' Hospital).[4] The management committee of the Conjoint Diploma subsequently agreed that the DA could be granted without examination

Date	NAME OF CANDIDATE	Fee	Surgeons' Examiners			Physicians' Examiners			RESULT
			Paper	Oral		Paper	Oral		
1942 December	Drumm, John Joseph	10.10.0							Rejected
	Graham, Frances Davidson	10.10.0							Rejected
	Hagan, Thomas John	10.10.0							Rejected
	Keegan, Leo Darley	10.10.0							Passed
	Kiernan, Patrick Wm.	10.10.0							Passed
	Kenny, Ethel Sheila	10.10.0							Passed
	Murphy, William Robert Harnett	10.10.0							Passed.
	Smith, Walter Dermot	10.10.0							Rejected
1943 February	The following were granted, without examination, but on payment of Ten Guineas each, the Diploma in Anaesthetics – Boyd, John Deane-Oliver, Silver Margaret Esther Gilmartin, Thomas James Murphy, Oswald Joseph Shaw, Richard William								

Results of the first Conjoint Diploma in Anaesthetics Examination, 1942 and 1943. Photograph by Bobby Studio.

until the end of 1944 to anaesthetists who had held appointments in recognised clinical hospitals in Dublin for a period of not less than ten years.

1943

In 1943, the Northern Ireland Anaesthetists Group of the British Medical Association (BMA) first met (see Chapter 15). There were 14 anaesthetists in total in the province, most of whom were also general practitioners. This group separated from the BMA in 1972 when it became the Northern Ireland Society of Anaesthetists.

157

1946: Section of Anaesthetics, Royal Academy of Medicine in Ireland
(see Chapter 16)
In 1945, Dr Thomas (Tommy) Gilmartin approached the Royal Academy of
Medicine in Ireland (RAMI) to form a section of anaesthetics. The Academy had
been founded in 1882 with the amalgamation of a number of medical societies
(Medical, Surgical, Obstetrical and Pathological) and received its 'Royal' prefix
in 1887 from Queen Victoria. It was similar to the RSM in that they were both
made up from groups of medical societies, though the RAMI antedates the RSM
by 25 years. The council of the Academy consented to the formation of a section
of anaesthetics with the proviso that at least 12 people would attend the first
meeting. Dr Thomas Percy Claude Kirkpatrick was elected president and
Gilmartin secretary of the section. The first scientific meeting was held on 12
December 1946 to commemorate the centenary of the first anaesthetic and Dr
Ivan Magill was invited to speak. His subject was 'Current Topics in Anaesthesia'
and his talk was published in the *Irish Journal of Medical Science* (*IJMS*) in
February 1947.[5] The meeting attracted over 100 delegates and was deemed a
great success. The specialty now finally had a forum for clinical and academic
meetings.

1946
It is worth noting that there were a number of other meetings held in 1946 to
celebrate the centenary of the discovery of anaesthesia, apart from the first
meeting of the Section of Anaesthetics of the Academy described above. The
'Clinical Club' met in RCSI on 15 October at which Gilmartin spoke on three
different anaesthesia topics: bronchoscopy and one lung anaesthesia, refrigeration
for anaesthesia and a report on his initial experience in using curare. The
centenary was also celebrated by the publication of a symposium on anaesthesia
in the October issue of the *Irish Journal of Medical Science*. .[7] The topics were:
'Tricloroethylene anaesthesia' by F.W.E.Wagner; 'Cyclopropane anaesthesia' by
John Boyd; 'Surgical anaesthesia' by T. Percy C. Kirkpatrick; 'The introduction
of ether and chloroform to Dublin' by John D.H. Widdess; 'Anaesthetic fatalities'
by J. Beckett; 'The status of the anaesthetist' by R.W. Shaw; 'Anesthesia in
abdominal surgery' by Victor O. McCormick; 'Anaesthesia in thoracic surgery'
by Tommy J. Gilmartin; 'Anaesthesia in neurosurgery' by Paul F. Murray;
'Anaesthesia in goitre operations' by Patrick Drury Byrne; 'Anaesthesia in
childhood' by Patrick J. Nagle; 'Intravenous anaesthesia' by Oswald J. Murphy
and 'Spinal anaesthesia with hypobaric percaine' by Patrick Kiely.

1950s

The Anaesthetists Group of the Irish Medical Association produced a report on anaesthetic services in Ireland in 1950 and this led to new contracts with proper payments to anaesthetists for their work in public hospitals. In the 1950s, a number of anaesthetists came together to form the Dublin Anaesthetists Travelling Club. Their objective was to educate themselves on new developments in the specialty by visiting hospitals in other countries and meeting with their overseas colleagues. They visited centres such as Liverpool in the UK and Nijmegen in the Netherlands. The membership was drawn from various Dublin hospitals but was confined to 12 members only. There were three meetings held each year, two at home and one abroad.[8] However, the minute book has not been found, so a complete list of the centres visited cannot be established nor the names of all the members. A similar development took place in Cork with the establishment of the South of Ireland Society of Anaesthetists in 1955 (see Chapter 17).

1960s–1990s

In 1960, the Faculty of Anaesthetists, RCSI was inaugurated (see Chapters 18 and 19). This subsequently became the College of Anaesthetists of Ireland in 1998. In 1964, Dr John Wharry Dundee was appointed as the first professor of anaesthetics in Ireland followed, in 1965, by the appointment of Tommy Gilmartin as associate professor at RCSI in Dublin.

In 1971, an out-of-town meeting took place in Galway, the precursor of the Western Anaesthetic Symposium which commenced in 1979 (see Chapter 20).

The Eastern Regional Anaesthetic Training Scheme was started in 1972 and in 1976, the first senior registrars were appointed. By 1980, there were four regional training schemes, the Eastern, Southern and Western regional training schemes as well as the Northern Ireland scheme. The Intensive Care Society of Ireland was founded in 1987 (see Chapter 21) and the Irish Board of Intensive Care Medicine was subsequently established in 1994. A few years later, in 1998, the first Diploma of the Irish Board of Intensive Care Medicine (DIBICM) was awarded. In the same year, Dr John Cooper convened a working group to establish a Diploma in Pain Management. Finally the College of Anaesthetists was founded in September 1998. It purchased number 22 Merrion Square as its new headquarters in 2000 (see Chapter 23).

Key Foundation Dates in the Twentieth Century

1893   Society of Anaesthetists in London

1908   Section of Anaesthetics, Royal Society of Medicine, London

1932   Association of Anaesthetists of Great Britain and Ireland (AAGBI)

1935   Diploma in Anaesthetics of the Royal College of Physicians of London and the Royal College of Surgeons of England

1942   Conjoint Diploma in Anaesthetics of the Royal College of Physicians of Ireland (RCPI) and the Royal College of Surgeons in Ireland (RCSI)

1943   Northern Ireland Anaesthetists Group of the British Medical Association, later the Northern Ireland Society of Anaesthetists

1946   Section of Anaesthetics, the Royal Academy of Medicine in Ireland (RAMI)

1947   Faculty of Anaesthetists of the Royal College of Surgeons of England

1950   Report produced on anaesthetic services by the Irish Medical Association

1955   South of Ireland Society of Anaesthetists

1960   Faculty of Anaesthetists, Royal College of Surgeons in Ireland

1961   First intensive care units, Mater Misericordiae Hospital, Dublin[9] and Royal Victoria Hospital, Belfast[10]

1964   First Professor of Anaesthetics, Northern Ireland (Queen's University Belfast) appointed

1965   First (Associate) Professor of Anaesthetics, Ireland (RCSI) appointed

1979   Western Anaesthetic Symposium

1986   First Professor of Anaesthetics, Ireland (RCSI) appointed

1987   Intensive Care Society of Ireland

1994   Irish Board of Intensive Care Medicine

1998   College of Anaesthetists of Ireland

2000   Purchase of 22 Merrion Square

References

1 'The origins of the COA and its Fellowship', available at rcoa.ac.uk/college-heritage (accessed 23 January 2021).

2 'Prof R.S.J. Clarke, 50 years en route to the square', Abstract from lecture, CAI Archives.

3 'Minute Book', Council, Heritage Collection RCSI, File RCSI/COU/28(1938–1960).

4 Examination office, CAI, record book, Conjoint Diploma in Anaesthetics.

5 Magill I.W., 'Current topics in anaesthetics', *Irish Journal of Medical Science*, 1947, 22, pp. 45–54.

6 Raftery H., 'Anaesthesia coming of age', *Irish Journal of Medical Science*, 1968, 1, pp. 523–530.

7 *Irish Journal of Medical Science*, 1946, 21, issue 10.

8 'Dublin Anaesthetists Travelling Club. News and Notices', *Anaesthesia*, 1982, 37, p. 1058.

9 Nolan M.E., *One Hundred Years: A History of the School of Nursing and of Developments at Mater Misericordiae Hospital 1891–1991*, Dublin: Goldpress Limited, 1991, p. 73.

10 Clarke R.S.J., *The Royal Victoria Hospital, Belfast: A History 1797–1997*, Belfast: Blackstaff Press, 1997, p. 214.

The Association of Anaesthetists of Great Britain and Ireland (1932)

John Cahill

The Association of Anaesthetists of Great Britain and Ireland (AAGBI) was founded in 1932 with **Henry Walter Featherstone (1894–1967)** as its first president. In an article in the inaugural edition of *Anaesthesia*, the AAGBI journal, launched in 1946 to mark the centenary of the first successful public demonstration of anaesthesia administered by William T. Morton in October 1846 in Boston Massachusetts, Featherstone recounted the reasons for establishing the AAGBI and its primary objectives.[1]

The first body to represent the interests of the emerging specialty of anaesthesia was the Society of Anaesthetists founded in London in 1893. The society endeavoured to promote and encourage friendly relations between anaesthetists and to address the practical and academic aspects of anaesthesia. In particular, the society lobbied for the inclusion of instruction on the administration of anaesthesia in the undergraduate medical curriculum, a proposal which was duly adopted by the Royal Colleges and the General Medical Council.[2] The ability of the Society to continue influencing the practical aspects of anaesthesia ended, however, in 1908 when it became a section, along with 22 others, in the newly formed Royal Society of Medicine and its activities were restricted to academic matters by charter.

Featherstone, who was the retiring president of the Section of Anaesthetics in 1932, saw the need for a new body that could represent the medico-political needs of the specialty and following a visit to North America and with strong support from the *British Journal of Anaesthesia*, he decided to take action: 'Accordingly, invitations were issued to one hundred anaesthetists on the staffs of the main teaching hospitals to attend a meeting for the purpose of forming an association which would meet the needs.' It is important to note that these were personal letters written by Featherstone to individual anaesthetists in the United Kingdom and in the then Irish Free State, inviting them to attend the meeting in London.[3]

There was widespread support for Featherstone's proposal. A preliminary meeting was held in London on 27 April 1932 and a provisional council was formed with Featherstone elected as the first president. The other 10 council members included Zebulon Mennell as honorary treasurer and W. Howard Jones as honorary secretary. A number of resolutions were passed including: 'That an association of anaesthetists be formed which will deal with the problems of the organisation of this branch of medicine' and 'That the title of the association shall be the Association of Anaesthetists of Great Britain and Ireland'. Writing in 1946 Featherstone stated:

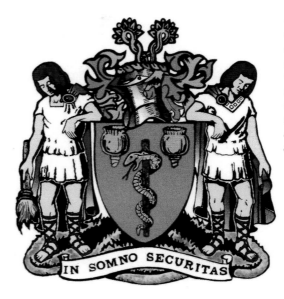

Coat of Arms of the Association of Anaesthetists of Great Britain and Ireland. Courtesy of the Association of Anaesthetists.

> The rather lengthy name – the Association of Anaesthetists of Great Britain and Ireland – was selected after careful reflection. To the writer, at first, the title 'Guild' appealed, for this emphasised the technical skill based upon training which specialists in anaesthetics must possess; but such a title would have been too stylistic. There was a general desire that colleagues in Éire should be able to join the Association and a number have done so.[1]

This inclusiveness and support for the specialty in Ireland was clearly present from the very outset and has continued ever since, and anaesthetists in Ireland have played their part in the affairs of AAGBI over the years.

The Provisional Council met on a number of occasions in May 1932 before the inaugural meeting on 1 July at which Featherstone, Mennell and Howard Jones were confirmed in their positions as president, honorary treasurer and honorary secretary respectively, and Joseph Bloomfield was elected as vice president. The rules of the new association were proposed, debated and passed and included its objectives which were to:

- Promote the development of this branch of medicine [i.e. anaesthesia]
- To coordinate the activities of anaesthetists
- To represent anaesthetists and promote their interests
- To favour the establishment of a Diploma in Anaesthetics
- To encourage friendship among anaesthetists

While each of these was hugely important to the future development of the specialty, the creation of a diploma in anaesthetics was perhaps the one that did most to put anaesthesia on an equal footing with other medical specialties, improve patient safety and provide a foundation for negotiating terms and conditions of employment for anaesthetists. Anaesthetic practice in Ireland was very similar to that in Britain at the time. At the time there was no recognised postgraduate qualification and outside the major teaching hospitals, most anaesthetics were administered by newly qualified housemen or by general practitioners. Discussions with the Royal College of Surgeons of England and the Royal College of Physicians of London on the introduction of a diploma examination began soon after the foundation of AAGBI and were led by Ivan Magill.

The regulations were finally agreed and published in the *British Journal of Anaesthesia*.[4] The first examination for the Diploma in Anaesthetics of the Conjoint Examining Board of the Royal College of Physicians of London and the Royal College of Surgeons of England, DA (D.A., R.C.P. and S. Eng.) was held in November 1935. There were two examiners and 46 successful candidates. The last Diploma examination took place in 1996 when it doubled as Part 1of the new three-part fellowship of the Faculty of Anaesthetists of the Royal College of Surgeons of England (FFARCS). The existence of a recognised postgraduate qualification in anaesthesia at the establishment of the National Health Service in the United Kingdom (UK) in 1948 was a major factor in ensuring that anaesthetists were recognised as consultants along with physicians and surgeons. The Irish DA was introduced in 1942[5] and continued until 1972 when it was replaced by the fellowship examination of the Faculty of Anaesthetists, Royal College of Surgeons in Ireland (FFARCSI).

The first member of AAGBI Council from Ireland was Dr James Beckett, anaesthetist to the Adelaide Hospital in Dublin. He served from 1936 to 1944 and was also a district representative, a post which was the forerunner of AAGBI's Linkman Organisation. At regular intervals since then, the names of anaesthetists from Ireland appear in the lists of council members and officers, notably that of vice president.

In the early years, the work of AAGBI on behalf of members in relation to medico-political matters and terms and conditions of employment in the UK had been equally relevant and applicable in Ireland but the introduction of the National Health Service in 1948 and the creation of the Voluntary Health Insurance Board (VHI) in Ireland in 1953 heralded the beginning of a progressive divergence in work practices, conditions of employment and remuneration in the two countries. The number of anaesthetists in the UK was also far greater than that in Ireland and with the passage of time, the association's work increasingly reflected these differences.

The growth and development of the specialty of anaesthesia in Ireland as evidenced by the inauguration of the Faculty of Anaesthetists, RCSI in 1960 and the establishment of the three regional training schemes, followed by the National Senior Registrar Rotation in 1976, all helped to heighten awareness of the need to re-harness the resources and know-how of AAGBI and direct them specifically at the difficulties members in Ireland were experiencing. The introduction of the common contract for consultants in April 1981 further underlined the need for a more focused approach in Ireland in order to address the medico-political needs of AAGBI members working in the Irish health service.

The foundation of the Irish Faculty was enthusiastically supported by AAGBI and deans of the faculty (and later, presidents of the Irish college) have been co-opted members of the council of the AAGBI from the outset. In October 1961, the AAGBI Annual Scientific Meeting was held at the Royal College of Surgeons in Ireland (RCSI) – it had never been held outside the UK prior to this – and was clearly as a gesture of support for the new faculty. The meeting opened with a state reception at the Municipal Gallery of Modern Art (now Dublin City Gallery The Hugh Lane) at which fellows of the Faculty of Anaesthetists, RCSI and members of AAGBI were received by Mr Seán MacEntee, Tánaiste and Minister for Health. The John Snow Lecture was delivered by Mr Erskine Childers, Minister for Transport and Power.[6,7] As well as a busy scientific programme at RCSI, there was a convivial lunch in the Guinness Brewery and a gala dinner at the Gresham Hotel attended by over 500 members and guests. The toast to AAGBI was proposed by Mr Donogh O'Malley, parliamentary secretary to the Minister for Finance; the president of AAGBI, Dr Ronald Jarman replied. The social programme included a special performance at the Abbey Theatre of *The Evidence I Shall Give* by Richard Johnson on the evening of Friday 20 October. .[8,9] The proceeds from the meeting were donated to the funds of the newly-formed faculty.[10]

Subsequent Annual Scientific Meetings of AAGBI were held in Belfast in

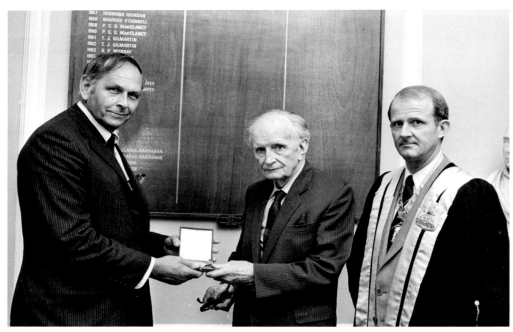

Professor Tommy Gilmartin receiving the John Snow Silver Medal from Dr Tom Boulton, President of the Association of Anaesthetists of Great Britain and Ireland at a meeting of the Faculty of Anaesthetists RCSI at the Royal College of Surgeons in Ireland, 27 September 1985. Courtesy of Bobby Studio.

1967 and 2001 and in Dublin in 1977, the latter jointly with La Société Française d'Anesthésie et d'Analgésie et d'Réanimation (SFAAR), the French Society of Anaesthesia, Analgesia and Intensive Care, when the John Snow Lecture was delivered by Dr T.K. Whitaker, and in Dublin again in 2008.

The Irish Anaesthetic Senior Registrar Group was founded in 1981 and quickly established friendly relations with its counterpart in the UK, the Junior Anaesthetists Group (JAG), now the Group of Anaesthetists in Training, (GAT). Since then, trainee anaesthetists in Ireland have been represented on the GAT Committee either by election or co-option and trainee anaesthetists from the UK have regularly attended the annual meetings of the Irish trainees. The Irish Senior Registrar Group subsequently became the Anaesthetists in Training in Ireland (ATI) and later the Committee of Anaesthesia Trainees (CAT) of the College of Anaesthetists of Ireland.

Despite the longstanding support and inclusiveness shown to anaesthetists in Ireland by AAGBI, it became clear over time that a separate forum to deal specifically with the needs of anaesthetists working in the Irish health service was required.

The lead in this regard came from the Faculty of Anaesthetists, RCSI in the person of Padraic Keane.

References

1   Featherstone H.W., 'The Association of Anaesthetists of Great Britain and Ireland. Its inception and purpose', *Anaesthesia*, 1946, 1, pp. 5–9.

2   Boulton T.B., *The Association of Anaesthetists of Great Britain & Ireland 1932–1992 and the Development of the Specialty of Anaesthesia*, London: Association of Anaesthetists of Great Britain and Ireland, 1999, p. 5.

3   *Ibid.*, p. 9.

4   Examining Board in England of the Royal College of Physicians of London and the Royal College of Surgeons of England, 'Regulations for obtaining the Diploma in Anæsthetics (D.A., R.C.P. AND S. Eng)', *British Journal of Anaesthesia*, 1935, 12, pp. 184–7.

5   'Royal College of Surgeons in Ireland Annual Report. 100th Annual Report to Council 1939–1959', Dublin: Catalogues and Collections at the Royal College of Surgeons in Ireland, p. 74.

6   'Association News', *Anaesthesia*, 1962, 17, p. 124.

7   'Minister praises anaesthetists', *Irish Independent*, 20 October 1961, p. 5.

8   Johnson R., 'The evidence I shall give. Abbey Theatre 1961. Notes', Abbey Theatre Archives, available at https://www.abbeytheatre.ie/archives/production_detail/3776/ (accessed 30 June 2021).

9   Coulter C., 'Courtroom drama at Abbey depicted institutional cruelty', *Irish Times*, 4 June 2009, available at https://www.irishtimes.com/news/courtroom-drama-at-abbey-depicted-institutional-cruelty-1.774891 (accessed 30 June 2021).

10   Boulton, *The Association*, p. 259.

The Standing Committee in Ireland of the Association of Anaesthetists of Great Britain and Ireland (1988)

John Cahill

Professor Padraic Keane was dean of the Faculty of Anaesthetists, RCSI from 1985 to 1988. A career-long AAGBI member, he was also a founding member of the Western Anaesthetic Symposium. In choosing a suitable venue to accommodate and entertain those attending the symposium, he simply drew on a little local knowledge, his sense of history and a touch of the exclusive, all of which pointed to Ballynahinch Castle, in Connemara, County Galway.

So it was at Ballynahinch Castle on 4 March 1987, when the scientific elements of the symposium had concluded, that Prof. Keane called a meeting to describe the outcome of informal discussions he had had with Prof. Michael Rosen, president of the Association of Anaesthetists of Great Britain and Ireland (AAGBI), regarding the need for an anaesthetic organisation in the Republic of Ireland which would represent anaesthetists in matters other than teaching and training, which were the responsibility of the Faculty of Anaesthetists, RCSI. An ad hoc committee was formed there and then and was given the task of consulting anaesthetists around the country so as to decide the best way forward. The committee met in Limerick in May and in Dublin in July of 1987. The July meeting was addressed by Prof. Rosen and at that point, it was clear that there was widespread support for an organisation which would represent the medico-political concerns of the specialty and which would have elected representation on a regional or health board basis.

The most pressing concerns of anaesthetists at the time were stated to be the structuring of consultant appointments, standards of equipment and monitoring, assistance for anaesthetists and anaesthesia fees in private practice. As a result of these meetings, a formal request was made to AAGBI Council to establish a 'Standing Committee in Ireland of the Association of Anaesthetists of Great Britain and Ireland' and Drs Des Riordan and P.J. Breen travelled to Bedford Square, London, the home of the association, for further discussions with the

THE STANDING COMMITTEE IN IRELAND OF THE ASSOCIATION OF ANAESTHETISTS (1988)

president, and honorary secretary, Dr Peter Morris.

Finally, at the October meeting of council that year and with the enthusiastic support of the president, council approved, in principle, the establishment of a standing committee in Ireland.[1,2] On 16 January 1988, the final meeting of the original ad hoc committee took place at RCSI, and the Standing Committee came into being with Des Riordan being elected convenor and P.J. Breen becoming honorary secretary.[3]

The new Standing Committee clearly took its duties very seriously. By the end of the year in which it had been established, it had met on eight occasions and two of these meetings, on 24 June and 25 November, were followed by open meetings, the latter becoming the Annual Open Meeting.

In 1990, the first elections were held with each of the eight health board areas electing members. The Eastern area elected four, the Southern two and each remaining area elected one. In 1991, the November open

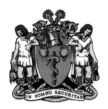

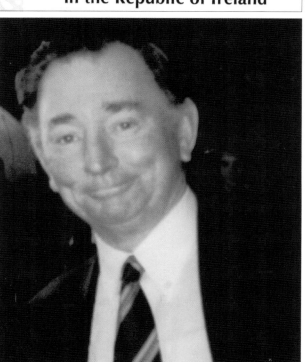

The Association of Anaesthetists of Great Britain and Ireland

Irish Standing Committee

National Survey of Ambulatory Anaesthesia in the Republic of Ireland

Report on a National Survey of Ambulatory Anaesthesia in the Republic of Ireland carried out by the Standing Committee in Ireland of AAGBI.

Dr Des Riordan, the first Convenor of the Standing Committee in Ireland of the Association of Anaesthetists of Great Britain and Ireland. Photo courtesy of Mrs Nano Riordan.

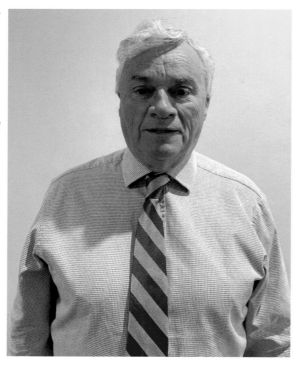

Dr P.J. Breen, the first honorary secretary of the Standing Committee in Ireland of the Association of Anaesthetists of Great Britain and Ireland

meeting was followed by an AAGBI seminar, a practice that continues to this day. The title of the first seminar was 'Litigation and the anaesthetist in Ireland'. It was chaired by Prof. Richard Clarke, the new dean of the Faculty of Anaesthetists, RCSI. The speakers included Prof. Alan Aitkenhead from Nottingham, Dr Roger Doherty of the Medical Defence Union, Dr Bill Wren who spoke on 'How not to get sued' and Prof. Padraic Keane, who advised on 'What to do if you are sued'.

The Constitution

The constitution for the Standing Committee was approved by council in 1991.[4] The document is based on AAGBI's own constitution but is a much slimmer volume and it sets down clearly the duties and responsibilities of the new committee and the means by which its objectives might be achieved.

The Standing Committee was to liaise with AAGBI Council, submit reports and make recommendations with regard to the practice of anaesthesia in the Republic of Ireland and generally to assist council in promoting the aims and ideals of the association. In other words, the primary function of the Standing Committee was and remains one of communication – firstly, with AAGBI members in Ireland, and secondly with council on their behalf. One of its hallmarks was its effort to be inclusive and to consult widely. Representatives from the Faculty of Anaesthetists, RCSI, from anaesthetists in training and from specialist societies were invited to join the Standing Committee and AAGBI members in Ireland were encouraged to stand for election to council. The constitution also set down the rules for the election of officers, the minimum number of meetings each year, voting procedures and a budget.

From the outset, those concerned with setting up the Standing Committee were convinced that regional representation would be more effective than representation on a national basis, even though this was the method operated by AAGBI itself and indeed the Faculty of Anaesthetists, RCSI. The eight health board areas were used as the electoral units, the number of delegates for each area reflected their different sizes and a simple method of ensuring elections were held each year was devised.

Since its foundation in 1932, the AAGBI has enjoyed considerable support in Ireland. Between 1936 and 1996, 16 members from Ireland were elected to council – eight from Belfast, including S. Morrell Lyons who served as president from 1994 to 1996, five from Dublin, four of whom served as vice president, two from Cork and one from Drogheda. The advent of the Standing Committee bolstered this support and resulted in an increase in membership, better communication with council and a greater awareness of the activities and ideals of AAGBI. The constitution requires the committee to meet at least three times each year and from the beginning, these meetings were planned so as to maximise the potential to engage members throughout the country and to stimulate interest in AAGBI. A schedule of meetings was established with two business meetings each year taking place outside Dublin, mid-week and within the working day. This approach was adopted to acknowledge the regional basis of the Standing Committee and to avoid the difficulties of travelling late in the evening after work, or at weekends when family commitments would suffer. The result was that within the first ten years of its existence, every health board area had hosted at least one meeting with the local representative taking responsibility for the arrangements. A third meeting, the Annual Open Meeting, would be held in Dublin over a weekend. This meeting has become very popular and well supported undoubtedly due to a combination of factors including a fixed date and venue, the attendance of AAGBI officers and administrative staff and the inclusion of AAGBI seminars as part of the open meetings.

Safe Service

The first AAGBI booklet which dealt exclusively with anaesthesia matters in Ireland was entitled *Anaesthesia in Ireland – the provision of a safe service*.[5] The chairman of the working party was Dr Pat Fitzgerald and it was published in May 1989. The booklet is important for two reasons – firstly, because it was the first of its kind dealing specifically with matters in Ireland, and secondly and perhaps more importantly, for the tone and nature of its content. The purpose of

AAGBI booklets has always been to provide reference points and benchmarks regarding standards of clinical practice and related matters for practising anaesthetists. This booklet, however, was written primarily for health board officials and hospital managers who, in the opinion of the working party, had little understanding of what anaesthetists did or what they required to do it safely.

The opening section sets the tone and painstakingly describes some different facets of hospital practice in which anaesthetists play a vital role: 'The role of the modern anaesthetist is much wider than the administration of anaesthesia in the operating theatre. It involves many areas of patient care [including] preoperative evaluation, obstetric anaesthesia, intensive care, resuscitation'.

The totally inadequate staffing levels in small anaesthetic units throughout the country, all of which were providing a 24-hour emergency service, which often included obstetric cover, was highlighted, as was the failure to recruit new consultants to these units. The need for proper consultation between hospital management and anaesthetists in drawing up job descriptions for consultant posts seems rather obvious from this distance, but clearly it was not happening at that time. Attention was also drawn to the uncommon but nonetheless totally unacceptable practice of engaging trainee anaesthetists in place of consultants – the working party stated that where a service cannot be delivered safely, it should be moved to another properly staffed location.

A section on administrators' attitudes to the specialty of anaesthesia was included, specifically at the request of the regional representatives. Nor was the working party afraid to take a potentially unpopular stance in the interest of patient safety. Insisting that all anaesthetic units must meet the minimum standards of staffing and equipment, it stated 'where this is not economically realistic for reasons of size or geographical location, these units should be closed, amalgamated or relocated'. The same comments were made in relation to substandard obstetric units and further, 'where an obstetric unit is identified as providing a substandard level of anaesthetic service, the public should be made aware of this and offered an alternative unit where a comprehensive service is provided'.

As well as setting out clearly the minimum standards of equipment, staffing and assistance for anaesthetists, the working party made three main recommendations:

1. A joint review of anaesthesia services by the Standing Committee and the Department of Health

2. The appointment of a national advisor on anaesthesia
3. A programme of study days for hospital administrators

Although there has never been a joint review of anaesthesia services in small units, the specialty is now much more likely to be consulted on matters pertaining to service development and planning and there is a greater awareness of the problems of small peripheral units. An advisor on medical manpower was indeed appointed in 1990 – Dr Bill Wren, who held the post for four years – but he was not replaced when he completed his tour of duty. For some years after 1989, a number of Department of Health officials and hospital managers took part in the regular seminars that followed the Annual Open Meetings and these proved fruitful and worthwhile encounters.

The second booklet produced by the Standing Committee, *Workload for Consultant Anaesthetists in Ireland*[11] was published in 1992. A revised common contract replacing the original contract of 1981 had just been offered by the Department of Health to consultants working in the public and voluntary health services. The contract included a number of new elements such as practice plans, work schedules, consultants in management and options on wholetime or part-time contract commitments. The Standing Committee booklet gave advice on all of these matters as well as sample weekly work schedules for anaesthetic departments of varying sizes, advice on contract choice and stressed the importance of teaching, training and continued medical education as part of a consultants scheduled work.

Voluntary Health Insurance Board (VHI)
If staffing and equipment were the most pressing clinical issues, the level of anaesthesia fees in private practice was, undoubtedly, the outstanding non-clinical concern. The levels of reimbursement by the Voluntary Health Insurance Board (VHI) – essentially the only private health insurer in the country at the time – were remarkably low and despite numerous attempts by individual clinicians to rectify this, the attitude of the VHI to anaesthetists was, at best, indifferent. There were also other developments at this time which only served to complicate matters.

Prior to 1988, the relationship between patients and clinicians in private practice was, in effect, a contract between the two with the patient accepting responsibility for the clinician's fee and then referring to their medical insurer (VHI) for reimbursement. This situation emphasised the doctor-patient relationship and put a certain distance between the profession and the insurance company.

The 1988 Finance Act, however, introduced the Professional Services Withholding Tax which meant, amongst other things, that the VHI now paid clinicians directly rather than reimbursing patients. VHI wasted no time in informing patients that the doctor had already been paid, which was only partly true, and this led to the practice of 'balance billing' which often annoyed and upset patients and proved difficult for anaesthetists with small private practices and those in rural communities.

In the early 1990s, the UK Monopolies & Mergers Commission was about to conclude that any agreement between private health insurers and representative medical organisations regarding fees – the British Medical Association (BMA) had, at the time, taken on the task of publishing anaesthesia fee schedules on behalf of AAGBI – would be anti-competitive and therefore illegal. Despite describing the decision as 'perverse', the BMA gave a voluntary undertaking not to publish any more fee schedules. In Ireland, the Standing Committee set up a fees subcommittee to engage directly with the VHI. The members of the subcommittee were Drs Aidan Synnott, P.J. Breen, John Dunphy and Tom Fogarty. Understandably, there was enormous frustration amongst anaesthetists and not a great deal of confidence that any measure of success could be achieved.

Early meetings with VHI did indeed prove to be disappointing and unproductive and at special open meetings in January 1991 and March 1993, the fees subcommittee advised members to reject the most recent offer from the insurer. A survey of members later in 1993 drew a 60 per cent response representing approximately 80 per cent of private practice in the country.

The survey demonstrated overwhelming support for the Standing Committee as the appropriate body to negotiate on behalf of anaesthetists. The range of fees that members indicated would be acceptable to them was very similar to that of AAGBI (no longer to be published!) and there was strong support for a proposal that in the event of an agreement being reached between the Standing Committee and VHI which proved acceptable to members, the signatures of those members accepting such an agreement would be held in trust by the Standing Committee

Finally, at a special open meeting in October 1994, despite a substantial amount of unfinished business (work on fees for intensive care had not even begun), the Standing Committee was prepared to recommend acceptance of the fee schedule which VHI was about to offer. The basis for this recommendation included: (1) a quadrupling of the global sum VHI was prepared to make available for anaesthesia; (2) acceptance by VHI that members of the fees subcommittee would oversee a redistribution of the funds over the various categories; (3) the introduction of a special reporting procedure to deal with unusual or problem cases and (4) a commitment to a review within two years in order to take account of medical inflation and other necessary adjustments. Acceptance of the VHI offer would mean an undertaking by members not to balance bill. When the committee completed its presentation and recommended acceptance, Dr Aidan Synnott famously added the caveat, 'but don't dismantle your billing systems yet'.

There was considerable and varying comment both at the special open meeting and immediately afterwards. No allowance had been made for the added complexity of paediatric and neonatal anaesthesia. The issue of pain procedures under general anaesthesia had not been addressed and members who worked exclusively in private practice believed the fee schedule to be totally inadequate. There was an interesting debate regarding three smaller benevolent societies whose dealings with anaesthetists had always been thoroughly professional and non-argumentative. The committee took the view that fees to members of these three societies should not exceed those agreed with VHI. Interestingly, not all anaesthetists accepted this. Nevertheless, by the time of the Annual Open Meeting that year, 90 per cent of anaesthetists had accepted the new schedule.[6]

After 1994, the fees subcommittee continued to engage in reviews with VHI every two to three years and although progress was slow and frustrating, the landmark gains of the 1994 agreement have largely been maintained. The advent in 1996 of a second health insurer, the British United Provident Association (BUPA), failed to have the anticipated positive effect and in a later rather ironic twist, the Competition Authority, after a prolonged investigation into how the Irish Hospital Consultants Association (IHCA) had engaged with VHI for the purposes of drawing up an agreed fee schedule, came to the conclusion that such actions amounted to price fixing and were in breach of Section 4 of the Competition Act of 2002. At that point, nobody seemed to know what the next legal move would be.

While dealings with VHI occupied much of the Standing Committee's time, there was considerable activity on other fronts including the production of various documents published by AAGBI on behalf of the Standing Committee. There was, of course, a continuous flow of publications by AAGBI on standards in clinical practice, and other documents which had equal relevance in Ireland

and the UK, or required no more than a short reference to highlight some slight difference. However the national surveys identified areas of clinical practice where there was significant variation.

National Surveys

The National Surveys are of interest not just for the information they contain but also for the extent to which the general membership contribute to data collection.

It had been the Irish Standing Committee's intention to include all aspects of anaesthesia practice in one large survey but this proved unmanageable, so the work was split into different sections, the first of which was the *National Manpower Survey* published in 1993.[7] This was probably the first time that up-to-date accurate information on the total number of anaesthetic units providing a 24-hour emergency service, their staffing levels and other details had been brought together in one publication. Consultant to trainee ratios were calculated, and the report included an estimate of the number of trainees required to bring staffing levels up to minimum standards in small peripheral units and also to allow for consultant retirements. Further national surveys followed – the *National Survey of Intensive Care Units*,[8] the *National Survey of Paediatric Anaesthetic Practice in General Hospitals in the Republic of Ireland*[9] and a *National Survey of Ambulatory Anaesthesia in the Republic of Ireland*.[10]

Although such surveys are an excellent method of producing a snapshot of data at a particular instant or over a short timeframe, they are very labour intensive and require a high response rate to have any real relevance. In all of these surveys, well over three quarters of the anaesthetic departments invited to take part returned complete data sets, which was a great compliment to the membership in general and to the perseverance of the Standing Committee.

Today these data are collected on a regular basis and published in annual reports by the College of Anaesthesiologists of Ireland (CAI), and specialist societies such as the Intensive Care Society of Ireland, and the Irish Paediatric Anaesthesia and Critical Care Society.

Medical Manpower

In April 1991, following discussions between Comhairle na nOspidéal, the Department of Health and the Postgraduate Medical and Dental Board, a collaborative study group on medical manpower in acute hospitals was established under the chairmanship of the Chief Medical Officer Dr Niall Tierney. The group was tasked with undertaking a comprehensive study of the number and distribution of consultants and non-consultant hospital doctors (NCHDs) in acute hospitals by specialty and geographic area and putting forward suggested courses of action designed to achieve an equitable mix and distribution of medical manpower throughout the country. The results of the group's deliberations were published in June 1993 in the document *Medical Manpower in Acute Hospitals – a Discussion Document*[12] which proposed (among other things) moving to a consultant-delivered service (for all specialties), reducing the number of trainees and the duration of training and increasing the number of consultants – all to be achieved over a 10-year period and in a 'cost neutral' way.

In responding to Dr Tierney's proposals, the Standing Committee pointed out that the specialty of anaesthesia already provided a consultant-delivered service in many areas and especially in small peripheral units and that the consultant to trainee ratio was one of the lowest of all the medical specialties and very close to the ideal of 1:1.[13]

Ten years later, in 2003, almost identical objectives were proposed in the report of the National Taskforce on Medical Staffing (Hanley Report)[14] with the added stimulus of the European Working Time Directive and all to be achieved in five years, with the emphasis on value for money rather than being cost neutral.

One notable difference between the two government publications was the fact that the Hanley Report did at least seek some input from the specialty by inviting Dr Jennifer Porter, consultant anaesthetist at the Midland Regional Hospital, Mullingar (and later consultant at St James' University Hospital, Dublin) and Dr Eamon Tierney, the then honorary secretary of the Standing Committee and consultant anaesthetist at Wexford General Hospital, to sit on the advisory panel.

Trainee Contribution

From the very outset, the Standing Committee realised the importance of including trainee representatives in its activities. The ad hoc committee set up in 1987 invited Dr Gerry Fitzpatrick (later consultant at Tallaght University Hospital and vice president of the College of Anaesthesiologists of Ireland) to join them as the first trainee representative and this approach has been maintained ever since. The contribution made by trainees to the general work of the committee has been considerable and they have been particularly active in representing the views and concerns of fellow trainees in Ireland; they have also developed strong links with their counterparts in the UK, the committee of the

Group of Anaesthetists in Training (GAT). In 1993, Dr Frances Colreavy was elected to GAT and represented trainees' interests at meetings of the National Training Committee of the Royal College of Anaesthetists in London while at the same time serving on the Standing Committee representing the interests of her colleagues in Ireland. Officers of the GAT Committee became regular guests of the Irish trainees at meetings in Ireland. Dr Colreavy's successors continued her good work in this regard and trainees in Ireland have been represented on the GAT Committee, if not by election, then as co-opted members.

Closer to home, the Standing Committee's attention was also drawn to the difficulties of trainee anaesthetists accompanying critically ill patients during interhospital transfer. There was a complete lack of any personal accident insurance cover for these trainees and the legal position of trainee doctors with temporary registration with the Medical Council was unclear.

Temporary registration in Ireland identified a single named location at which the doctor could work but the validity of registration when the doctor was literally between two hospitals had never been clarified. From initial discussions with the Medical Council, it was clear that the council had never been asked to consider this problem before but without much delay, the practical view was taken that the ambulance was, in effect, an extension of the base hospital until it had arrived at the receiving hospital.

Mishaps to doctors during the transfer of critically ill patients are thankfully very uncommon but do happen and the lack of proper insurance cover added another layer of anxiety and uncertainty. The Standing Committee discovered that health boards had little knowledge of or interest in the problem but by late 1997, following representations from the Standing Committee, Irish Public Bodies Mutual Insurance Ltd was about to offer an insurance policy to all health boards specifically to deal with the problem. It was finally solved in 1999 by AAGBI when it introduced insurance cover for all members engaged in caring for ill patients anywhere in the world. The significance of this development was acknowledged by Dr John Loughrey, chairman of the Anaesthetists in Training in Ireland at their annual meeting in Dublin in December 1999.

Honours and Awards
The AAGBI Council of the association may choose to acknowledge the work of members in a variety of ways. Honorary membership is the oldest honour, dating from the inaugural meeting of the association in 1932.

The first anaesthetist in Ireland to be awarded honorary membership was

Dr Thomas J. Gilmartin in 1976. Profs John Dundee and Richard Clarke were similarly honoured in 1988 and 1994 respectively.

In 1997, Dr Bill Wren became an honorary member while in 2002, Prof. Padraic Keane's contribution was recognised in the same manner.

The Pask Certificate of Honour is named after Prof. Edgar Alexander Pask, whose courage and bravery as an experimental physiologist in the Royal Air Force during World War Two is well documented.[15] It was instituted to honour those who have rendered distinguished service, either with gallantry in the discharge of their clinical duties or to the specialty of anaesthesia as a whole or to AAGBI itself.

In 1985, Dr Wilfred Maurice Brown was awarded the certificate for his services to anaesthesia in Northern Ireland and four years later, Dr Eugene Egan, a graduate of University College Cork, received the honour for his work in anaesthesia in Tanzania. In 2000 and 2004, Drs P.J. Breen and Dr Sean McDevitt were similarly honoured. Both Dr Breen and Dr McDevitt are past convenors of the Standing Committee.

While not identified in the official list, it is clearly a huge honour for any particular city to be chosen to host the Annual Scientific Meeting or Annual Congress as it is now known. This is the AAGBI's showcase event and is probably the largest anaesthetic meeting in Britain or Ireland, attracting well over 600 delegates. Prior to the formation of the Standing Committee, AAGBI Annual Scientific Meetings had been held in Dublin in 1961 and 1976, so the decision by council to bring the Annual Congress to Dublin once again in 2007 can be seen as a vote of confidence in and an acknowledgement of the work and professionalism of the Standing Committee, the convenor Dr Ellen O'Sullivan and honorary secretary Dr Rory Page.

The Standing Committee and *Anaesthesia News*
Since its establishment in 1988, the Standing Committee has enjoyed an extremely good and very productive relationship with *Anaesthesia News*, the official AAGBI newsletter. The willingness of the editors to accept and publish reports of various meetings and important anaesthetic events in Ireland with the newsletter's characteristic humour and ingenuity (during the editorship of J Edmund (Ed) Charlton, 1992–6, the March edition of *Anaesthesia News* appeared as the *Annual Irish Issue* with a green masthead!) has been of enormous assistance to the Standing Committee in its efforts to communicate widely and raise the association's profile in Ireland.[16–18]

References

1 Association of Anaesthetists of Great Britain and Ireland Council Minutes, October 1987, p. 4, item 7.
2 *Ibid*. December 1987, p. 4, item 5.
3 Working Party to establish the Standing Committee in Ireland of the Association of Anaesthetists of Great Britain and Ireland, minutes of the meeting 16 January 1988, London: Association of Anaesthetists of Great Britain and Ireland.
4 *Constitution of the Standing Committee in Ireland of the Association of Anaesthetists of Great Britain and Ireland*, London: Association of Anaesthetists of Great Britain and Ireland.
5 *Anaesthesia in Ireland – the provision of a safe Service*, London: Association of Anaesthetists of Great Britain and Ireland, 1989.
6 Standing Committee in Ireland of the Association of Anaesthetists of Great Britain and Ireland, minutes of the Annual Open Meeting 19 November 1994, London: Association of Anaesthetists of Great Britain and Ireland.
7 Standing Committee in Ireland of the Association of Anaesthetists of Great Britain and Ireland, *National Manpower Survey*, London: Association of Anaesthetists of Great Britain and Ireland.
8 Standing Committee in Ireland of the Association of Anaesthetists of Great Britain and Ireland, *National Survey of Intensive Care Units*, London: Association of Anaesthetists of Great Britain and Ireland.
9 Standing Committee in Ireland of the Association of Anaesthetists of Great Britain and Ireland, *National Survey of Paediatric Anaesthetic Practice in General Hospitals in the Republic of Ireland*, London: Association of Anaesthetists of Great Britain and Ireland.
10 Standing Committee in Ireland of the Association of Anaesthetists of Great Britain and Ireland, *National Survey of Ambulatory Anaesthesia in the Republic of Ireland*, London: Association of Anaesthetists of Great Britain and Ireland.
11 Standing Committee in Ireland of the Association of Anaesthetists of Great Britain and Ireland, *Workload for Consultant Anaesthetists in Ireland*, London: Association of Anaesthetists of Great Britain and Ireland, 1992.
12 'Medical Manpower in Acute Hospitals – A Discussion Document', available at http://hdl.handle.net/10147/46291 (accessed 30 June 2021).
13 Standing Committee in Ireland of the Association of Anaesthetists of Great Britain and Ireland and the Board of the Faculty of Anaesthetists of the Royal College of Surgeons in Ireland, *Response to the Discussion Document Medical Manpower in Acute Hospitals*, London: Association of Anaesthetists of Great Britain and Ireland.
14 'Report of the National Task Force on Medical Staffing (Hanley Report)', available at https://www.gov.ie/en/publication/8736d0-report-of-the-national-task-force-on-medical-staffing-hanly-report/?referrer=/wp-content/uploads/2014/03/report-of-the-national-task-force-on-medical-staffing-hanly-report.pdf (accessed 30 June 2021).
15 'Obituary. Professor E.A. Pask.', *Anaesthesia*, 1966, 21, pp. 437–39.
16 *Anaesthesia News*, 1995, 92, pp. 1–2.
17 *Anaesthesia News*, 1996, 104, pp. 1–4.
18 *Anaesthesia News*, 1997, 116, pp. 1–4, 7.

Chapter 15

The Northern Ireland Anaesthetists Group of the British Medical Association/The Northern Ireland Society of Anaesthetists (1943)

Joseph Tracey, Declan Warde

Minute Book (1963–77)

In the early 1940s, there were a number of doctors in Northern Ireland with an interest in anaesthesia, although the majority of these were general practitioners and only worked part-time in the specialty. These included: Drs Evelyn Allen; Olive Anderson; Olive Darling, DPH (Diploma in Public Health); James Heney, DA (Diploma in Anaesthetics); Stafford Geddes, DA; John Houston, DA; Vida Lemon, DA; John Macauley, DA and Maurice Woods, DA, who were all general practitioners. Heney was also an assistant anaesthetist and tutor in anaesthetics at the Royal Victoria Hospital, Belfast. The others anaesthetists were full time: John Boyd MD, who was a paediatric anaesthetist; James Elliott, MD, DA, who went full time in 1943; Florence McClelland, DA, DRCOG; and Victor Fielden who was a lecturer in the Department of Therapeutics at Queen's University Belfast (QUB) and was full-time anaesthetist at the Royal Victoria Hospital (RVH). Fielden had been appointed at the turn of the century and retired in 1936 but continued working as an honorary visiting staff member during World War Two until shortly before his death in 1945. Wilfred Maurice Brown wrote later about the working conditions of anaesthetists in the 1940s, stating that none of the part-time anaesthetists:

> had any staff status and were more or less permitted to work in hospital on a grace and favour basis. They were sometimes called clinical assistants. All the hospitals were voluntary and none of the staff was paid (except the Health Service £50 per annum), hence the reason for so many GP/anaesthetists. The GP/ anaesthetist could survive on the income from his practice but the

full time anaesthetist had to make do with any crumb which fell
from the surgeons [*sic*] private operating table[1]

Florence McClelland visited both Liverpool and Edinburgh in spring 1942
to take short intensive courses in anaesthesia. When she came back and told her
colleagues about what she had learned, they asked her to give them a talk on the
recent advances. This was the beginning of regular meetings between colleagues
where each one in turn would give 'a dissertation on some personal recent
anaesthetic experience, problem, disaster or discovery'. These meetings were, in
effect, the early beginnings of the Northern Ireland Anaesthetists Group of the
British Medical Association.[1]

The first recorded meeting took place on 11 June 1943 and John Boyd was
the first honorary secretary. In the beginning, the meetings were relatively small
with a core group of Boyd, Elliott, Lemon, MacAuley, McClelland and sometimes
Hamilton but after a while, the numbers increased so that by 1946, there
averaged about 10 to 12 attendees. The meetings were held in a small room in
the Whitla Institute, College Square North in Belfast. Wilfred Brown, in his notes
concerning the difficulties encountered by anaesthetists during the 1940s, said
that:

> At the time there were few anaesthetic machines at the Royal
> Victoria Hospital, one frequently chained it to the theatre to
> prevent it being purloined by a colleague during the night.[1]
>
> The specialty continued to grow and expand and with it the
> number of attendees at the meetings. Fortunately with the advent
> of the NHS in 1948 the anaesthetists in Northern Ireland who
> had a DA or an MD or other higher qualification were eventually
> recognised by the Northern Ireland Government as consultants
> and awarded a salary and position in NHS hospitals[1]

Dr Wilfred Maurice Brown who wrote the account of the early days of the
specialty in Northern Ireland became a member of the group in 1946 when he
succeeded Fielden at the RVH. A Queen's University graduate, he was the first
consultant anaesthetist to be appointed to the hospital after World War Two. He
had served with the Royal Navy during the war and had suffered severe facial
burns after his ship was torpedoed in the Mediterranean. He then trained in
anaesthesia under Dr Ivan Magill at the Westminster Hospital in London before

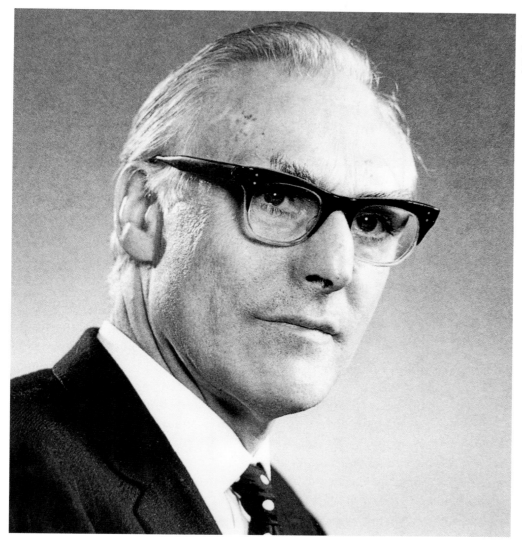

Wilfred Maurice Brown. Courtesy of Belfast Health and Social Care Trust.

returning to Belfast to take up his consultant post. He retired in 1976.[2] The original minute book of the Northern Ireland Anaesthetists Group was unfortunately lost and so he provided an account of the early days to be inserted into the new minute book which commenced in 1963.

1963

The Annual General Meeting (AGM) of the Northern Ireland Anaesthetists Group took place on 27 May 1963 in the medical tutorial room, Institute of

Clinical Sciences (which is located at the Royal Victoria Hospital, Belfast). The chairman at the time was J.F. (Minty) Bereen and the honorary secretary was S. Harold S. Love, both of whom stood down from their respective offices. Following an election, Douglas Wilson was appointed chairman and David Wilson Barron as honorary secretary. The incoming committee was made up of Bereen, J.W. Dundee, S.H.S. Love, W.J. Love, G.W. Black, J.C. Hewitt and R. Armstrong. Harold Love, who had been secretary since 1959, presented the group with a new minute book and requested that future minutes be typed. There were two case presentations after the AGM by Dr R.M. Nicholl and Dr Roy Bolton. There were three further meetings in 1963 in October, November and December.

1964

Harold Love showed a film and gave a talk on paediatric dental anaesthesia at the January meeting. The annual Registrars' Prize, which took place in February, was won by Henry Craig with a paper on 'Muscle pain following suxamethonium'. The group decided at that meeting that they 'should press for the creation of a University chair in anaesthesia' and also that the Association of Anaesthetists of Great Britain and Ireland (AAGBI) should consider Belfast as a venue for future meetings. In March, Dundee presented on a new intravenous anaesthetic agent, FBA 1420, and described the chemistry and pharmacology of the eugenol derivative. In April, there was a visit to Altnagelvin Hospital, Derry which started with a tour of the operating theatres, followed by a sherry reception at noon and then lunch. Dr Atwood Beaver from the National Hospital for Nervous Diseases in London gave a talk on 'The functions and running of a Respiratory Unit' at the academic session in the afternoon. The honorary secretary, in his annual report, pointed out that the same third of the membership had been paying their subscription and thus had effectively been subsidising the other two thirds for the preceding 10 years. It was decided at a later meeting that the annual subscription should, in future, be paid by banker's order. The bank balance was £16. The annual dinner was held at the Old Inn, Crawfordsburn, (dress was formal). The after-dinner talk was given by Mr Maurice Miles, conductor of the City of Belfast Orchestra.

Dr James Elliott was elected chairman at the June meeting with Barron continuing on as secretary. In November, the chairman paid tribute to John Boyd, who had been the first honorary secretary of the group (in 1943) and proposed that he became an honorary life member. They also considered a memorandum on anaesthetic fees for private patients and set up a subcommittee to make recommendations.

1965

The Registrars' Prize in February was won by Dr W.B. Loan who presented 'Morphia versus Omnopon'. The 21st anniversary of the group was celebrated at the annual dinner at the Old Inn on 28 May; tickets were £3 for consultants and £2 for registrars. The academic session beforehand was addressed by Dr J.D. Robertson from Edinburgh on 'Breathing – is it worth it?'. The honorary secretary's report proposed that, in future, the Registrars' Prize should consist of both a medal and cash. The new method of collecting subscriptions was very successful with a 90 per cent payment rate, the bank balance had increased to £56. Dr A. Armstrong was appointed chairman at the June meeting, Barron as secretary and Elliott, Dundee, Love, McNeilly, Bingham, Orr and R. Armstrong as committee members. A new subcommittee was formed to advise the Central Midwives Board of Northern Ireland on equipment and drugs. The group held a joint meeting in December with the obstetricians and paediatricians, at which Dr M.A. Lewis and Dr J. Moore described their experiences in Scandinavia and Scotland respectively.

1966

Dr J.B. Wyman spoke in March on 'Epidural anaesthesia in labour'. The theme in November was 'Recent advances in circulatory pharmacology' with talks by Prof. I.C. Roddie and K.J. Hutchison. A total of eight meetings were held during the year

1967

The year started in BMA House with a talk by Dr G.W. Stephen from Edinburgh on research he had carried out at the University of Pennsylvania on the respiratory effects of premedication. The Registrars' Prize was won in February by Dr S. McDowell for a paper on 'Neostigmine resistant curarisation'. The main speaker before the annual dinner was Dr John Bunker from Stanford University, Palo Alto on 'Metabolic effects of anaesthetics and liver dysfunction'.

The AGM was held in October and the outgoing chairman, Dr Wilfred Maurice Brown, was presented with a new badge of office by Dr Vida Lemon. The badge had cost £100. Brown then presented the badge to the incoming chairman, Dr W.F.K. Morrow. Richard Clarke took over as honorary secretary.

Insignia of Northern Ireland Anaesthetist's Group. Courtesy of John Darling.

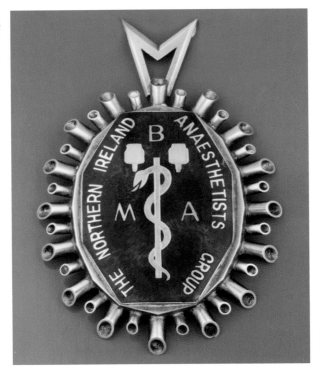

1968

The new year began at the Wellington Park Hotel with a talk on 'Intensive therapy' given by G.T. Spencer from St Thomas' Hospital in London. The winner of the Registrars' Prize was Dr Coppel for his paper on 'Anaesthesia for the repair of cleft palates in infants'. In October, R.A. Hearn spoke on 'Reversal of curare' and the year finished in December with Prof. Martin Isaac from India who spoke on 'Some observations on anaesthesia for poor risk patients in the tropics'.

1969

Wing Commander John Ernsting spoke in February at the Wellington Park Hotel on 'Hypoxia and its management in aircraft'. This was followed in April by a talk by Prof. R.L. Katz from New York on the 'Clinical pharmacology of muscle relaxants'. It was reported at the AGM in May that the group had received a letter from Dr Aileen Adams, honorary secretary of the AAGBI, regarding the representation of provincial anaesthetic organisations at the association. The October meeting took place in BMA House on the Ormeau Road where Dr M.K. Sykes, senior lecturer in anaesthesia at the Hammersmith Hospital in London gave a talk titled 'Hypoxaemia and hypotheses'.

1970

The honorary secretary's annual report noted a large increase in the numbers attending the meetings. This was felt to be as a result of several of these being 'patronised' by pharmaceutical firms or equipment companies. This, in turn, helped the committee to bring in more visiting speakers. There were now 62 members of the group and the society's bank account had £148 cash in hand.

Harold Love was appointed chairman and Gerry Black as secretary. The members of the committee were James McNeilly, T.A. Brown, J. Cooper, I. Carson, Sylvie Browne, Dundee, Clarke and Hazlett. The year was characterised by the large number of visiting speakers. For example, in September, there were three speakers from North America, D. Eastwood on 'Toxicity and anaesthetics', M. Herlich on 'Ketamine' and J. Steinhaus on 'Cough'. After that, speakers included Mark Swerdlow from Salford Royal Hospital who spoke on 'Neurosurgery in intractable pain', R.A. Miller from the Clinical Research Centre at Northwick Park on 'Anaesthesia in the sitting position for neurosurgery' and finally, in December, Peter Baskett from the Bristol Royal Infirmary gave a talk on 'Developments on the use of Entonox'.

1971

W.R. Gilmore was appointed chairman at the AGM in May and J. Moore took over the role of honorary secretary. Membership of the group had increased to 80. Barron and Love were appointed as members of council of the AAGBI. There was again a large number of visiting speakers this year. W.S. Wren from Dublin spoke on 'Post-operative cyanosis in infants', W.D. Wylie from St Thomas' Hospital gave a talk on 'Medico-legal aspects of medicine', D. Churchill-Davidson, St Thomas' Hospital, on 'Clinical use of muscle relaxants', A.C. Ames from Neath General Hospital on 'Parenteral nutrition' and Andrew Hunter from Manchester on 'Keeping the brain in order'.

1972

At the AGM on 30 May, the honorary secretary reported that there had been seven meetings in the past year. The group continued to have generous sponsorship from many companies and the bank account had a positive balance of £173. The group was incensed at the low level of Distinction awards held by anaesthetists in Northern Ireland and decided to write to the Minister of Health and Social Services. It was also decided, after much discussion, that the Northern Ireland Anaesthetists Group should become independent of the British Medical Association. Dr Armstrong proposed that the name be changed to the Northern Ireland Society of Anaesthetists (NISA) and this was accepted unanimously. The first meeting of this new body, NISA, took place on 16 October 1972. There was a debate on the change of name and also on the fact that the group was leaving the BMA. James McNeilly objected, stating that inadequate notice had been given. He outlined the advantages of remaining within the BMA, such as the availability of a venue for meetings at BMA House and the free secretarial help. David Barron replied that the Medical Association was in fact 'pruning' its subcommittees and that they would have had to leave eventually. It was decided to have an extraordinary general meeting of the group which took place in November. Denis Coppel proposed that the original decision be endorsed and this was seconded by James Elliott. There were a number of visiting speakers in 1972: Prof. Gordon McDowell who spoke on 'Hypotension and cerebral blood flow' and Surgeon Commander Mackay from the Royal Naval Research Centre on 'Hyperbaric oxygen therapy and decompression problems'.

1973

At the AGM in June, the honorary secretary reported that the finances were in a healthy state and that there had been seven meetings during the year with four visiting speakers. It was proposed that there should be a new structure to the committee with 11 members in all. This would consist of a chairman, vice-chairman, secretary and assistant secretary, one member from each of the new area hospital groups (four in all), two representatives of the junior anaesthetists and one representative from the QUB Department of Anaesthetics.

Speakers during the year included Dr T.B. Boulton from St Bartholomew's Hospital on 'Outpatient dental anaesthesia', Dr M.W. Johnstone from the Royal Infirmary, Manchester on 'The choice of inhalational anaesthetic agents', Dr George Robertson from Aberdeen on 'Methoxyflurane and renal function', Dr John Griffin from the Department of Health and Social Security (DHSS) in London on 'Requirements for clinical trials in new drugs' and Prof. B.R. Simpson from London Hospital on 'The impact of Marcaine on regional anaesthesia'.

1974

The AGM took place at Craigavon Hospital in County Armagh. The honorary secretary reported that holding the meetings in hospitals had been popular with the membership. The year had a significant number of well-known speakers from the UK as well as others. They included Dr D.B. Scott from the Royal Infirmary in Edinburgh, Dr Jackson Rees from Liverpool, Dr A.A. Spence from Glasgow on 'Hazards of anaesthesia', Dr Leo Strunin on 'The liver and anaesthesia', Dr M.D. Vickers from Birmingham, Dr Peter Horsey and Dr Sheila Kenny from Dublin who gave a talk titled 'The petals unfold'.

1975

It was reported at the AGM that there were seven meetings in total during the year and there was £163 in the account. It was agreed that the names of the chairmen should be inscribed on the chain of office. Overseas speakers included Dr Gillian Hanson from Whipps Cross Hospital, London on 'Septic shock' and Prof. M.K. Sykes of the Hammersmith Hospital, also in London. The Registrars' Prize was won by Dr I.O. Samuel for 'Circulatory effects of morphine after open heart surgery'. Dr William S. Wren, the dean of the Faculty of Anaesthetists, RCSI, attended the meeting in April along with Dr John R. McCarthy.

1976

The AGM was held in October and the exiting committee was re-elected. The Registrars' Prize was won by Dr Rajinder Mirakhur. The November meeting took place in Craigavon where the new 'Omagh' ambulance was inspected. Speakers that year included Dr J.D. Havard on 'Medico-legal aspects of anaesthesia', Dr Derek Carson on 'The Forensic aspects of civil unrest' and Dr J. Bolt from Guernsey on 'Underwater medicine'.

1977

An extraordinary meeting of NISA took place in June to consider the implications of the allocation of merit awards in the province by the Anaesthetic Committee of the Northern Ireland Council for Medical Education. It resolved that NISA 'wishes to express profound disquiet at the lack of recognition afforded by the Distinction Awards Committee to several of its members'. It went on to state that this lack of recognition had a deleterious effect on the morale of local anaesthetists, many of whom were working in difficult and often dangerous working conditions. The resolution was forwarded to the Merit Awards Committee. The visiting speakers included Dr Colin Wise from Wales, Dr P. Keane from Galway and Dr R.J. Weir from the DHSS in London.

Minute Book (1978–April 1991)

Some presentations at NISA meetings were on subjects that were far removed from the day-to-day practice of anaesthetists, but may have been all the more interesting for that reason. In February 1978, for example, Dr Richard Clarke spoke on old churches and their graveyards; he was followed in October of the same year by Dr Liam McCaughey who provided an account of his expedition to the Himalayas. The latter meeting also included further discussion on how to work to increase the number of Merit awards made to anaesthetists in Northern Ireland.

A significant change in the society's constitution took place in September of the following year when Dr Harold Love proposed:

> In view of the present large size of the society, its community of
> spirit and its high purpose in the promotion of learning, that its
> dignity and stature would be most appropriately acknowledged
> by designating its chief officer President rather than Chairman.

It was envisaged that each holder of the new office would deliver a presidential address during his or her term, although this would not be mandatory. The meeting minutes record that the proposal was seconded by Dr Robin King and warmly adopted by all present. Dr Gerald Black, a consultant colleague of Dr Love's at the Royal Belfast Hospital for Sick Children, became the society's inaugural president at the same meeting. His presidential address, delivered in October 1980 was titled '20th century vapours' – a subject on which he was an acknowledged expert.

While most speakers at NISA meetings are based in Britain or Ireland, this is not always so; the May 1980 meeting featured two lecturers who had each travelled from North America – Dr Alan 'Al' Conn of the Hospital for Sick Children in Toronto, Canada spoke on his specialist subject of near-drowning while Dr Maxwell Weingarten from Milwaukee, USA delivered a talk on the use of mass spectrometry in the operating theatre.

At that time, society members regularly discussed its finances and also various aspects of their working conditions and professional status. The secretary/treasurer's report for the 1980/81 session reported a significant escalation in the cost of meetings, especially where catering and travelling expenses were concerned. Some sponsors were unable to meet the full cost of meetings. There were presentations in 1980 on the 'New consultant contract' and the 'Anaesthetic manpower situation in Northern Ireland' while in October 1981, Dr John Nunn, dean of the Faculty of Anaesthetists of the Royal College of Surgeons of England, presented a paper on 'The Faculty, past, present and future'. There was an exchange of views at this meeting on the merits or otherwise of a possible future College of Anaesthetists. Eighteen months later, Prof. Michael Vickers of the Welsh National School of Medicine in Cardiff addressed the members on 'The future of the specialty of anaesthesia'. In late

1982, the honorary secretary drew the members' attention to a memorandum from the Department of Health on Maternal and Infant Care. Dr James Moore informed the meeting that the document had been drawn up without consultation with anaesthetists and although it stressed the importance of teamwork in maternal and infant care, the part played by anaesthetists was not mentioned. The secretary was asked to write to the Department of Health to express the dissatisfaction of the society's members with the report.

A special general meeting was held in April 1985 in order to discuss major changes to the society's constitution so that it would become a registered medical society, thereby allowing tax relief for the members' subscriptions and for interest earned by the society's funds. The proposed changes were approved. Later that year, the congratulations of the society were conveyed to Dr John Alexander, consultant anaesthetist at Belfast City Hospital, who had recently been honoured with the position of honorary surgeon to Her Majesty Queen Elizabeth II, the first time that such an honour had been bestowed upon an anaesthetist from Northern Ireland.

A Registrars' Prize meeting had been held annually for many years. Following Prof. John Dundee's retirement, it was re-named the Dundee Medal competition and continues to be one of the highlights of the society's year to this day. As the 1980s drew to a close and the final decade of the twentieth century commenced, its meetings continued to attract regular attendances of 70 or more. Members were attracted by visiting speakers of the calibre of Dr J.D. Morrison of Halifax, Nova Scotia (January 1989, 'Anaesthesia in Canada'), Prof. Brian Craythorne of the University of Miami (April 1990, 'Anaesthesia happenings in the USA today') and one year later, Prof. Herman Turndorf of New York ('Epidural narcotic relief of postsurgical pain').

This account was sourced from the minute books of the British Medical Association – Northern Ireland Anaesthetists Group 1963–1991, which were saved by Prof. Howard Fee 'from being dumped in a skip'.[3] The society's minute book for the period October 1991–8 was unavailable at the time of writing.

References

1   Brown W.M., 'Introduction in the "British Medical Association – N.I. Anaesthetists Group Minute book" for the years 1963–77', available to view at the Public Record Office of Northern Ireland (PRONI).
2   Clarke R., *The Royal Victoria Hospital, Belfast: A History 1797–1997*, Belfast: Blackstaff Press, 1997, p. 209.
3   Personal communication from Prof. Howard Fee.

Chapter 16

The Section of Anaesthetics, Royal Academy of Medicine in Ireland (1946)

John Cahill

The Academy of Medicine in Ireland was formed by the amalgamation of four Dublin Medical Societies (the Surgical Society of Ireland, the Medical Society of the King and Queen's College of Physicians of Ireland, the Pathological Society and the Dublin Obstetrical Society) on 22 October 1882 at a meeting in Dublin at the Royal College of Surgeons in Ireland (RCSI). The new Academy had a president – the first being John Thomas Banks, Regius Professor of Physic at Trinity College Dublin – and a council. Members of the four founding societies became fellows. Each society became a section with its own president and council. Two further sections were included later that year, for State Medicine and Anatomy & Physiology.

On 28 October 1887, the Academy became a Royal Academy, leave to do so having been granted by Queen Victoria. Its purpose was to provide a forum for the exchange of scientific knowledge by reading of papers, demonstration of clinical signs, presentation of pathological specimens and the promotion of debate and discussion between all areas of medicine and allied sciences.

To begin with, the business of the Academy was run by the president and general council consisting of six fellows, the officers and a representative from each section. No further sections were added for over 40 years but from 1930 onwards, many more came into existence and there are now more than 20. Consequently, an executive committee was established to deal with the day-to-day business. At the time of writing, the General Council meets three times during the academic year and the Executive Committee meets monthly.[1]

The Section of Anaesthetics was established in 1946, the centenary year of the first successful public demonstration of anaesthesia in October 1846 in Boston, Massachusetts. Following discussions between Dr Thomas J. Gilmartin and Mr Adams A. McConnell, president of the Academy, permission was granted to establish a section of anaesthetics at a meeting of the General Council on 6 April 1946.

The initial meeting of the section took place on 13 September 1946. The first section president was Dr Thomas Percy Claude Kirkpatrick; Dr Gilmartin became honorary secretary. Council members included the officers and Drs Victor O. McCormick, George Pugin Meldon, Oswald J. Murphy and Richard W. Shaw. The first scientific meeting was held on 12 December 1946 and was addressed by Dr (later Sir) Ivan Magill.[2] He spoke on 'Current topics in anaesthesia'. The session was opened by Mr McConnell, followed by Mr John J. Fitzsimons, president of the Surgical Section then by Dr McCormick and finally Dr Gilmartin.

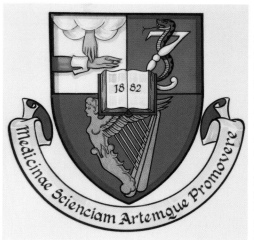

The Section of Anaesthetics of the Royal Academy of Medicine in Ireland. Detail from the Royal Academy of Medicine in Ireland Grant of Arms, 1991 (RCPI Archive – RAMI/1/2). Reproduced by permission of the Royal Academy of Medicine in Ireland.

In his address, Ivan Magill thanked the Academy for the honour of making the inaugural address to the Section of Anaesthetics and quipped that even if 'a prophet has no honour in his own country' apparently an anaesthetist has.

He noted that the Academy had been in existence long before its counterpart in London, the Royal Society of Medicine, and referred to the leaders of medical science in Ireland – Stokes, Graves, Colles, Freyer, McCarrison and Millin, all of whom, he said, had added to the lustre of Irish medical schools and would be famous for all time in medical history.

The meeting attracted over 100 delegates and was deemed a great success. From then on, meetings were held regularly, usually on clinical topics.

For almost 15 years, until the establishment of the Faculty of Anaesthetists, RCSI in 1959, the Section of Anaesthetics was the only all-Ireland academic forum run by anaesthetists for anaesthetists. Over the ensuing decades, many prominent researchers were invited to speak at its meetings. One of the first was Mr Charles King (1951) who spoke on 'The history and development of anaesthetic apparatus'. He presented the Academy with a book by George Foy entitled *Anaesthetics Ancient and Modern*.

Prof. Cecil Gray from Liverpool (1951) and Prof. Henry Beecher from Massachusetts General Hospital (1951) spoke on 'Cardiac surgery' and 'Pain and pain relief', respectively. In 1956, Dr L.A. Boeré of Leiden, Holland delivered a lecture on hypothermia. Other prominent speakers were Prof. James P. Payne

Out of town meetings of the Section of Anaesthetics proved to be very popular.

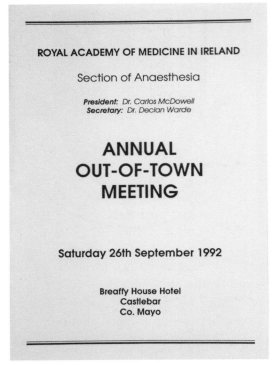

ROYAL ACADEMY OF MEDICINE IN IRELAND

Section of Anaesthesia

President: *Dr. Carlos McDowell*
Secretary: *Dr. Declan Warde*

ANNUAL OUT-OF-TOWN MEETING

Saturday 26th September 1992

**Breaffy House Hotel
Castlebar
Co. Mayo**

(1960) from London and Prof. Cornelis Ritsema Van Eck (1961), president of the World Federation of Societies of Anaesthesiologists (WFSA)[3] who presented an address 'On a respiratory centre', in which he described the unit functioning in the University Hospital in Groningen, Holland. Dr Bjorn Ibsen of the Commune Hospital, Copenhagen outlined the manner in which continental anaesthesia had developed and matured. He spoke first on anaesthetic departments and then on recovery rooms. In 1963, Dr Eric Nilsson and Dr Allan Brown described a new anaesthetic technique when they presented papers on neuroleptanalgesia.

In 1955, a joint meeting of the section and the Northern Ireland Anaesthetists Group of the British Medical Association was held under the chairmanship of the then president, Dr Patrick Drury Byrne. Four papers were presented and a dinner was held to celebrate the occasion.

The lectures given at the section meetings varied widely as a sample of titles demonstrates: 'Analgesia on demand' (1978), 'Smoke inhalation' (1979), 'Clinical use of the mass spectrometer' (1979), 'Transcutaneous O_2 tension monitoring' (1983).

The development of the Regional Anaesthetic Training Schemes and National Senior Registrar Rotation by the Faculty of Anaesthetists, RCSI in the 1970s gave rise to an increase in the number of anaesthetic trainees and the Section of Anaesthetics proved a popular forum for presenting interesting clinical cases and research projects and for competing for the prestigious Registrars' Prize. Newly appointed consultants who had completed fellowships abroad were also invited to speak about their experience overseas and present the results of their research work. The section also held out-of-town meetings and joint meetings in conjunction with anaesthetic departments around the country including those in Cork, Limerick, Sligo and Drogheda.

In 1987, at the request of the president of the section, Prof. Anthony J. Cunningham, its name was changed to the 'Section of Anaesthesia'.

The *Irish Journal of Medical Science*

The *Irish Journal of Medical Science* (IJMS) is the official organ of the Royal Academy of Medicine of Ireland (RAMI) and over the years, it has diligently published accounts of meetings of the Section of Anaesthetics and individual papers. As such, it can rightfully be considered an integral part of the history of the Section of Anaesthetics of RAMI. The journal was founded in 1832 as *The Dublin Journal of Medical and Chemical Science* by Robert John Kane and is the oldest medical periodical in Ireland.[4,5]

Kane's original plan was to publish a scientific journal dealing with chemistry and chemical interactions but he was persuaded to broaden the scope to include medicine, and on 1 March 1832, there appeared the first number of the *Dublin Journal of Medical and Chemical Science, exhibiting a comprehensive view of the latest discoveries in Medicine, Surgery, Chemistry, and the collateral Sciences.* It contained three sections: Original Communications, Bibliographical Notices and Scientific Communications.

Over its long and distinguished career, the journal has been published under a number of different titles – the *Dublin Journal of Medical Science* from 1836 and the *Dublin Quarterly Journal of Medical Science* from 1846. By 1869, the editor, Dr James Little, was able to report that 'at the present time its circulation, not only at home, but in England, on the Continent, in America, and in the British Colonies, is greater than at any previous period.'

In 1872, it appeared as the *Dublin Journal of Medical Science* (again) and was published monthly. Finally, in March 1922, the title changed to the *Irish Journal of Medical Science* (IJMS) which became the official organ of the Royal Academy of Medicine in Ireland.

The entire issue of the journal for October 1946, just one month after the first meeting of the Section of Anaesthetics, was given over to anaesthesia. It contained 12 papers all by leading anaesthetists of the day with one exception – 'Spinal anaesthesia with hypobaric percaine'[6] written by Mr Patrick Kiely, professor of surgery at University College Cork and consultant surgeon at the Bon Secours Hospital, the South Charitable Infirmary and the Mercy Hospital, Cork.

The professor based his comments about spinal anaesthesia on 'personal records of between 1,000 and 1,200 cases operated on by this method in the past seven and a half years'. It was his confirmed opinion that operating was much easier, haemorrhage less, shock less and the mortality decidedly lower with this method than with general anaesthesia and he listed 66 operations carried out by him in 1945 using hypobaric percaine, also administered by him. One third of these procedures involved upper abdominal incisions and there was one death. On the phenomena noticed during spinal anaesthetic, he commented, 'Faintness, pallor, sweating, vomiting, fallen blood pressure, air hunger, and inability to cough in very high anaesthesia due to paralysis of the intercostal muscles are the changes most commonly observed', and he continued, 'they generally tend to pass off in from 12 to 20 minutes, and are to a large extent preventable by the preliminary injection of ephedrine (gr. 1½ for an adult)'.

He went on to state that it was, however, his practice to 'employ general anaesthesia' for all the short simple cases (hernia, appendicectomy) and to use hypobaric percaine for all the more difficult operations.

He listed some of the practical difficulties in administering spinal anaesthetics – failure to enter the theca due to osteoarthritis or obesity; failure to obtain a good flow of cerebrospinal fluid (CSF) in elderly debilitated patients; and failure to obtain satisfactory analgesia due to a faulty drug or insufficient dose. Should the anaesthesia turn out to be imperfect, 'it was wise' he stated, 'to reinforce the spinal with local, gas and oxygen, or even a general anaesthetic as thought fit'. The only common sequel of spinal anaesthesia in his experience was headache for which 'hypertonic derivation by 6 ozs. of a 50 per cent solution of magnesium sulphate into the rectum is the best method; aspirin may be given as well'. His five contra-indications to spinal anaesthesia were operations above the diaphragm, pyaemia, pregnancy, malignant disease and shock, especially wound shock due to haemorrhage. In keeping with the times, there was no mention of intravenous access, supplemental oxygen or routine monitoring of vital signs.

Other articles of interest to anaesthetists but written by non-anaesthetists also appeared in the journal. In 1960, Prof. Eoin O'Malley, professor of surgery at University College Dublin, set out his views on modern anaesthesia[7] and stated confidently that 'The patient will seldom recall enough of his experience at their (anaesthetists) hands to enable him to offer useful comment. The surgeon, however, is more vocal and in a position to be either critical or appreciative.' He considered the control of ventilation during anaesthesia to be a major advance but that the expanding list of anaesthetic drugs brought with it a multiplicity of unwanted side-effects and posed a serious problem. Acknowledging that postoperative derangements of water and electrolyte balance (la maladie postopératoire) were largely due to surgery, anaesthetists were invited to also take their share of the blame. Extracorporeal circulation and oxygenation and hypothermia offered an exciting view of the future:

> with respiration, circulation and metabolism, to all intents and purposes, abolished – no longer would they need attention or control; having ceased, they cannot go wrong. If the problem of getting a patient into and out of this state with safety could be solved, it would seem to be the answer.

O'Malley concluded in complimentary fashion, predicting: 'Spectacular advances in anaesthesia can be anticipated through greater understanding and application of the fundamentals of physiology and biochemistry. Now that anaesthesia (or anaesthesiology) has become established as such a virile and progressive science, it is only right that Irish anaesthetists should have taken the step which they took in founding the Faculty of Anaesthesia.'

Presidential Addresses
Presidential addresses, traditionally given at the end of each term of office and published in the *Irish Journal of Medical Science*, contain a good overview of the developments and progress of anaesthesia as well as the aspirations and concerns of its practitioners.

In his 1950 address, 'Present and future of anaesthesia and the anaesthetist', Dr Victor McCormick, consultant anaesthetist at Sir Patrick Dun's Hospital Dublin, considered developments of the previous 25 years.[8] The introduction of endotracheal intubation, cyclopropane and Waters' carbon dioxide absorber were to the fore; in his opinion, the development of thoracic surgery was one of the finest examples of co-operation between the surgeon and the anaesthetist with each recognising their dependence on the other and each allowing the other the opportunity to perform their task efficiently and without interference. Operating lists had become longer and more complex and he commented, 'it is now a matter of course that the anaesthetist should not make his first contact with the patient on the operating table, nor should he say good-bye to him when he leaves the table'. The working conditions and pay for anaesthetists had, however, not kept pace with the increased clinical demands and he was concerned that young Irish graduates with an interest in anaesthesia would simply go abroad in search of better opportunities and working conditions.

Dr Sheila Kenny, consultant anaesthetist at the Adelaide Hospital, Dublin, chose the inscription on the crest of the Association of Anaesthetists of Great Britain and Ireland (AAGBI) 'In Somno Securitas' as the title of her presidential address (1960).[9] She modestly included herself in the older category of anaesthetist, largely self-taught and clinically based, and acknowledged the younger group whose training had given them a thorough understanding of basic sciences, and who were therefore better equipped to understand the findings of research. Safety in anaesthesia is the goal that all clinicians and researchers aspire to, hence the title of her address. To emphasise her point, she discussed various aspects of patient physiology which anaesthetists attempt to control during surgery but her section 'Control of respiration' is especially interesting. The introduction of muscle relaxants and tracheal intubation meant that the anaesthetist took over ventilation of the patient. The effectiveness of manual ventilation was (and still is) notoriously unreliable, nor was there a proven method of choosing the correct ventilator settings for each individual patient so the hazards of serious hypo- or hyperventilation and their attendant physiological disturbances were very real. Dr Kenny described how, with the help of a young medical student who designed and built a portable ventilator and a grant from the Medical Research Council of Ireland, she was able to monitor the patients' minute ventilation, oxygen saturation, capillary pH and carbon dioxide tension by means of a Wright's Anemometer, a Cox's Oximeter and an Astrup Micromethod Analyser. 'By the use of these instruments,' she continued, 'I hope to find the optimal level and rate of ventilation, and to discover what exactly hyper- and hypoventilation mean for each patient'. She may well have been one of the older self-taught generation of anaesthetists but her understanding of patient safety and how it might be ensured was remarkable for its time.

'Anaesthesia coming of age' was the title of the address given by Dr Hugh Raftery (1968), consultant anaesthetist at St Vincent's Hospital, Dublin.[10] He reviewed some of the significant events of the years since the formation of the Section of Anaesthesics and, in particular, noted the death in 1954 of its first president, Dr T.P.C. Kirkpatrick, the establishment of the Faculty of Anaesthetists, RCSI in 1960, the Annual Scientific Meeting of the Association of Anaesthetists of Great Britain and Ireland (AAGBI) in Dublin in 1961 and the foundation of the first chair in anaesthesia in Dublin in 1965 with Dr Gilmartin as professor.

In his review of recent and future developments in clinical practice, Dr Raftery took the title of the very first address to the section by Prof. Ivan Magill in 1946, 'Current topics in anaesthesia', and posed the question of what these were in 1968. Patient monitoring devices, computerisation and teaching and training in anaesthesia were prominent in his discussion. He noted that 'The range of electronic apparatus available to monitor every conceivable vital process is vastly impressive, as is the great skill shown in its design and the ease with which it can be used' but he warned, 'no machine can replace a lively mind, alert for any departure from normal, which can usually be seen clinically in a qualitative way if full quantitative correction demands biochemical control'.

He believed that computers would have a major role to play in storing all kinds of medical information and with an astute eye to the future, suggested that anaesthesia take the lead and design a common standard anaesthetic record for the whole country suitable for computer storage. He 'was glad to report' that servo control of anaesthesia had been unsuccessful so far but considered computers may have an important role to play in intensive care.

Cardiac Arrest

On 5 April 1958, a joint meeting of the Sections of Anaesthetics and Surgery was held.[11] The topic of the meeting was cardiac arrest with Drs G. Raymond (Ray) Davys and Alexander McA Blayney, consultant anaesthetists at St Vincent's and the Mater Misericordiae Hospitals respectively, describing the causes and management and Messrs Nigel Kinnear and J. Augustine 'Gussie' Mehigan, consultant surgeons at the Adelaide and St Vincent's Hospitals, respectively, speaking on the role of surgeons in such an emergency. The meeting confined its deliberations exclusively to cardiac arrest in the operating theatre.

The three basic principles of maintaining the airway, cardiac massage and defibrillation were described in detail but the means of applying them were vastly different to the methods used today.

Diagnosing a cardiac arrest was considered to be the responsibility of the anaesthetist by confirming the absence of a carotid pulse 'and ECG evidence, if available'. The time of the arrest was recorded, all anaesthetic drugs discontinued and 100 per cent oxygen administered. An ECG machine and defibrillator were sent for 'if required'. The surgeon was requested to perform a thoracotomy and to massage the heart directly even if the abdomen was open – the landmark publication on closed cardiac massage did not appear until 1960.[12] The chances of a good outcome depended on the duration of hypoxia immediately before the arrest and the time it took the surgeon to establish an adequate cardiac output as judged by the anaesthetist palpating the carotid pulse.

Key points made by the speakers included:

- Once effective massage is started the emergency is over.
- Ventricular fibrillation is easily diagnosed .... when the pericardium is opened.
- Again there is no need to panic; an adequate circulation can be maintained by cardiac massage.
- Even if you do not possess a defibrillator, there is plenty of time to borrow one from a nearby hospital.
- A single shock brought directly from the mains in the most simple manner has been used with dramatic success, when no proper defibrillator was available. This state of affairs should not, however, arise as there should be at least one defibrillator available for every group of hospitals, and if the commercial models prove too expensive, the apparatus is easily made in a hospital workshop.

The importance of drill and exercise was emphasised – 'We are bound to prepare ourselves so that we may be able to diagnose the condition with confidence and to act at once'.

A lively discussion followed the formal presentations with many contributions from the floor. Dr William 'Bill' Wren described the difficulties of diagnosing and treating cardiac arrest in small babies and the challenges presented by cardiac arrest in the dental surgery were discussed. Mr T.C.J. O'Connell, consultant surgeon at St Vincent's Hospital, struck a sombre note reminding those present that it was possible to restart a heart and circulation even when catastrophic brain anoxia had occurred.

Safety in Anaesthesia

Just two years after the establishment of the Section of Anaesthetics, the need to systematically investigate the causes of mortality and morbidity associated with anaesthesia had been articulated when Dr Kathleen Bayne, a graduate of Trinity College and consultant anaesthetist at the Royal Victoria Eye and Ear Hospital, Dublin, proposed that:

the Council of the Section should establish a Statistical Research Sub-Committee which would be charged with the responsibility of collecting from the members particulars of their experience and of collating the results for further scientific study of fatality and mortality under anaesthesia. The data, under particular sub-headings, could be assigned to selected members of the Academy for special investigation, the provisional conclusions being communicated to and discussed at such a meeting as this.[13]

Both Sheila Kenny and Hugh Raferty were acutely aware of the importance of safety in anaesthesia and discussed the topic in their presidential addresses – Kenny considered safety to be the goal that all clinicians and researchers aspire to and Raftery proposed a common standard anaesthetic record for the whole country suitable for computer storage

In 1987, almost 40 years after Bayne's proposal, Professor Anthony Cunningham asked 'Anaesthesia in Ireland 1987 – how safe is it?'.[14] 'Safer than twenty years previously', he concluded, and quoted a mortality rate directly due to anaesthesia of approximately one in 10,000 anaesthetics from French and American studies. Despite the lack of published figures from Ireland, he did not believe there was any specific reason why Irish anaesthetic mortality and morbidity should differ significantly from other developed Western nations, but he lamented the lack of any epidemiological studies into morbidity and mortality associated with anaesthesia in Ireland and urged that this omission be rectified.

The inaugural national medical scientific meeting was held by the Academy in 1992. Research papers and poster presentations from all the medical specialties and allied sciences were invited. Anaesthesia and intensive care

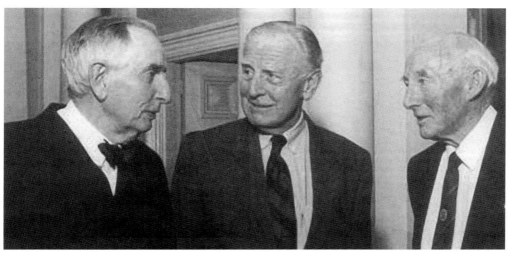

The Inaugural William S. Wren Lecture. Dr Wren is pictured with his colleagues Dr Don Coleman (l) and Dr Des Gaffney (r). With kind permission Bobby Studio.

Presidents, Section of Anaesthetics, Royal Academy of Medicine in Ireland

1946–8	Dr T. Percy Kirkpatrick	1974–6	Dr John R. McCarthy
1948–50	Dr Victor O. McCormick	1976–8	Dr Deirdre Pepper
1950–2	Dr Richard W. Shaw	1978–80	Dr John Goodbody
1952–4	Dr Thomas J. Gilmartin	1980–2	Dr Hugh J. Galvin
1954–6	Dr Patrick Drury Byrne	1982–4	Dr James Gardiner
1956–8	Dr Patrick J. Nagle	1984–6	Dr Desmond Riordan
1958–60	Dr Sheila Kenny	1986–8	Prof. Anthony J. Cunningham
1960–2	Dr Joseph A. Woodcock	1988–90	Dr Patrick Fitzgerald
1962–5	Dr Raymond Davys	1990–2	Dr Carlos McDowell
1965–7	Dr Alexander MacA. Blayney	1992–4	Dr Lesley Fox
1967–9	Dr Hugh Raftery	1994–6	Dr Vincent Hannon
1969–72	Dr Edmund J. Delaney	1996–8	Dr Eamon Tierney
1972–4	Dr John Conroy	1998–2000	Dr Sean McDevitt

medicine contributed over a dozen items to the first meeting and continued to contribute in a major way to subsequent national medical scientific meetings.[15,16]

The first eponymous lecture of the Section of Anaesthesia, 'Inhalational anaesthesia in children – the first 150 years' was delivered on 26 November 1997 by Dr Declan Warde in recognition of the outstanding contribution made by Dr William 'Bill' Wren (1929–2006) to anaesthesia in Ireland.

References

1   Royal Academy of Medicine in Ireland – History of RAMI, available at https://www.rami.ie/about/n (accessed 30 June 2021).

2   Magill I.W., 'Current topics in anaesthesia', *Irish Journal of Medical Science*, 1947, 22, pp. 45–54.

3   Dorlas J.C., 'Dr. Cornelis R. Ritsema van Eck: A Many-Sided Pioneer', in J. Rupreht, M.J. van Lieburg, J.A. Lee and W. Erdmann (eds), *Anaesthesia – Essays on Its History*, Berlin Heidelberg: Springer-Verlag, 1985, pp. 54–8.

4   Kirkpatrick T.P.C., 'An account of the Dublin medical journals', *Dublin Journal of Medical Science*, 1915, 140, pp. 1– 3.

5   Mullen J., Wheelock H., 'The Dublin Journal of Medical and Chemical Science catalogue. 2010', available at https://web.archive.org/web/20110818164338/http://irserver.ucd.ie/dspace/bitstream/10197/2487/3/ResearchPaperDublinJournalMedicalChemicalScience.pdf (accessed 30 June 2021).

6   Kiely P., 'Spinal anaesthesia with hypobaric percaine', *Irish Journal of Medical Science*, 1946, 21, pp. 704–10.

7   O'Malley E. 'A surgeon's view of modern anaesthesia', *Irish Journal of Medical Science*, 1960, 35, pp. 435–8.

8   McCormick V.O., 'Present and future of anæsthesia and the anæsthetist', *Irish Journal of Medical Science*, 1950, 25, pp. 193–200.

9   Kenny S., 'In Somno Securitas', *Irish Journal of Medical Science*, 1960, 35, pp. 297–309.

10 Raftery H., 'Anaesthesia coming of age', *Irish Journal of Medical Science*, 1968, 1, pp. 523–30.

11 Davys R., Kinnear N., Blayney A.M. and Mehigan J.A., 'Cardiac Arrest', *Irish Journal of Medical Science*, 1958, 393, pp. 414–25.

12 Kouwenhoven W., Jude J. and Knickerbocker G., 'Closed chest cardiac massage', *Journal of the American Medical Association*, 1960, 173, pp. 1064–7.

13 Bayne K., 'Statistical research in anaesthetics', *Irish Journal of Medical Science*, 1948, 23, pp.166–8.

14 Cunningham A.J., Editorial, 'Anaesthesia in Ireland, 1987 – How safe is it?, *Irish Journal of Medical Science*, 1987, 156, pp. iii–iv.

15 'Inaugural National Scientific Medical Meeting', *Irish Journal of Medical Science*, 1993, 162, pp. 56–7.

16 *Ibid.*, pp. 113–16.

Chapter 17

The South of Ireland Society/ Association of Anaesthetists (1955)

John Cahill

The South of Ireland Society of Anaesthetists was founded in Cork on Saturday 19 March 1955. Dr Eugene Thomas was elected president, Dr Timothy Stanislas Reynolds vice president and Dr Edward Guest Hobart honorary secretary and treasurer. A committee of six members was also elected: Drs Daniel Coleman, John Bourke, Maurice Flynn, Mary Solan, Maura O'Driscoll and John O'Sullivan.

The business of the inaugural meeting included agreeing that the group be called 'The South of Ireland Society of Anaesthetists', that the annual subscription would be two guineas, and that the society's year would commence on 5 April. Society meetings would be held once per month with a quorum of five members but the president could call an extraordinary meeting at any time on the request of a member. Other rules could be drawn up by the committee from time to time as considered necessary. The founding of the new society was communicated to the honorary secretaries of the Association of Anaesthetists of Great Britain and Ireland (AAGBI).[1] the Anaesthetists Group of the Irish Medical Association and the Royal Academy of Medicine in Ireland. The members decided to meet again on 7 May 1955, but matters progressed rather more rapidly than anticipated and an extraordinary meeting was called for Saturday 4 April.

The subject that occasioned the first extraordinary meeting was the advertising of a post of consultant anaesthetist at one of the hospitals in Cork city. In the opinion of the members, the salary on offer was inadequate. The minutes do not state what this was but a number of initiatives were taken including suggesting to the hospital authorities that an annual salary of £1,250 would be appropriate, and putting a notice in the public press inviting anyone interested in the post to contact the society before applying. The hospital subsequently agreed to pay the new salary but any satisfaction was diminished when it became clear that an appointment had been made without re-advertising the post. This meant, of course, that a number of potential applicants who had taken notice of the society's concerns had not been interviewed. Despite this frustration, it was decided to close

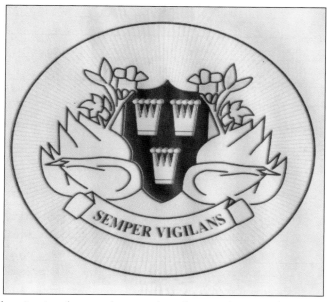

Crest of the South of Ireland Association of Anaesthetists.

discussions on the matter and to invite the newly appointed consultant to become a member, which he duly did. His name appears in the list of those present at a meeting on 15 December that year and he became president two years later.

The business of the society over the next number of years was taken up largely by discussions about and attempts to influence the terms and conditions of employment of consultant anaesthetists in Cork and further afield, and a close working relationship developed with the Anaesthetists Group of the Irish Medical Association (IMA). Health matters in general were entering a new and tumultuous phase at that time and the 1953 Health Act was central to the heated medico-political discussions that were taking place. The Department of Health became a standalone department in January 1947[2] – previously health matters were handled by the Department of Local Government and Public Health. A government white paper published in 1947, 'Outline of proposals for the improvement of the health services', contained in the 1947 Health Act[3] set out the plans for universal social insurance and a health service mirroring the new National Health Service recently introduced in the United Kingdom (UK). The sustained opposition of religious and medical representatives to the proposals including the fall of the inter-party government and the resignation of the Minister of Health in 1951 are well documented.[4–6]

The 1953 Health Act was a very much watered-down version of the original proposals but it did extend free medical care to a significant proportion of the population. This would have a significant impact on the incomes of general practitioners as well as hospital consultants since the number of patients liable for doctors' fees would be greatly reduced at a time when pay and conditions of employment for hospital consultants were still being negotiated. The medical profession generally was suspicious of 'socialised' medicine and the prospect of being a salaried civil servant was seen as a threat to professional independence. The IMA was in favour of voluntary private health insurance which, indeed, came to pass with the establishment of the Voluntary Health Insurance Board (VHI) in 1957. The minutes of the society reflect the concerns of its members in this regard, as shown by this extract from a meeting of 12 April 1956:

> A discussion took place on the proposed payment of anaesthetists and the terms thereof, under the new Health Act. The Hon Sec was instructed to write to Doctor T Gilmartin (anaesthetists' representative at the IMA) to elicit information on a number of obscure points
>
> • The method of payment for an anaesthetist doing two theatres at one time.
> • Whether pre operative and post operative examinations are included in anaesthetic sessions.
> • Whether entitled patients under the scheme who decide to go into semi-private or private wards were liable personally for anaesthetic fees.
> • The question of notional sessions: Whether an anaesthetist who is engaged to do a session or sessions every week is to be paid if there happens to be no operations at these times though he has to be on call.
> • The position of holiday & sick leave.[7]

To this list can be added concerns about payment for midwifery cases in nursing homes and for anaesthetics given in dental surgeries – the society suggested a maximum fee of £2. 10s .0d for public patients and a minimum of 2 guineas for private patients – and fees for what is now called monitored care. The first clinical meeting of the new society took place on Saturday 24 March 1956 at University College Cork (UCC). The guest speaker was Prof. William Mushin of Cardiff Royal Infirmary who gave an illustrated account of his recent visit to Brazil. He had been invited there to advise on anaesthetic services in that country, and he described the social and clinical aspects of medicine in general and anaesthesia in particular. Prof. Mushin was entertained to lunch and dinner over the weekend by members of the society. The total bill for the meeting came to £29.10s.1d, including travelling expenses and accommodation for Prof. Mushin.

Meetings did not become annual events immediately; the second took place on Saturday 14 June 1958, again at UCC. Notification had been sent to the Royal Academy of Medicine in Ireland and to anaesthetic colleagues in Galway and Limerick. The meeting included a film on hypotensive anaesthesia and the speakers on the day were all members of the society. The topics included 'Difficulties in relation to anaesthesia, Dr Maurice Flynn', 'Dental anaesthesia, Dr Don Coleman', 'Caesarean section, Dr John D Bourke' and 'Experimental work, Dr Richard Walsh'.

Prof. Sir Robert Macintosh was the guest speaker at the clinical meeting held in December 1960. He was welcomed with a sherry party in the UCC staff room attended by 60 guests on the evening of 1 December. He gave an informal talk at the Imperial Hotel the following day which was followed by dinner. On 3 December, Prof. Macintosh demonstrated the new Nuffield ether vaporizer on three patients at the North Infirmary, Mr John Kiely operating. Total expenses for the meeting came to £75. 2s. 2d

The society had enjoyed a steady first five years and the 1960s saw further consolidation and development. Despite the small number of members, no more than a dozen, the business of the society records some noteworthy events, both local and international. A bank account was opened at the Munster & Leinster Bank on Patrick Street, Cork, the society's financial year was to begin in January rather than April and most significantly perhaps, at a meeting held on 5 October 1962 at the Victoria Hospital, Cork, the name of the organisation was changed from the South of Ireland Society of Anaesthetists to the South of Ireland Association of Anaesthetists (SIAA).[8]

In 1960, the former Belgian Congo gained independence and became a republic but almost immediately descended into civil war. A United Nations peacekeeping force was deployed; it included an Irish contingent in which two SIAA members, Drs Daniel Delaney and Tony MacSullivan served. Their colleagues in SIAA acknowledged this and agreed that the two should be exempt from paying their annual subscription while on military duty.[9] Thankfully, they were welcomed home safely later the same year.

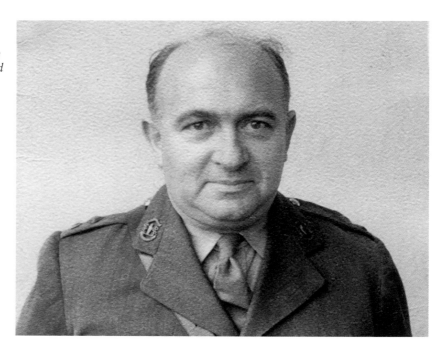

Dr Daniel Delaney, President of the South of Ireland Association of Anaesthetists 1969–1972. With kind permission of Maurice and Philomena Delaney.

The SIAA had been made aware of the preliminary discussions in 1958 that ultimately led to the founding of the Faculty of Anaesthetists, RCSI and had supported and contributed to these.[10] The faculty was formally inaugurated on 8 July 1960 with Dr T.J. Gilmartin as the first dean.[11] Dr Don Coleman, who was president of SIAA at the time, became a foundation fellow along with Drs John D. Bourke and Brendan Lyne.

The main business of SIAA, however, remained the terms and conditions of employment for anaesthetists, and the close working relationship with the Anaesthetists Group of the IMA continued to develop. Matters did not always go smoothly, however. A report by the group recommending an annual salary of £2,500 rising to £3,500 seemed acceptable but a passage in the same report[12] which stated that 'consultant anaesthetists should hold the FFARCSI or other approved higher qualification', but which failed to mention the DA gave the impression, that in the opinion of SIAA at least, county anaesthetists were not of the same calibre as their colleagues in the city hospitals. Not surprisingly, an indignant response[13] was dispatched to Dr Kevin O'Sullivan, honorary secretary of the Anaesthetists Group at the IMA.

SIAA officers were keen to become involved in teaching undergraduate students at UCC and in 1961, discussions took place between Dr Coleman and

Dr Bernard F. Honan, incoming dean of medicine. A programme of undergraduate teaching was established but by 1966, it was considered to be in a 'parlous condition'. In early 1967, meetings took place between the SIAA and the dean of medicine at UCC, Prof. Denis O'Sullivan, in order to agree the content and timing of six lectures in anaesthetics to be given to third-, fourth- and final-year medical students,[14] and when the professor of surgery, Michael P. Brady, set up a curriculum subcommittee, the SIAA was invited to nominate two members.[15] Consultant anaesthetists delivering lectures to undergraduate medical students were recognised as part-time lecturers in anaesthesia (Department of Surgery, UCC), a situation which continued until the appointment of Prof. George Shorten as the first professor of anaesthesia and intensive care medicine at UCC in 1997.

Notwithstanding these other activities, the Annual Clinical Meeting and dinner remained the centrepiece of the SIAA's calendar, and minutes from 1962 describe many of the features of these meetings. The invited speaker for the Annual Clinical Meeting was Dr Gordon Jackson Rees of the Department of Anaesthesia at Liverpool University. The title of his talk, which he illustrated with slides, was 'Some aspects of paediatric anaesthesia':

> On Friday 30 March 1962 Dr Jackson Rees was entertained to dinner in the Cork & County Club at 7.30 pm by the members of the Association and their wives. In all there were fifteen persons present.
>
> The following morning, he was given a guided tour of two Cork hospitals, the Bon Secours Hospital and St Stephen's Hospital, Sarsfield's Court. He expressed particular interest in the neonatal ward at the Bon Secours Hospital and in certain cardiac operations carried out by Mr M Hickey, FRCS, at St Stephen's Hospital.
>
> The clinical meeting began at 5pm following afternoon tea. A stenographer recorded the proceedings in shorthand, for which she received 3 guineas, and a typed copy of Dr Jackson Rees' talk was later made available. Approximately thirty persons attended the meeting from counties Waterford, Cork, Kerry, Limerick, Clare, Tipperary, Kilkenny and Dublin. The dean of the Faculty of Anaesthetists, RCSI, Dr T J Gilmartin was also in attendance.

The annual dinner was held that evening in the Metropole Hotel. There were 38 guests. The president of the association, Dr Don Coleman, proposed the toast 'Ireland', and the dean of the Faculty of Anaesthetists, RCSI, Dr Gilmartin proposed 'The Association'. Dr Jackson Rees and Mr M Hickey also spoke.

At the request of the president, Dr M Flynn entertained the company by playing the piano.

On Sunday April 1st, Dr Jackson Rees was seen off at Cork Airport by the president and the Honorary Secretary of the Association.

Total costs for the meeting came to £114. 4s. 3d (including £0. 17s. 6d for a projector), leaving a final balance of £0. 13s. 1d.

Despite the enthusiasm and tenacity of the SIAA officers, however, momentum began to wane during the 1970s and a number of meetings, including two AGMs [May 1974 and May 1978], were postponed as a quorum had not been reached. However, there were a number of significant developments in the Irish health service in the 1970s and 1980s which had the effect of reinvigorating the SIAA.

The 1970 Health Act introduced eight new health boards, replacing the far more numerous and much smaller health authorities which served the functional areas of city and county councils. The act also established Comhairle na nOspidéal, a statutory body responsible for advising government on the appropriate number of consultants and senior registrars in all medical specialties. On the recommendation of Comhairle, as it was known, the number of consultant appointments in anaesthesia began to increase.[16] The new Cork Regional Hospital (now Cork University Hospital) opened in 1978. The hospital, considered to be 'state of the art' was referred to locally as the 'Wilton Hilton'. The Faculty of Anaesthetists, RCSI established three regional anaesthetic training schemes in Dublin, Galway and Cork and when the National Senior Registrar Training Scheme was set up in 1976, Cork Regional Hospital was part of this rotation. The introduction of the first Common Contract for consultants in 1981[17] standardised terms of employment and remuneration for all medical consultants in public hospitals and removed a range of anomalies and inequities which heretofore were contested locally by bodies such as SIAA.

The arrival in the southern health board area of a new generation of anaesthetists, both consultant and trainee, led to a significant rise in SIAA membership and the content and format of the clinical meetings reflected this.

Specialist areas of clinical practice and research were new topics at SIAA seminars, often led by newly-appointed consultants. At a joint meeting with the Section of Anaesthetics of the Royal Academy of Medicine in Ireland held on 8 April 1979 the pioneering work on malignant hyperpyrexia led by Prof. James Heffron of the Department of Biochemistry, UCC and Dr Mary Lehane, consultant anaesthetist at Cork Regional Hospital was presented. On 23 October 1982 a seminar on pain medicine was organised by Dr Tom Fogarty, a colleague of Dr Lehane's at Cork Regional Hospital.

Notwithstanding this very welcome influx of 'new blood', the founding SIAA members took time to pay tribute to one of their number, Dr Edward G. Hobart, a founding member and officer, when, on the occasion of his retirement from clinical practice, he was made an honorary life member of SIAA at a 'very pleasant function at the Cork & County Club on May 25th 1980'. The association also celebrated its 21st birthday with a clinical meeting and dinner at UCC in May 1978 (despite the fact that SIAA was founded in 1955!). Local speakers included Prof. Denis O'Sullivan, Dr Dan O'Mahony, Mr John Bartholomew (JB) Kearney and Dr Mary Lehane. The guest speaker was Prof. Mike Rosen of the Cardiff Royal Infirmary.

Annual Clinical Meetings were held in a number of venues outside Cork, including Waterford, Kilkenny, Limerick, Killarney and Kinsale. A Friday evening component, the Abbott Lecture, was introduced, at which non-medical topics as diverse as local history, architecture, politics, and veterinary medicine were presented by local experts. In the early1990s, the May guest lecture was named the Janssen Lecture in recognition of the support the company had given to SIAA over the years. These lectures were delivered in the case study room at UCC. The 1991 Janssen Lecture was given by Dr Anita Griffith, a newly-appointed consultant anaesthetist at the Mercy Hospital. The title of her lecture was 'Postoperative delirium in the elderly patient'. Trainees were given a permanent slot at the annual meetings from 1989 onwards, in the first instance by means of an essay competition and in later years by a Registrars' Case Presentation forum. The first winning essay was entitled 'A suitable time to introduce anaesthetics' and was read by its author, Dr George Shorten.

The association also entertained a number of anaesthetic societies from the UK at its annual meetings – the Society of Anaesthetists of the South West Region, SASWR (1981), the Society of Anaesthetists of Wales (May 1979 & October 1996) and the South Yorkshire Anaesthetists Society (October 1994). A return visit by SIAA to Bristol in 1988 for a joint meeting with SASWR proved to be a most enjoyable and successful occasion not least because Dr Frances O'Donovan, a UCC graduate and anaesthetic trainee, captured the President's Prize with a witty and highly entertaining account of a year she spent training in anaesthesia at the Centre Hospitalier du Kremlin-Bicêtre in Paris entitled 'The French connection'.

As the date of its 40th anniversary approached – April 1995 – SIAA affairs appeared to be on a very sound footing. At the annual dinner in October 1990, the chain of office was worn for the first time by Dr Seamus Hart, president of the South of Ireland Association of Anaesthetists. The chain of hallmarked silver had the names of all previous presidents inscribed on it and carried a medallion, also of hallmarked silver, bearing the SIAA emblem depicting the three kingdoms of Munster (Thomond, Ormond and Desmond) and the flower Atropa belladonna flanked by two swans.

Elected representation on the board of the Faculty of Anaesthetists, RCSI had always been an important issue for SIAA. Drs Coleman (1967 & 1980), Gaffney (1970) and O'Brien (1983) had all been successful candidates from the Southern Health Board area but as the number of fellows in other parts of the country increased, particularly in Dublin, success in faculty elections became much more difficult.

In order to address this challenge, a faculty election subcommittee of SIAA was established in January 1990 with immediate results. Dr Seamus Hart was elected in May 1990 and was followed by Dr Pat Fitzgerald in 1991, Dr Peter Kenefick in 1995 (having had to contend with a postal strike in 1993 and a narrow defeat in 1994) and Dr John Cahill (1998). Dr John McAdoo was elected to the Council of the College of Anaesthetists of Ireland (2002) and went on to become president in 2006.

The establishment of the Standing Committee in Ireland of AAGBI in 1988 and its cordial interactions with SIAA led to some significant developments. SIAA had contributed to the fundraising efforts of AAGBI in support of the move to its new home at 9 Bedford Square, London in 1985[18] and in 1995, SIAA and AAGBI jointly sponsored Dr Eamon Tierney, consultant anaesthetist at Wexford General Hospital, when he took part in the annual anaesthetic officer refresher course in Uganda.

The AAGBI stand, replete with various association publications, including booklets published on behalf of the Irish Standing Committee, became a feature at the SIAA Annual Clinical Meeting. In addition, Dr Wendy Scott, consultant anaesthetist at Milton Keynes Hospital, attended on a number of occasions as a representative of AAGBI Council but also as a guest of SIAA.

Private practice fees for anaesthetists had been a contentious issue for many years. Perhaps the most significant issues (and there were many!) related to the low level of remuneration available to anaesthetists ('the shilling on the surgeon's guinea') and the fact that there was just a single insurer, VHI. Despite considerable efforts by Don Coleman working through the IMA's Fees Committee and subsequently the Irish Medical Organisation (IMO) over many years, there had never been an agreement on a schedule of fees for anaesthetists and VHI published its own fee schedules on a 'take it or leave it' basis. The lack of an agreement with VHI and the reticence of many anaesthetists to 'balance bill' patients for the difference between what VHI allowed and what the specialty considered an appropriate fee meant that the situation was unclear and unsatisfactory for both patients and anaesthetists.

The presence of the Standing Committee in Ireland of AAGBI, however, meant that anaesthetists were now in a position to negotiate directly with VHI as a single body representing anaesthetists alone. The efforts of the Irish Standing Committee led by Drs Aidan Synnott, John Dunphy, P.J. Breen and Tom Fogarty resulted in the first ever agreement with VHI on a schedule of private practice fees for anaesthetists. The agreement was by no means perfect – discussions relating to the subspecialty areas of intensive care and pain medicine had been deferred – but when the proposed schedule was presented to anaesthetists at a special open meeting of the Standing Committee in October 1994 it was overwhelmingly accepted.[19]

The 1995 Annual Clinical Meeting celebrated the 40th anniversary of the South of Ireland Association of Anaesthetists.[20] The meeting was held in October in Cork and was a joint meeting with the Society of Anaesthetists of Wales (SAW) led by their president, Dr Seiriol Davies, secretary Dr Jeanne Seager and treasurer Dr Graham Arthurs. The Friday evening Abbott Lecture was delivered by Mr Liam Guerin, a well-known veterinary surgeon in Cork who spoke about his experiences dealing with a variety of animals, large and small, at the Fota Wildlife Park on the outskirts of the city. The speakers at the scientific meeting on Saturday included Prof. Stephen F. Dierdorf, Indiana University School of Medicine Indianapolis and Drs Seiriol Davies, Howell Davies, Eamon Tierney, David O'Flaherty and Inder Bali. The Registrars' Prize competition was won by Irene Leonard, anaesthetic registrar at the Mater Misericordiae Hospital, Dublin. The gala dinner that evening was graced by no less than three presidents, S. Morrell Lyons, president of the Association of Anaesthetists of Great Britain and Ireland, Seamus M. Hart, president of the South of Ireland Association of

213

Presidents of the South of Ireland Society of Anaesthetists

1955–7	Dr Eugene Thomas	1974–5	Dr Richard Walsh
1957–9	Dr Richard Walsh	1975–8	Dr Desmond Gaffney
1959–60	Dr John Bourke	1978–80	Dr John Casey
1960–1	Dr Daniel Coleman	1980–6	Dr Daniel Coleman
1961–3	Dr Maurice Flynn,	1986–9	Dr Rory O'Brien
1963–8	Dr Daniel Coleman	1989–91	Dr Jerry Twomey
1968 –9	Dr Desmond Gaffney	1991–4	Dr John Walsh
1969–72	Dr Daniel Delaney	1994–6	Dr Seamus Hart
1972–4	Dr Maurice Flynn	1996–8	Dr Patrick Fitzgerald

Anaesthetists and James Seiriol Davies, president of the Society of Anaesthetists of Wales. The principal guests, however, were three of the four surviving founding members of the SIAA, Drs Maura O'Driscoll, Maurice (Mossy) Flynn and 'Don' Coleman. Dr Mary Solan, unable to attend due to ill health, was toasted in her absence. Dr Flynn, responding to the toast, said how delighted he was to be there and then quipped, 'at my age I'm delighted to be anywhere'.

This account of the South of Ireland Association of Anaesthetists is based on the original minute book of SIAA which contains the handwritten records of the ordinary and annual general meetings of SIAA from March 1955 to February 1994. The minute book is available for reference purposes at the archives section of the library at University College Cork. An electronic version of the minute book can also be accessed at www.ucclibrary @ucc.ie

References
1   'Association News', *Anaesthesia*, 1955, 10, p. 32.
2   Ministers and Secretaries (Amendment) Act, 1946, available at
3   www.irishstatutebook.ie/eli/1946/act/38/enacted/en/print.html (accessed 30 June 2021).
4   Health Act 1947, available at www.irishstatutebook.ie/eli/1947/act/28/enacted/en/html

(accessed 30 June 2021).

5 Counihan H.E., 'The Medical Association and the Mother and Child Scheme', *Irish Journal of Medical Science* 2002, 171, pp. 110–15.

6 Wren M.-A., *Unhealthy State. Anatomy of a Sick Society*, Dublin: New Island, 2003, pp. 25–43.

7 Wren M.-A., '100 years of bishops and doctors', *Irish Times*, 2 October 2000, p. 13.

8 Minutes of the meeting of the South of Ireland Society of Anaesthetists April 21th 1956.

9 Minutes of the meeting of the South of Ireland Society of Anaesthetists October 5th 1962.

10 Minutes of the meeting of the South of Ireland Society of Anaesthetists May 4th 1962.

11 Minutes of the meeting of the South of Ireland Society of Anaesthetists November 21st 1958.

12 Gilmartin T.J., 'The Faculty of Anaesthetist of the Royal College of Surgeons in Ireland', *Irish Journal of Medical Science*, 1960, 419, pp. 483–4.

13 'Association News. Anaesthetists Report', *Journal of the Irish Medical Association*, 1962, 30, pp. 107–9.

14 Minutes of the meeting of the South of Ireland Association of Anaesthetists October 5th 1962.

15 Minutes of the meeting of the South of Ireland Association of Anaesthetists May 11th 1967.

16 Minutes of the meeting of the South of Ireland Association of Anaesthetists October 3rd 1969.

17 Twomey C., 'Comhairle Na n'Ospideal and health service reform', *Irish Times*, 4 July 2003, p. 17.

18 'Annual Report of Central Council 1981', *Irish Medical Journal*, 1982, 75, pp. 129–31.

19 Minutes of the meeting of the South of Ireland Association of Anaesthetists, 21 March 1986

20 Minutes of the Annual Open Meeting of the Standing Committee in Ireland of the Association of Anaesthetists of Great Britain and Ireland, November 19th 1994.

21 *Anaesthesia News*, 1996, 104, pp. 1–4.

Chapter 18

The Faculty of Anaesthetists, Royal College of Surgeons in Ireland: The Early Years, 1959–1970

Joseph Tracey

From the minute books of the Council, Royal College of Surgeons in Ireland and of the Faculty of Anaesthetists, Royal College of Surgeons in Ireland:

At a council meeting of the Royal College of Surgeons in Ireland (RCSI) on May 8th 1958 Mr Thomas Bouchier-Hayes raised the question of the granting of an FFA (Fellowship of a Faculty of Anaesthetists) by the college. The Registrar was asked to see if any correspondence had been received about it. The Education committee of RCSI met on July 8th 1958 and it was noted in the minutes that 'Letters were received from the Queen's University of Belfast and a Dr. Pais asking the college to give an FFA. It was decided as a first step to obtain a legal opinion as to whether the College has the power to do so.'[1]*

At the next committee meeting held in October 1958, it was reported that in the opinion of legal counsel, Mr Frank Fitzgibbon, under the existing charters and bye-laws, the council of RCSI had full powers to create a Faculty of Anaesthetists and to award a fellowship of the faculty. It was again suggested that the advice of the English college should be sought. The council set up an advisory committee of anaesthetists and Dr Joseph 'Joe' Woodcock was

---

*A search of the Irish and British Medical Directories failed to find the Dr Pais who had written to RCSI. He was subsequently identified in the minute books of the Faculty of Anaesthetists, RCSI when discussing his letter from Singapore to the new faculty in 1961 requesting that he be considered for a fellowship without examination. His persistence was rewarded as he was one of the group conferred with a fellowship, without examination, in June 1964.

appointed secretary with the correspondence addressed from his home in Rathgar, Dublin. The earliest letter was dated 8 January 1959 notifying the committee of a meeting on 14 January at the Royal College of Surgeons in Ireland (RCSI) on St Stephen's Green. The group seems to have spent a lot of time discussing who should be considered as foundation fellows of the proposed new faculty and duly submitted a preliminary list to the RCSI Council. It also submitted a report from Woodcock with advice on the setting up of a faculty. In May 1959, the council declared that:

> it is now recommended that the Council inaugurates a Faculty of Anaesthetists and that an advertisement be put in the journals stating that a number of Fellowships will be awarded to those who have an Irish D.A. and a further five years experience or who have had comparable experience and that persons who wish their claims to be considered should give particulars to the Registrar.[1]

This faculty would be the first one created by the Royal College of Surgeons in Ireland. At a further meeting in November 1959 the council recommended that the South African Society of Anaesthetists could send in names for consideration for the FFA.

The first meeting of the Board of the Faculty of Anaesthetists, RCSI was held on Tuesday 15 December 1959 in the Council Room at RCSI at 5.00 p.m. The dean of the faculty, Dr Thomas James Gilmartin, was appointed in the first instance by the RCSI president and council. He then read the notices directing that the meeting be convened and stated that the following had been appointed to the board:[2]

Dr Thomas James Gilmartin	Dean
Dr Victor Ormsby McCormick	Vice Dean
Dr Desmond J. Riordan	(College representative)*
Dr Geoffrey Raymond Davys	
Dr Patrick Joseph Drury Byrne	
Dr John Wharry Dundee	

---

*The college representative, Dr Riordan , was a radiologist and would subsequently become the first dean of the Faculty of Radiologists, RCSI. His son Desmond would also qualify in medicine, and was appointed as a consultant anaesthetist at the Charitable Infirmary, Jervis Street. He served as honorary secretary to the board and was the founder of the Irish Standing Committee of the AAGBI.

Dr Ethel Sheila Kenny
Dr Samuel Harold Swann Love
Dr Paul Finbarre Murray
Dr Patrick Joseph Nagle
Dr Joseph Augustine Woodcock

Woodcock was then appointed as honorary secretary. A letter was read from the registrar of the college indicating that the number of fellowships without examination should be about 40, and that the time for application for such a fellowship was to be extended to the end of the year at the request of the South African Society of Anaesthetists.[3] No explanation was given as to why the RCSI Council was so concerned about South African anaesthetists. The registrar stressed in his letter that the word 'Membership' should not be used otherwise the letters MFA might be assumed as a qualification and this might suggest to the uninitiated that they were half-way towards their fellowship. (It is ironic that the College of Anaesthesiologists of Ireland has recently introduced the Membership examination replacing the Primary as a step leading to the award of the fellowship.) It was agreed that the new faculty would be housed within the RCSI building. The dean then thanked the members of the advisory committee who had not been appointed to the board (Drs Conroy, Walsh and Glynn). The vice dean then drew lots to determine the number of years each member should serve before seeking re-election. The results were as follow:

Kenny – one year, for re-election 1961
Love – one year, for re-election 1961
McCormick – two years, for re-election 1962
Nagle – two years, for re-election 1962

1960
Dean Dr Thomas James 'Tommy' Gilmartin 1960–4
The next meeting of the board took place on Tuesday 19 January 1960. The first item on the agenda was to write and congratulate Sir Ivan Magill on the honour (Knight Commander of the Victorian Order) bestowed on him in the New Year honours list. The question of foundation fellowships or fellowships without examination and who should receive them was something which occupied the board for the first few years of its existence and which was documented time and time again in the minute books. The matter was discussed at the January meeting

and it was decided that fellowships should be awarded to distinguished anaesthetists of senior consultant status, who were actively involved in the anaesthetic 'milieu', who were members of learned scientific societies, had contributed to the literature or were members of academic department or lecturers. It was proposed that foundation fellowships be awarded to all members of the board. Other fellowships were to be awarded to some English and South African anaesthetists (five South Africans in total) as well as Dr Don Coleman and Dr J.D. Bourke from Cork.

A second list was then submitted for consideration for fellowship by election (Drs Gerry Black, Alex Blayney, Johnny Conroy, Eddie Delaney, J. Desmond Gaffney, Kevin P. O'Sullivan and Una B. Byrne to name just a few). The committee eventually decided on three lists of names: List 1 would be persons proposed as foundation fellows, List 2 included those proposed for fellowship by election and the third list included names of those who would be considered for fellowships at a later date. Some names could be promoted from one list to another. All of these lists had to be approved by the council of the college.

There were two other areas discussed at most board meetings: (i) the choice of speakers and topics for the Annual Scientific Meeting and (ii) the regulations for the examinations and the eligibility criteria for examiners. Dundee from Belfast was chairman of the Examination Group and was the person to lead the development of the examinations over the first few years. It was decided that the first Annual Symposium should be held on 24 and 25 May (this date was changed later) and that the proposed registration fee should be 30 shillings. Traditionally the annual conference of the college is still held in May. It was also decided that the first fellowship examination would be in two parts, the Primary examination and Final fellowship examination, and would be held in March 1961. The examination fees would be 10 guineas for the Primary exam, 20 guineas for the Final exam and 20 guineas for the Diploma. There would be a fee of 25 guineas for the foundation fellows. The Finance Committee of the college (RCSI) recommended that all fees obtained on behalf of the faculty for fellowships should be placed in a separate account by the RCSI registrar, that this account could be inspected by the dean and faculty board at any time and that the board would be consulted on matters relating to its disposal. It was announced that the first honorary fellowship should be conferred on Sir Ivan Magill. The committee also discussed more mundane matters such as the type and number of gowns required for the conferrings, who would be wearing gowns and who would attend.

There were further discussions about the examinations. The Primary would be only slightly different from the Primary fellowship exam of the Royal College of Surgeons in Ireland in that there would be a substantial amount of pharmacology with rather less anatomy. The other subjects would be physiology and pathology. Dundee felt that the Final examination should consist of two papers, two orals and a clinic in line with the English exam. The president of RCSI had assured the dean that the Irish exam would be similar to the English equivalent in every way.

There were a number of discussions at RCSI Council meetings about the new faculty. It was agreed that the president would admit the new fellows on Friday 8 July and that the college would host a sherry party for the new conferees as well as lunch and afternoon tea. It was also agreed to obtain an estimate on the cost of 15 gowns which would be similar to the surgical fellows' gowns but with a double blue stripe. The council agreed to confer three honorary fellowships.[1] The board was informed at the June meeting that Magill would not be able to attend the conferring due to other commitments.

The Faculty of Anaesthetists, RCSI was formally inaugurated by Mr Thomas George Wilson, president of RCSI, at a meeting held in the college on 8 July 1960. The first board was convened and the first conferring of fellowships of the new faculty took place. There were a total of 37 doctors conferred as foundation fellows including all members of the board (see Appendix 1). It is difficult to ascertain the criteria used in deciding who would be foundation fellows apart from the obvious one being members of the first board of the faculty. There were a large number from England and South Africa as well as some from further afield. The conferring took place in the presence of members of the Council of the Royal College of Surgeons in Ireland, the dean, vice dean and members of the board of faculty. It had been originally intended that the first honorary fellowship should be conferred on Magill but as he was unable to attend, the decision was made to confer it on Dr John Gillies. His citation was read by the vice dean, Victor McCormick. Gillies had served as a combatant in World War One and was decorated for gallantry in the field. He qualified in medicine in Edinburgh after the war and had a distinguished career in anaesthesia; he was a founder member of the Faculty of Anaesthetists of the Royal College of Surgeons of England (RCSEng), was a council member and president of the Association of Anaesthetists of Great Britain and Ireland and a founder member of the World Federation of Societies of Anaesthesiologists (WFSA). The second honorary fellowship was conferred on Dr Geoffrey Organe, Dean of the Faculty of

Anaesthetists, RCSEng at the time and who was also a WFSA founder member. His citation was read by Drury Byrne. Dr Organe, in turn, presented the new faculty with an illuminated scroll and a history of the Royal College of Surgeons of England by Sir Zachary Cope.[5] On Saturday 9 July 1960, the faculty began its academic life with a scientific meeting on 'Levels of anaesthesia'. It was opened by the dean.

Programme
- Dr Thomas Gilmartin, Dean, Opening remarks, 'History of anaesthesia'
- Dr Victor McCormack showed a film, 'Classical assessment of depth of anaesthesia'
- Prof. Cecil Gray, 'Changing concepts of levels of anaesthesia'
- Dr Barry Wyke, 'Neurological analysis of the stages of anaesthesia'
- Dr John Dundee, 'Pharmacological action of anaesthetics in relation to clinical effect'
- Prof. David Mitchell, 'The place of antidotes in reversal'
- Prof Eoin O'Malley, 'A surgeon's view on modern anaesthesia'

The Dean and Board of
Faculty of Anaesthetists
of the
Royal College of Surgeons of England
send their warmest greetings
on the occasion of the Foundation of the
Faculty of Anaesthetists
of the
Royal College of Surgeons of Ireland
They wish the Dean and Board of their sister Faculty a long and successful history of service to anaesthesia, and look forward to a happy and fruitful association with their colleagues in the Irish Faculty in the years ahead

8th July 1960

Scroll presented to the Faculty of Anaesthetists, RCSI by the Faculty of Anaesthetists, RCSE in July 1960. Courtesy of Bobby Studio.

There were 107 attendees and the proceedings were chronicled in a commemorative issue of the *Irish Journal of Medical Science* in November 1960.[3]

The conference dinner that night was attended by the dean, the vice dean and members of the board, the two new honorary fellows, Organe and Gillies, Mr Tom Wilson (president of RCSI), the college vice-president Mr Nigel Kinnear and the conference speakers Cecil Gray, Barry Wyke, David Mitchell and Eoin O'Malley. The dinner was described by the dean, Gilmartin, as follows : 'The dinner, one of the most expensive in the history of the college, was a Lucullian feast and was enjoyed equally by gourmet and gourmand'.[4]

The Faculty still had no room of its own in RCSI but was assigned its own secretary. Regulations for the examinations were drawn up and discussions were commenced with the English college on reciprocity. It was decided that the first sitting of the Primary exam would take place in June 1961 and that of the Final in December. The Education Committee was asked to organise lectures and training. As regards finances, the RCSI Council stipulated that the faculty could have a separate bank account but that it would remain under the control of the college registrar. This was the start of a long-running battle over the faculty finances which would not be fully resolved until the 1990s.

It was decided that a total of 45 names from List 2 would be submitted for fellowship by election. The Council of RCSI wrote to the board to say that no more applications for fellowship without exams would be accepted after two years from the inauguration of the faculty.

1961

The second Annual Scientific Meeting and the AGM took place on 3 June 1961. The day began at 11 a.m. when 44 new fellows were admitted to the faculty (see Appendix 2) and then an honorary fellowship was conferred on Sir Ivan Magill (see Chapter 24) by the president of RCSI. This was followed by the AGM at midday. The scientific meeting took place in the afternoon with lectures on the theme of obstetrical anaesthesia. Speakers included Drs Alan D.H. Browne MD, FRCOG (Dublin), R.J. Hamer Hodges FFARCS (Portsmouth), Arthur P. Barry MD FRCOG (Dublin), Charles A.G. Armstrong MB DA FFARCSI (Mid Ulster Hospital) and John Dundee FFARCSI (Belfast). The first anniversary dinner was held that evening and was catered for by the Dolphin Hotel with musical entertainment by a Miss Watkins.

The complete minutes of the board meeting held on 18 October 1961 are quoted below as they give an interesting description of an historic day in the story of the faculty, (probably written by the dean):

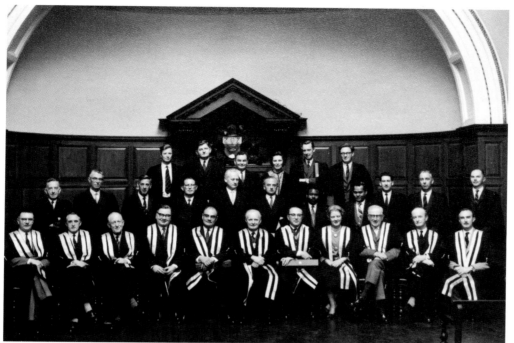

Conferees and Board of Faculty of Anaesthetists, RCSI, 1962. Photograph by Lafayette.

On Wednesday 18th October 1961 at four o'clock in the afternoon Members of the Board of the Faculty of Anaesthetists, RCSI assembled in the Colles Room of the college. The purpose for which the gathering took place was in order that the eminent Irish anaesthetist, Sir Ivan Magill, Knight Companion [*sic*] of the Victorian Order, could present to the dean, for the faculty to which he had been elected as an honorary fellow, a chain of office for the dean of that faculty. The medal finely wrought in silver gilt is the work of Mr Fitzpatrick, Silversmith of Anne Street. It is universally admired no less for its size, than for its delicate and intricate workmanship, including as it does in bands of silver gilt, an elegant achievement of the College Arms graven in enamel. Sir Ivan, having been welcomed by the dean of the faculty in terms suitable to the occasion, before presenting the chain of office, proceeded to speak of the great honour done to him in making him an honorary fellow of the new faculty. He then presented the medal to the dean, who having spoken his thanks, and emphasised the honour he felt in being the first to bear this fine

223

emblem of his office, then invited the distinguished company, including as it did Mr Nigel Kinnear, President of RCSI, Lady Magill, Mrs Victor McCormick, the dean of the Faculty of Anaesthetists of the Royal College of Surgeons of England and all members of the Board, to an adjoining table where champagne and other tokens of festivity were consumed in quantities adequate to the generous gift and importance of the occasion.[5]

This event was timed to coincide with a meeting of the AAGBI held in Dublin that year.

In November 1961, the first Primary examination for fellowship of the Faculty of Anaesthetists, RCSI was held. The candidates were examined in anatomy, pathology, physiology and pharmacology. Dr Edgar Alexander Pask was the examiner in physiology and Dundee in pharmacology. There were 25 candidates of whom six passed. The faculty board conceded on the point that it was only allowed to nominate examiners as it was the Council of RCSI who actually appointed them. This was to be a bone of contention for a number of years and wouldn't be resolved until 1978.

1962

At its first meeting in 1962, the board continued to press the college for its own accommodation. Mrs Angela Butler was appointed as the secretary to the board of the faculty and a list of examiners was submitted for approval. For the Final FFARCSI, this included Prof. W.W. Mushin, dean of the English faculty, Gilmartin, dean of the Irish faculty, V.O. McCormick and the surgeon Mr J.A. Mehigan. Dundee raised the subject of tuition for the Fellowship examination and McCormick discussed possible courses.

The annual meeting took place on 1 June 1962 and followed the format from the previous year (i.e. conferring, AGM, scientific meeting and annual dinner). Honorary fellowships were conferred on three distinguished anaesthetists: Prof. Ritsema Van Eck from the Netherlands who was president of the World Federation of Societies of Anaesthesiologists (WFSA) at the time, Prof. William Woolf Mushin, dean of the Faculty of Anaesthetists of the Royal College of Surgeons of England and professor of anaesthetics at the Welsh National School of Medicine in Cardiff, and Prof. Cecil Gray from the University of Liverpool who is acknowledged as being largely responsible for the introduction of muscle relaxants such as curare into the practice of anaesthesia in the British Isles. A further 46 fellows were admitted to the faculty (see Appendix 2).

The theme of the Annual Scientific Meeting that year was paediatric anaesthesia.

Programme
- Dr Gilmartin (Dean), 'Introduction'
- Dr Gerald R Graham (Great Ormond Street), 'Anatomical and

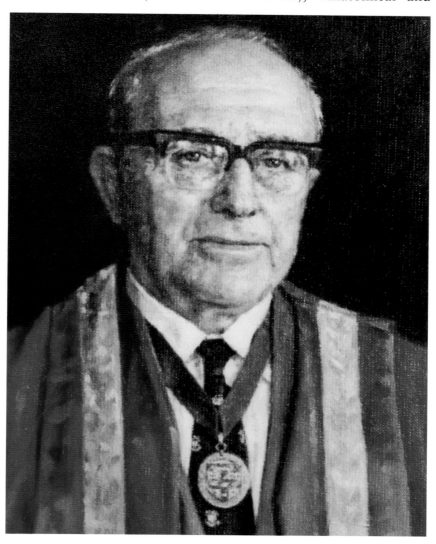

William Woolf Mushin, Welsh National School of Medicine. Courtesy of the Royal College of Surgeons in Ireland.

Cecil Gray,
University of
Liverpool.
Courtesy of the
Royal College of
Surgeons in
Ireland.

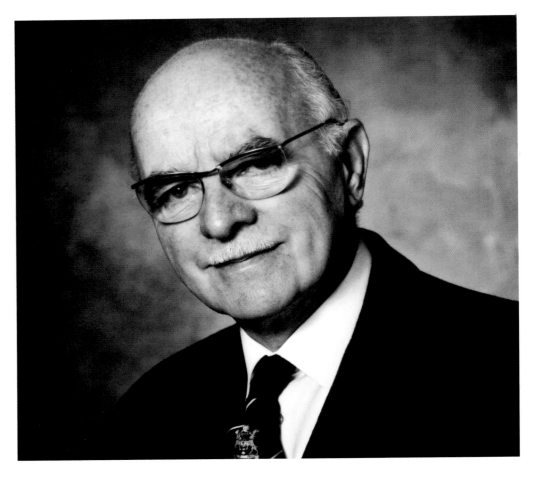

physiological factors in paediatric anaesthesia'
- Dr Sheila Anderson (Great Ormond Street), 'Preoperative assessment and premedication in paediatric anaesthesia'
- Dr Alan L. Stead (Alder Hey Children's Hospital, Liverpool), 'Anaesthetic management of the neonate'
- Dr I.J. Carre (Royal Belfast Hospital for Sick Children), 'Fluid balance in paediatric surgery'
- Dr John R. McCarthy (Our Lady's Hospital for Sick Children, Dublin), 'Neonatal asphyxia'
- Dr Harold Love (Royal Belfast Hospital for Sick Children), 'Paediatric outpatient dental anaesthesia'

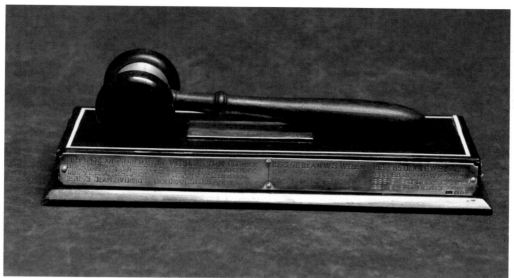

Gavel presented to the Faculty of Anaesthetists, RCSI by Cecil Gray.
Courtesy of Bobby Studio.

The faculty dinner was more expensive that year, costing seven shillings and sixpence per guest. Guests at the dinner that night included the Tánaiste and Minister for Health Seán MacEntee and Mrs MacEntee, Minister for Education Dr Hillery and Mrs Hillery, as well as the new honorary fellows Mushin, Gray and Van Eyck. Mr Nigel Kinnear, president of RCSI and Mrs Kinnear, Dr Jarman, president of AAGBI and Dr Maurice Cara, president de l'Association des Anesthésistes Français also attended.

The final board meeting of the year was again taken up with the problem of examiners being appointed by RCSI Council and not by the faculty board, the members of which were keen that the awarding of fellowships without examination could be extended out to five years from the foundation of the faculty. In November, Prof. Cecil Gray of Liverpool presented a ceremonial gavel to the faculty on behalf of himself, John Gillies of Edinburgh, Geoffrey Organe of London and William Mushin of Cardiff, all of whom had been conferred with honorary fellowships.

1963

In April 1963, the board proposed to the president and RCSI Council that the creation of a chair in anaesthesia in the college should be considered. The college representative, Riordan, suggested that it was a good time to raise the matter as the appointment of new professors was being discussed at that time. The council later pointed out that if such an appointment were to be made, it would not be remunerated. The college bye-laws would also have to be amended.

The board discussed and then agreed to Gilmartin doing an extra year as dean as 'a lap of honour' and that McCormick should continue as vice dean for another year. This was the only time that the post was held for four years; all subsequent deans had a tenure of three years.

The Annual Scientific Meeting was held on 7 June 1963. The first fellowships by examination were conferred by Mr Terence Millin, president of RCSI. Three fellows were conferred in person and a further four in absentia. The theme of the annual meeting was respiratory insufficiency.

Programme
- Dr G. Ray Davys (St Vincent's Hospital), 'Introduction'
- Dr Richard S. Clarke (QUB), 'Cases of respiratory insufficiency'
- Dr J. Howell (Royal Infirmary, Manchester), 'Diagnosis of respiratory insufficiency'
- Dr E.A. Cooper (Royal Infirmary, Newcastle), 'Principles of management'
- Dr Robert C. Gray (QUB), 'Respiratory problems in the treatment of tetanus'
- Prof. William W. Mushin (Royal Infirmary, Cardiff), 'Apparatus for ventilating'

One of the outstanding features of the meeting was the display of ventilating apparatus for use in cases of respiratory insufficiency. The exhibition was organised by Woodcock who acknowledged the assistance he had received from Medical Gases Ltd. The annual dinner was held that evening and was attended by 190 fellows as well as the distinguished guests. The proceedings of the meeting were included in the first edition of the new *Journal of the Royal College of Surgeons in Ireland,* published in December 1963. The dean of the faculty was automatically appointed to the editorial board.

Arrangements for postgraduate tuition for the faculty examinations were reviewed and recommendations sent to council.

1964
Dean Dr Joseph 'Joe' Augustine Woodcock, 1964–7
The board proposed that it should have representation on the RCSI Council. The college replied that this was not possible under the bye-laws. The council agreed

to the nomination of Mushin and Gilmartin as examiners in anaesthetics for the Final FFARCSI examination. Where the Primary exam was concerned, Dundee and Prof. Leonard Abrahamson would examine in pharmacology, Profs. F. Kane and Edgar Pask (Newcastle-upon-Tyne) in physiology and Prof. Irvine and Dr W.R. Lamb in anatomy. Dundee presented his observations on the Primary examination and a number of changes which he considered to be essential to the smooth running of the exam. He proposed that the written exams take place on Thursday and Friday followed by the orals on Monday and Tuesday. He also suggested that a maximum of 16 candidates should be examined per day and also an increase in the number of examiners. These proposals were submitted to RCSI Council for approval. Dundee was also critical of the Primary fellowship course which was deemed to be unsuitable and badly organised.

At the Annual Scientific Meeting in June, honorary fellowships were conferred on Henry Beecher, who was professor of research in anaesthesia at Harvard University and also chief of anaesthesia at the Massachusetts General Hospital in Boston, and Sir Robert Reynolds MacIntosh, the first professor of anaesthesia in Britain. The two conferees, in turn, presented the faculty with a pair of candelabra (purchased in Limerick at a cost of £55). Joseph Woodcock was elected dean and Sheila Kenny vice dean. The board wrote to council of the college recommending that the number of elected members to the board of the faculty be increased from 10 to 12 in order to ease the work of board members.

The First Academic Posts

Dr John Wharry Dundee who was a foundation fellow of the faculty and a consultant anaesthetist at the Royal Victoria Hospital, Belfast was appointed professor of anaesthetics at Queen's University Belfast in 1964, thus becoming the first professor of anaesthetics in Ireland. He had founded the Department of Anaesthetics at Queen's in 1958. Later that year (1964), Tommy Gilmartin was appointed lecturer in anaesthetics at the Royal College of Surgeons in Ireland.

1965

The board adopted regulations on the training of anaesthetists. There were no requirements for sitting the Primary examination. Candidates for the Final had to have completed not less than three years' whole-time appointments in anaesthesia, two years of which had to have been spent in a recognised training hospital, before being allowed to sit the examination. The Royal College of Surgeons of Australasia and the College of Surgeons of South Africa had both written requesting reciprocity with the Irish faculty examinations.

The board introduced stricter criteria on the recognition of hospitals for training:

> The visiting anaesthetic staff would have to consist of a minimum of two consultants, of whom at least one had the FFARCSI. Their duties should be arranged so as to provide adequate time for instruction and supervision. There should be an adequate record system. There should be regular Clinico-Pathological conferences. There should be an anaesthetic room for induction of anaesthesia and adequate facilities for Post-operative recovery. There should be adequate library facilities.

Some members of the board felt that it was time to abolish the DA as they were concerned that it would be accepted as equivalent to the FFARCSI in local authority appointments. RCSI Council approved the proposed increase in the number of elected members to the board from 10 to 12. It was decided that all fellows (by examination) who were living in Ireland would have to pay an annual retention fee of five guineas. An intensive one-week course in the basic sciences as related to anaesthesia was organised in October at the RCSI.

The Annual Scientific Meeting was held on 4 June with a symposium on 'Pain'. Gilmartin was appointed associate professor of anaesthetics at the Royal College of Surgeons in Ireland in October 1965, the first such academic appointment in the Republic of Ireland. It was also decided at the October board meeting to award an honorary fellowship to Edgar Alexander Pask but it was never conferred as he died in May 1966 before the annual meeting and conferring. In response to a request from the masters of the Dublin maternity hospitals, the board recommended a new syllabus for consideration by An Bord Altranais on analgesia in labour. The recommendations included guidelines on the use of pethidine and of trichloroethylene inhalers.

1966

The topic for the Annual Scientific Meeting on 4 June 1966 was 'Intensive care'.

Programme
- [Speaker name unknown], 'Planning of intensive care units'
- Prof. John Robinson, 'Respiratory and metabolic disorders'

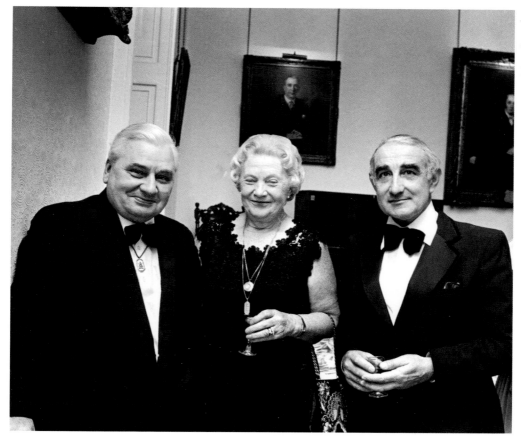

Joe Woodcock, Inagh Woodcock and Robin King. Courtesy of Bobby Studio.

- Dr G.V. Barton, 'Value and limitations of monitors in I.C.U.'
- Dr Donald Campbell, 'Acute trauma'
- Dr Sean Blake and Dr A. McA. Blayney, 'Management of cardiac disorders'
- Dr Gibson, 'Cross infection and sterilisation of instruments'

As in previous years, the main concerns of the board were examinations, appointments of examiners and the anaesthetic training programme. The anaesthetic trainees were now able to avail of a weekly seminar which had been organised by Dr Eddie Delaney of Dr Steevens' Hospital but only eight of the 25 trainees were able to attend on a regular basis. Dr Kevin O'Sullivan had compiled a list of training posts in Dublin teaching hospitals and Woodcock had proposed a pilot training scheme. This rotation was between the Charitable Infirmary

(Jervis Street), St Laurence's Hospital, the Coombe Lying-in Hospital and Our Lady's Hospital for Sick Children (Crumlin).

The board had a number of discussions with the RCSI registrar on the appointment of examiners as there was lack of clarity about who could apply. It was proposed that all fellows should be circulated when the appointments were scheduled to take place and that examiners should be appointed for a period of three years rather than the current system which only allowed for a one-year appointment which was unsatisfactory. The flat fee of £15 per examiner was no longer adequate and should be changed to four guineas a day. The examiners appointed for the Primary exam that year were Pask, Kane and Dr R.S.J. Clarke in physiology and Dundee, Abrahamson, Mitchell and Dr G.W. Black in pharmacology. There were also four examiners in anatomy and two in pathology. There were three examiners appointed in anaesthetics for the Final fellowship examination: Gilmartin, Mushin from Cardiff and Love. The majority of anaesthetists who were appointed as examiners in physiology and pharmacology were working in Northern Ireland. There were a number of applications received requesting fellowship without examination (from Drs H. Joseph Galvin, David F. Hogan, Dermot McCarthy and John V. McCooey). Love spoke at the board meeting in June saying that it seemed to him a pity that the board consisted mainly of members from Dublin and Belfast, and that he would like to see a better representation from the provinces. Provincial anaesthetists should be invited to apply and they might be further encouraged if travelling expenses were paid.

1967
Dean Dr Geoffrey Raymond 'Ray' Davys, 1967–70
It was decided to initiate a 'Kirkpatrick' Lecture in honour of Dr T. Percy Kirkpatrick, a distinguished early Irish anaesthetist. The first lecturer was Victor McCormick and his topic was 'Dr T. Percy C. Kirkpatrick'. The board agreed that there would be no further fellowships without examination. A number of changes in the Primary FFARCSI examination were made in order to conform with the new English examination and maintain reciprocity. These changes included having a choice of questions in pharmacology and physiology, although some would be compulsory. It was also recommended that there should be 16 examiners, eight anaesthetists and eight specialists in the basic sciences, e.g. physiology and pharmacology. Woodcock finished his term of office as dean and was replaced by Ray Davys. Dundee was elected vice dean and Dr Johnny

Conroy as honorary secretary. Dr Don Coleman from Cork was elected to the board , the first member from Munster. The college registrar informed the board that the college was looking for space to house the faculty and that the payment of travelling expenses was also being considered.

Annual Scientific Meeting
Pre-operative assessment
- Dr Derek Wylie, 'Introduction'
- Dr Donald Campbell, 'Pulmonary function'
- Dr Richard Clarke, 'Cardiovascular function'
- Dr William O'Dwyer, 'Renal function'
- Dr Sheila Sherlock, 'Hepatic function'
- Dr ?, 'Anaesthetic drugs and the liver'
- Prof. T.M. Jenkins, 'Endocrine function'

Delaney organised a new programme of lectures for the trainees commencing on 16 October and running to the middle of December. The course fee was 5 guineas. Subjects covered included: 'Functional anatomy' by Dr P. Hill; 'The EEG' by Dr J. Kirker; 'The anatomy of the sympathetic and para-sympathetic systems' by Dr B. Weeks; 'Drugs acting on the synaptic and myoneural junction' by Dr F. Curtin; 'Anatomy of the lungs' by Dr B.P. Rooney; 'Pulmonary function' by Dr B. McGovern; and 'Pulmonary haemodynamics' by Dr G.F. Gearty.

1968
Further changes were made in the Primary fellowship examination. Anatomy and pathology were to be replaced by a new subject, clinical measurement. A third of the marks would be allocated to each of the three subjects: physiology, pharmacology and clinical measurement. There was a lot of discussion about how the faculty could be more inclusive of provincial anaesthetists. This had been raised originally by Love who felt that the board was composed mainly of members from Dublin or Belfast. It was felt that there should be a meeting of the faculty held in a country venue and both Athlone and Limerick were suggested. The first Registrars' Essay Prize of £21 was won by Dr S.A. McDowell of Belfast for his paper 'Muscle relaxants and prolonged apnoea'. A second prize of 5 guineas was sent to Dr Padraic Keane of Galway for his essay 'A physiological approach to induced hypothermia'. The vice dean mentioned that Dr Joseph Ozinsky, a fellow of the faculty from South Africa, had given the anaesthetic for

the first heart transplant at Groot Schuur Hospital in Cape Town.

At the annual meeting held in May an honorary fellowship was conferred on Dr Patrick Shackleton (citation read by Drury-Byrne). Shackleton, President of AAGBI at the time, was a descendant of Abraham Shackleton who in 1726 had founded the school at Ballytore, County Kildare where both Napper Tandy and Edmund Burke were educated. He was also related to Sir Ernest Shackleton, the Antarctic explorer. Later on in the proceedings, Shackleton, in turn, presented the John Snow Medal of the Association of Anaesthetists of Great Britain and Ireland to Mr Erskine Childers TD, Minister for Transport and Power.

A post-world congress meeting and tour was held in Dublin on 15 and 16 September, organised by Kevin O'Sullivan on behalf of the board. This included a trip to the Abbey Theatre, a tour of the country and a visit to Belfast where they heard a number of papers on 'Anaesthesia and alcohol'.

An honorary fellowship was conferred on Prof. Eric Neilssen (citation read by Sheila Kenny). Dr John Conroy read a paper on 'Smoking and anaesthetic risk'. Dr Derek Wylie, dean of the Faculty of Anaesthetists of the Royal College of Surgeons of England, was invited to attend the November board meeting. He gave a talk on the Royal Commission on Medical Education (the Todd report) which recommended that the three years of general professional training should be mainly devoted to the specialty but six months to a year could be spent working in another branch of medicine.

1969
The out-of-town meeting took place in Limerick in April 1969 and was organised by Dr Val McDermott. The AGM and conferring of fellowships took place on Friday 23 May, followed by the Annual Scientific Meeting on 24 May 1969. Speakers included Dr John Reid from Glasgow who spoke on 'Parenteral nutrition'. Gilmartin attended a meeting in London of the new Central Committee for specialist training in anaesthesia. The faculty received new gowns for conferrings and submitted a final list of anaesthetists for fellowships without examination. The total number of fellows of the faculty was about 360 but not all were paying their annual subscription. It was decided that six years of training would be required for anaesthesia.

1970
At the Annual Scientific Meeting in May 1970, the programme was as follows. Programme:

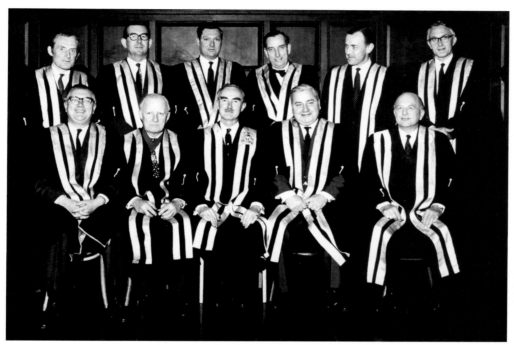

Board of Faculty of Anaesthetists, RCSI, 1969. Front row (left to right): John Dundee, Tommy Gilmartin, Ray Davys (Dean), Joe Woodcock, William Bingham. Back row (left to right): Johnny Conroy, Kevin O'Sullivan, Eddie Delaney, Don Coleman, William Wren, Harold Love. Photograph by Lafayette.

- Commander E.P. Barroxl, 'Underwater medicine'
- Dr I. Ledingham, 'Basis for oxygen therapy'
- Dr P. McGovern, 'Oxygen tension in infants'
- Dr S. Morrell Lyons, 'Operative and post-operative oxygen tension'
- Dr D. Seigne, 'Oxygen therapy and equipment'
- Prof. E. Gaffney, 'The story of O_2'

Five firms exhibited at the trade show associated with the meeting.

An honorary fellowship was conferred on Dr Ronald Jarman who in 1935 had been one of the first anaesthetists in the British Isles to use thiopentone. He had been awarded the Distinguished Service Cross (DSC) for bombing and sinking a German submarine when he was just 19 years of age. His citation was read by O'Sullivan. There were two other recipients of honorary fellowships that year, Prof. Robert Dunning Dripps from the University of Pennsylvania and Major General Keith Stephens, their citations being read by Dundee and J.C. Hewitt respectively.

Wren referred to the desirability of the dean of the faculty presiding at conferrings rather than the president of RCSI.

John Dundee replaced Ray Davys as dean of the faculty at the board meeting on 6 October 1970. Gilmartin presented a report from the London meeting of the Joint Committee for Higher Training of Anaesthetists. It was noted that many Dublin hospitals might not meet the training requirements proposed by the Joint Committee but Love suggested that a group of hospitals might jointly be able to do so. There was continued discussion about the examinations. The Dublin and London examinations now had the same entrance requirements and London was keen to continue with using exchange examiners between the two faculties. Bingham pointed out that there was a preponderance of examiners from Northern Ireland. It was suggested that examiners should be appointed for a period of three years and it was also proposed that a Multiple Choice Question (MCQ) examination should be introduced into the Primary exam.[6]

The Kirkpatrick Medal was struck in silver at a cost of £70 for the die and £5 per medal. Ray Davys presented Mr T.C.J. O'Connell of St Vincent's Hospital with the medal after he delivered the second Kirkpatrick Lecture in November 1970.

References

1 Minute book, Council of the Royal College of Surgeons in Ireland, File RCSI/COU/28(1938-60), available from Heritage Collections, RCSI.
2 Minute book 1, Board of the Faculty of Anaesthetists, RCSI, available from CAI.
3 *Irish Journal of Medical Science*, 1960, 35, pp. 483–538.
4 Minute Book 1, Board of the Faculty of Anaesthetists, RCSI, p. 18, available from CAI.
5 *Ibid.*, p. 35.
6 Minute Book 2, Board of the Faculty of Anaesthetists, RCSI, p. 9, available from CAI.

Chapter 19

The Faculty of Anaesthetists, Royal College of Surgeons in Ireland: From Faculty to Independent College

Joseph Tracey

1971

Dean Prof. John Wharry Dundee (1970–3)

Two scientific meeting were held in 1971, an out-of-town meeting and the Annual Scientific Meeting.

Programme:

Scientific Meeting, Galway, 17 April 1971

- Formal opening by the Dean
- Dr L. Coppel (Belfast) led a discussion following a film on 'The use of ketamine'
- Dr Padraic Keane (Galway), 'Haemodynamic changes in hypovolaemic shock'
- Dr James Moore (Belfast), 'A review of modern obstetric practice'
- Dr Peter Baskett (Bristol) 'Developments in Entonox'
- Dr Cyril Scurr (London), 'Discussion, Post-graduate training in anaesthesia'[1]

Annual Scientific Meeting, 29 May 1971

Intensive care – the present position

- Introduction by the Dean, Prof. J.W. Dundee (Belfast)
- Dr Richard Nolan (Dublin), 'Clinical management in the adult'
- Dr Des Gaffney (Cork), 'Mechanical ventilation'
- Dr E. Sherwood Jones (Liverpool), 'The therapeutic team'
- Dr Sam Kielty (Belfast), 'Clinical management in the infant'
- Dr Geoffrey Spencer (London), 'Ethical considerations'[2],

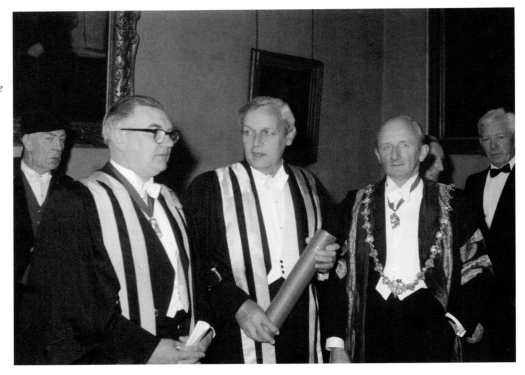

Dr Derek Wylie (who co-authored the textbook *A Practice of Anaesthesia* with Harry Churchill-Davidson) was conferred with an honorary fellowship at the May meeting. An agreement was reached with RCSI that the dean would henceforth admit new fellows at the conferring in the presence of the president of RCSI whereas previously it had been the president who had admitted them.

Dr Malachy Powell, deputy chief medical officer at the Department of Health, in a meeting with Davys and Wren in December 1970, proposed the development of a structured training programme for anaesthetists. The department had clearly stated that it did not wish to usurp or interfere in the role of the faculty but that it had the money and wished to assist the faculty in developing such a scheme.[3] The Department of Health wanted the faculty to propose a training scheme, designating what hospitals would provide the training and submit concrete proposals by July 1971. The board agreed that the Fellowship of the Faculty of Anaesthetists, RCSI (FFARCSI) was essential for a consultant post and that training should be divided into two periods, one prior to and one post-FFARCSI. There should be more posts recognised for the pre-fellowship programme than for post-fellowship specialist training. It also agreed that a specialist was one who had: (1) general professional training, (2) a fellowship in anaesthetics and (3) who had completed the three-year specialist programme. In response to this request, the board felt that there should be input from the various groups that would be affected and decided to convene a new forum, the Medical Advisory Committee (MAC) to advise the board on the planning and structure of a comprehensive training scheme. The MAC would consist of: (1) one anaesthetist from each of the three hospital regions, (2) a representative from the Section of Anaesthetics of the Royal Academy of Medicine in Ireland, (3) a representative from both the Irish Medical Association and the Irish Medical Union, and (4) two representatives from the board of the faculty.[4]

Continued consultant education appeared for the first time on the agenda and Dr Bingham suggested that consultants should be allowed to take a sabbatical once in six years.

In 1971, the conflict in Northern Ireland was at its worst and so special arrangements were made for examiners coming from Northern Ireland if travel across the border became impossible. A pairing system was agreed with Ray Davys as a substitute for Harold Love, Sheila Kenny for Richard Clarke and Hugh Raftery for John Dundee.

At the October board meeting, the registrar of RCSI, Dr Harry O'Flanagan, gave an outline of the revenue accruing to the faculty. The average income from the examinations from 1968 to 1971 was £4,150 with £350 from conferring, totalling an average yearly income of £4,500. On the expenditure side, the examiners' fees came to £1,500 per annum (p.a.), charges from RCSI for the use of the examination hall and secretariat amounted to £1,000 p.a. and the salary and pension for the secretary to the faculty was approximately £1,500 p.a. The board members felt that the charge by RCSI for the use of the examination hall and office was excessive and would not sign off on the accounts.[5]

A letter was received from the Minister of Health, Mr Erskine Childers, stating that approval was given by the Department of Health for attendance at the Annual Scientific Meeting. This included:

> the grant of leave, with pay, payment of travelling expenses and subsistence allowance and payment of the course fee. You may take it that there is no question of the usual facilities not being extended to those who attend the symposium next year.[6]

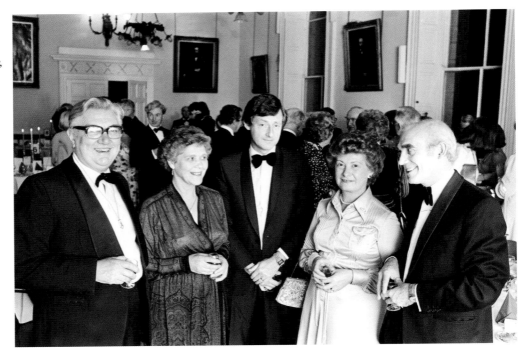

(Left to right)
John Dundee,
Sally Dundee,
Myles MacEvilly,
Arlene Kielty,
Sam Kielty.
Courtesy of
Bobby Studio.

1972

Because of increased numbers attending, the Annual Scientific Meeting was held at the Belfield campus of University College Dublin (UCD). The board meeting, conferring and Kirkpatrick Lecture were all held at the usual venue in RCSI. The anniversary dinner, however, took place at the Burlington Hotel as the RCSI venue was not available at the weekend. Honorary fellowships were conferred on Dr Harry Seldon (editor of *Anesthesia & Analgesia*) and Dr Kevin McCaul, dean of the Faculty of Anaesthetists, Royal Australasian College of Surgeons.[7] The third Kirkpatrick Lecture was given by Prof. John Biggart of Queen's University Belfast.

Annual Scientific Meeting, 20 May 1972

09:30	Introduction by the Dean, Prof. J.W. Dundee (Belfast)
09:40	Dr Ian Carson, 'Intravenous agents'
10:20	Dr Alan Dobkin (New York), 'Inhalational agents'
11:40	Dr Henry Blake (Dublin), 'Obstetric practice'
12:20	Dr John Hedley-Whyte (Harvard), 'Cardiac and pulmonary failure')

240

14-30   Dr Padraic Keane (Galway), 'Malignant hyperpyrexia'

15-10   Dr Leo Strunin (London), 'Organ toxicity'

It was agreed that there would be one last group to receive a fellowship by election and notices had been placed in the journals giving six months' notice to this effect. In all, 18 names were submitted by the Educational Subcommittee and were agreed upon by the board but with Davys and Woodcock dissenting.

Verbal and written complaints were received about the structure of the Final fellowship examination. It was felt that there was too much emphasis on non-anaesthetic subjects, there being one complete paper on medicine and one on surgery with no choice of question on either. Coleman protested at the absence of examiners from outside Dublin or Belfast.

A meeting took place in February to which all consultant anaesthetists had been invited. The following were nominated to the new MAC: Drs R. Walsh (Cork), A. Kennedy (Cork), A. Bourke (Castlebar), D. Kelly (Ballinasloe), D. Bourke (Portlaoise), J. Shanahan (Waterford), J.R. McCarthy (Dublin), K.P. O'Sullivan (Dublin), D.G. Coleman (Cork) and J.V. McDermott (Limerick). The dean and honorary secretary were ex-officio members of the committee. The total number of training posts in the country, including both senior house officers (SHO) and registrars, was 28, of which 13 were in the regions and the remainder in Dublin.[8] The deans of three of the medical schools nominated representatives to sit on the MAC. These were Gilmartin for RCSI, Colm. Breslin for UCD and Des Gaffney for UCC.

1973
Dean Dr William 'Billy' S. Wren, 1973–6

Annual Scientific Meeting, 19 May 1973
- Dr Michael Johnstone (Manchester), 'EKG in Anaesthesia'
- Prof. Armen Bunatin (Moscow), 'Computer analysis of the effects of Ketalar on haemodynamics'
- Mr Alan Crockard (Belfast), 'The brain-damaged patient'
- Dr Declan Tyrrell (Dublin), 'Neuromuscular disorders and anaesthesia'
- Dr Henning Poulsen (Aarhus), 'The anaesthesiologist in emergency aid'
- Prof. N.W. Craythorne (Cincinnati), 'The next ten years in American anaesthesia'

Honorary fellowships were conferred on Dr Alfred Lee, co-author with Richard

Atkinson, of one of the best-known textbooks in the specialty, *A Synopsis of Anaesthesia*, and on Dr Bjorn Ibsen, considered to be the founding father of intensive care medicine.[9]

Dr M.D. Vickers had written to Gilmartin to state that the Joint Committee for Higher Training was considering requests from centres that wished to be considered for higher training. The point was raised that, at that time, there were no trainees in Ireland who were designated as senior registrars but that this was simply a question of title as many of the fourth- and fifth-year registrars were, in fact, senior registrars. At a meeting with Comhairle na nOspidéal later that year, it was agreed that an establishment of ten senior registrars would be adequate in the Republic. The board noted however that there were 11 in Northern Ireland at the time. The Comhairle agreed that a training period of six years was necessary to achieve consultant status and that the Fellowship of the Faculty of Anaesthetists, RCSI (FFARCSI) was the recognised qualification.[10]

A number of joint meetings took place between the English and Irish faculties in order to develop multiple choice questions (MCQs). These meetings were attended by Drs A. Hunter, A. Thornton, J. Woodcock and J.S. West. Each member of the board and each examiner had been requested to submit 10 questions on either physiology, pharmacology or clinical measurement to the common pool. The MCQ section would be introduced at the May 1974 Primary examination. It was proposed that there would be 20 questions in each of the three subsets, making a total of 300 items. The new marking system was 50 per cent for viva, 25 per cent for MCQ and 25 per cent for the essay.[11] The format for the exam would be three MCQ sessions of one hour each in the morning and the essay session lasting two and a half hours in the afternoon. This should take place on a Thursday with the orals and clinical examinations starting on the following Monday.[12] Dr Niall Tierney, from the Department of Health, attended the meeting of the MAC. It was agreed that this committee would henceforth consider higher training as well as pre-fellowship training.

Gilmartin and McDermott were nominated by the Irish Medical Association (IMA) to the Section d'Anaesthésiologie et Réanimation of the European Union of Medical Specialists (UEMS). The faculty board agreed to fund a delegate to UEMS meetings when the agenda had sufficient academic content. Gilmartin was also nominated as vice president of the Association of Anaesthetists of Great Britain and Ireland. Wren was installed as dean of the faculty at the September meeting of the board, replacing Dundee.

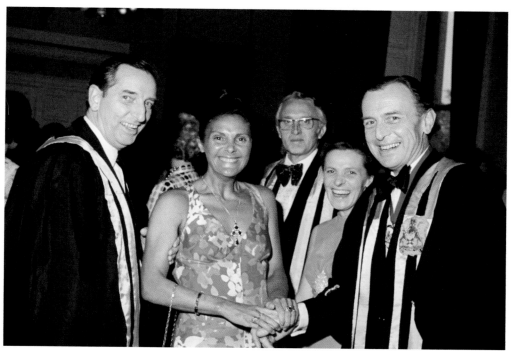

(Left to right)
Don Coleman,
Monique
Coleman, Harold
Love, Maev
Wren, William
Wren (Dean).
Courtesy of
Bobby Studio.

1974

The elections to the board, conferring and Kirkpatrick Lecture took place on Friday 17 May followed a day later by the scientific symposium, honorary conferring and annual dinner.

Annual Scientific Meeting
Morning session
Environmental hazard to operating room personnel
- Dr M.D. Vickers (Birmingham), 'Pollution'
- Dr Alastair Spence (Glasgow), 'Epidemiological study of morbidity and mortality'
- Dr C.J. Hull (Newcastle), 'Electrical hazards'
- Prof. Ellis N. Cohen (Stanford, California), 'The effects of trace anaesthetics on the health of operating room personnel'

Afternoon session
Aspects of ventilation
- Dr Alfredo Arias (Madrid), 'pCO_2 homeostasis in mechanical ventilation'

243

- Dr Marian Rice (Dublin), 'PEEP, the present position'
- Prof. J.F. Nunn (Northwick Park), 'Air versus oxygen during anaesthesia'[13]

The fee for the scientific symposium was £10. Honorary fellowships were conferred on Prof. Alexander Forrester from Glasgow, Prof. Jacques Boureau from Paris and Dr Alfredo Arias. Citations were read by Love, Coleman and McCarthy. The Kirkpatrick Lecture was delivered by Gilmartin on 'Realism in anaesthesia'.

The dean reported that the Council for Postgraduate Medical and Dental Education and Training had accepted the faculty as the suitable body to control training in anaesthetics in Ireland and had also approved the faculty training scheme. The recommendations for the General Professional Training Programme had been sent to the Department of Health (DOH). The DOH accepted the proposals but stated that all posts in the General Professional Training Scheme would be designated as 'Senior House Officer'. The board agreed to cover the cost of an overnight stay for members based in Northern Ireland as it was too dangerous at the time for them to travel home late at night. The faculty inspected those hospitals recognised for either general or higher professional training.[14]

1975

The theme for the Annual Scientific Meeting held in May was 'The anaesthetist and the sick child'. The speakers were Dr Robert Moors Smith (Boston), Dr Jack Downes (Philadelphia), Dr Suutarinen (Finland), Mr Barry O'Donnell (Dublin) and Dr Kevin P. Moore (Dublin). An honorary fellowship was conferred on Prof. Emanuel M. Papper from New York.

Comhairle nOspidéal had the statutory function of regulating appointments of senior registrars (SRs) and had allowed six training posts of three years each. It stipulated that for a consultant post, the appointees had to possess a fellowship in anaesthesia and have had six years of training in the specialty.

The Diploma in Anaesthetics (DA) came up for discussion at regular intervals. The faculty wanted it abolished as the fellowship was now considered the specialist qualification. The examination (DA) was, however, controlled by the Conjoint Board of the Royal Colleges of Physicians and Surgeons in Ireland and not by the faculty. The problem had arisen again as Directives 2 and 3 from the European Economic Community (EEC) allowed for migration of labour between all countries in the community and it had been suggested that three years' training and the holding of either the fellowship or the DA might be sufficient for admission to the Specialist Register. Although the faculty wrote to RCSI Council expressing their disapproval of the exam, the latter had replied that it was still considered to have a role and would continue.[15]

The board received a letter from Sir Geoffrey Organe informing them that preliminary discussions were underway in England on the formation of a separate College of Anaesthetists in the UK. This led to discussion about how the Irish faculty could break from RCSI to become an independent college. However, it would be another 23 years before this would come to pass.

1976
Dean Dr S. Harold Love, 1976–9
The AGM, conferring and board dinner took place on Friday 14 May, followed by the Annual Scientific Symposium and the annual dinner on the Saturday.

Annual Scientific Meeting, Saturday 15 May 1976
Therapeutic problems
- Dr Denis Moriarty (Dublin), 'New trends in monitoring'
- Prof. Brian Dalton (Boston), 'Therapeutic problems and coronary heart disease'
- Prof. Guy Vourc'h 'Cardiovascular accidents during pneumoencephalography'
- Prof. Harvey Shapiro (Pennsylvania), 'Anaesthetic protection for the brain'
- Prof. B. Craythorne (Miami), 'Letter from America'[16]

A new body known as the Irish Medical Council (IMC) was to be formed which would have full power in relation to education at undergraduate and postgraduate level, to maintain discipline and give recognition of specialist training. The board felt that that there should be representatives of specialist groups such as the Faculty of Anaesthetists, RCSI on this new body. It would replace the Medical Registration Council and would be responsible for keeping the General Medical Register and a Specialist Register. It was proposed that the IMC would recognise the appropriate training bodies that could recommend inclusion of names in the Specialist Register. In the opinion of the board, the position of the faculty and the Joint Committee of Higher Training would remain unaltered.

The Comhairle and the Department of Health refused to sanction new posts to facilitate the appointments of the six SRs. The Eastern Regional Training

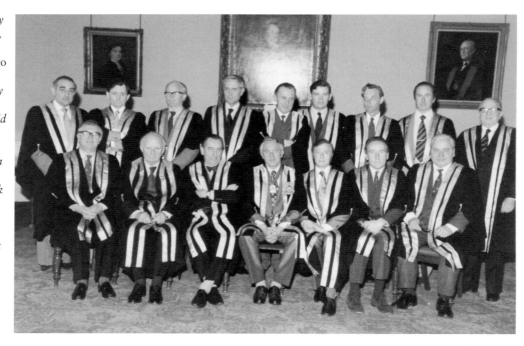

Board of Faculty of Anaesthetists, RCSI, 1977. Front row (left to right): John Dundee, Tommy Gilmartin, Don Coleman, Harold Love (Dean), John R. McCarthy, Colm Breslin, Joe Woodcock. Back row (left to right): Robin King, Des Riordan, Robert Gilmore, Gerry Black, William Wren, Declan Tyrrell, John Goodbody, Richard Nolan, William Bingham. Courtesy of Bobby Studio.

Scheme agreed to release three of their general professional training posts to allow the appointments. The new SR posts would be at the Mater Misericordiae Hospital and the Royal City of Dublin Hospital Baggot Street (a combined post) Our Lady's Hospital for Sick Children, Crumlin and between Jervis Street and St Laurence's Hospitals (also a combined post). Dr Keane hoped that it would be possible in the near future to appoint an SR to the Western Regional Training area.[17] A fourth senior registrar was appointed to St Vincent's Hospital, Dublin. Drs Sean McDevitt, Myles MacEvilly, and William O'Brien were the first three appointed as SRs with Dr Ron Kirkham being appointed to the fourth post a few months later.

The dean proposed to Prof. Gordon Robson, Dean of the Faculty of Anaesthetists of the Royal College of Surgeons of England, that the Irish faculty should have more representation on the Joint Committee for Higher Anaesthetic Training. The Council of RCSI agreed to the abolition of the DA with the final examination for the diploma being held in November 1976.

1977

The AGM took place on Friday 20 May followed by the Kirkpatrick Lecture which was given by Dr Tom Walsh, the Wexford anaesthetist who was one of the founders of the Wexford opera festival. The talk was titled 'The Wexford festival – an historical appraisal'.

Annual Scientific Meeting, Saturday 21 May 1977
- Dr J.E. Riding (Dean, London), 'The anaesthetist and the pain clinic'
- Dr K. Lilburn (Belfast), 'A new concept of ketamine'
- Prof. Andrew Thornton (Sheffield), 'A new era in toothpulling'
- Dr Robin King (Craigavon), 'Surgery and the pill'
- Dr J.E. Riding (London), 'So you want to write a paper'
- Dr William O'Brien (Cork/Dublin), 'Anaesthetic training in Canada and Ireland'
- Prof. J. Dundee, Dr S.B. Johnston (Belfast), 'Demonstration on audio-visual aids'

A joint meeting of the Association of Anaesthetists of Great Britain and Ireland (AAGBI) and the Société Française d'Anesthésie d'Analgésie et Réanimation was held in RCSI on Friday 30 September. An honorary fellowship was conferred at the meeting on Dr Cyril Scurr who was president of AAGBI at the time. His citation was read by Dundee. Prof. J. Lassner from the French society was also conferred with an honorary fellowship and Wren read his citation. The John Snow Lecture was delivered by Dr T.K. Whitaker, chancellor of the National University of Ireland, titled 'Anaesthesia in the EEC'.

Wren and Coleman attended the foundation meeting of the European Academy of Anesthesiology in Paris with 25 countries being represented. A second meeting was held in Dublin in September. Gilmartin and Wren were elected as honorary members of the Union Française d'Anésthesie-Réanimation. Prof. Myron B. Laver from Harvard came to Dublin in October as visiting professor to all three medical schools. The DOH agreed that SR posts would be supernumerary to the general professional training posts. An analysis of the MCQ results by Black and then a second analysis by Kirkham (SR) had found that it would be a good screening test of who should progress to the orals and written papers. Black stated that, in London, there was agreement that such a screening test was fair to the candidates and helped the examiners.

1978
The board meeting, conferring and AGM were on Friday 19 May; the scientific symposium took place a day later. An honorary fellowship was conferred on Prof.

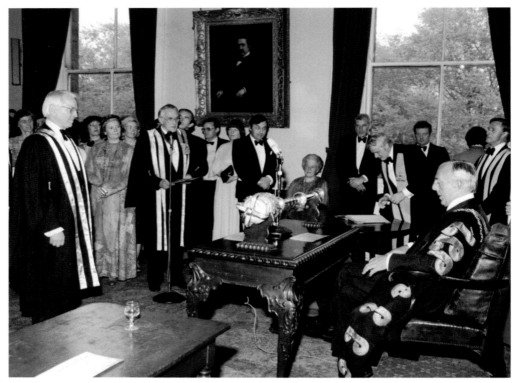

Pomp and ceremony, RCSI, 20 May 1978. President of RCSI Stanley McCollum is seated on the right with the ceremonial mace on the table in front of him. Harold Love is reading the citation for the conferring of an Honorary Fellowship of the Faculty of Anaesthetists, RCSI on Marion Thomas Jenkins from the Parkland Memorial Hospital, Dallas. Courtesy of Bobby Studio.

Marion Thomas Jenkins from Parklands Memorial Hospital in Dallas, Texas. He was the doctor who tried to resuscitate President John Fitzgerald Kennedy after he was shot and who later pronounced him dead. Two days later, he was also on duty when Lee Harvey Oswald was shot. The dean, Harold Love, read the citation.

The theme of the Annual Scientific Meeting was 'Anaesthesia and the elderly'.

- Prof. Marion Jenkins (Dallas), 'Preoperative preparation of the elderly patient'
- Prof. Cedric Prys-Roberts (Bristol), 'Cardiovascular problems'
- Dr Margaret Branthwaite (London), 'Respiratory problems'
- Dr Alastair Spence (Glasgow), 'Post-operative respiratory care of the elderly'
- Prof. Kevin O'Malley (Dublin), 'Drug responses in the elderly',
- Dr Richard Assaf (Dublin), 'Anaesthesia for the urological patient'
- Dr M. Hyland (Cork), 'Post-operative confusion in the elderly'

There was a general discussion at the board meeting in March on the faculty's frustration with RCSI regarding representation. The college president felt that the board's request to have a representative on council was unlikely to succeed. Dundee was particularly incensed that he had to apply to the president and vice president to be appointed to the Court of Examiners for the fellowship of the Faculty of Anaesthetists, RCSI. It was felt that it should be 'subject to the appointment being made by the Faculty'. Three options were proposed for the future of the faculty. It could join the newly created Royal College of Anaesthetists in England, it could remain as it was as a faculty of RCSI or it could consider forming an independent Irish College of Anaesthetists. It was suggested that the proposals should be put to a referendum of all anaesthetists in Ireland. The dean called a special meeting later in March to try to defuse the situation. It was agreed that the board would appoint its own examiners and also the chairman of the examination conference. The formal letter of complaint to the RCSI president was withdrawn but the views of the board would be passed on to him informally.[18]

On 5 September 1978, the first general assembly of the European Academy of Anaesthesiology took place in Paris.[20] There were 42 founder academicians, six of whom were from Ireland: Love, Gilmartin, Woodcock, Coleman, Wren and Dundee. Wren was elected as secretary to the new body.

1979
Dean Dr John R. McCarthy, 1979–82
The Annual Scientific Meeting took place on Saturday 19 May with the theme 'Medical problems in anaesthesia'.

- Prof. N.C. Nevin (Belfast), 'Genetic factors in anaesthesia'
- Dr F.R. Ellis (Leeds), 'Inherited muscle disease'
- Dr J. Curran (Cork), 'Anaesthesia, hypertension and myocardial ischaemia'
- Dr M. Ivor Drury (Dublin), 'Diabetes update'
- Prof. M. Fitzgerald (Dublin), 'Medical problems in the ventilated patient'
- Prof. J. Norman (Southampton), 'Acid-base imbalance'
- Prof. F.F. Foldes (New York), 'Use of muscle relaxants in patients with altered sensitivity'

An honorary fellowship was conferred on Prof. F.F. Foldes before the annual dinner held in RCSI. The citation was read by Dr J. Moore. The American

Marian Rice, the first woman elected to the Board of Faculty of Anaesthetists, RCSI, 1978. Courtesy of Bobby Studio.

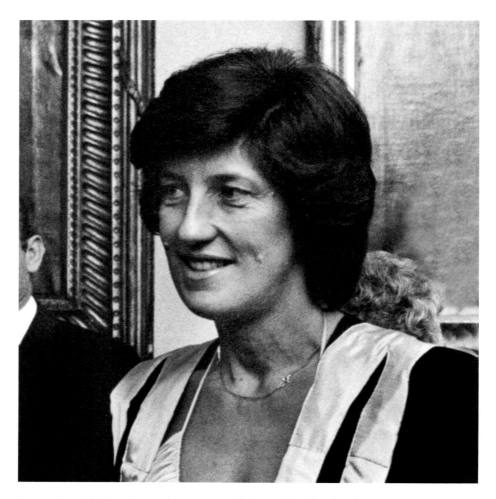

ambassador Mr William Shannon and his wife Elizabeth were in attendance at the reception.

The new IMC was created by statute law and had the power to create and maintain a register of specialists. This function would be carried out through the Postgraduate Medical and Dental Board which would decide which bodies (e.g. the faculty) were appropriate for the purposes of 'granting evidence of satisfactory completion of training'.[21] The board of faculty deemed its Medical Advisory Committee to be the appropriate group for this function. The faculty was finally given an office, designated as being solely for use of the dean, in the RCSI building. Dr John R. McCarthy replaced Love as dean at the September board meeting.

1980

The board meeting, conferring and AGM took place on Friday 16 May followed by the Annual Scientific Meeting one day later.

Practical problems in anaesthetic practice[22]
- Dr Liam McCaughey (Craigavon), 'Influence of previous drug therapy'
- Dr Cyril Scurr (London), 'Problems of difficult intubation'
- Dr M. Weingarten (Milwaukee), 'Closed circuit anaesthesia'
- Dr Sam R. Kielty (Belfast), 'Abdominal surgery in the infant'
- Dr John B. Magner (Dublin), 'Management of aortic aneurysms'
- Dr A.W. Conn (Toronto), 'Practical problems of raised intra-cranial pressure'

An honorary fellowship was conferred on Prof. Gordon Robson and the citation was delivered by Wren. The 21st Faculty Anniversary Dinner was held in the Banqueting Hall, RCSI on Saturday 17 May and was attended by the Minister of Health, Dr Michael Woods. Dr Tom Walsh, co-founder of the Wexford opera festival, was conferred with an honorary fellowship in December. His citation was also read by Wren.

The report from the National Anaesthetic Training Programme stated that there were a total of 64 anaesthetists in training. Additional SR posts had been approved at the Richmond Hospital (Neurosurgery); Our Lady's Hospital Crumlin (Paediatrics); The Regional Hospital, Wilton, Cork; The Regional Hospital, Galway; and St Vincent's Hospital, Dublin. There were, at that time, 13 SRs in total.

The faculty had three regional training committees (Eastern, Southern and Western) which were 'chaired' by Wren, Gaffney and Keane respectively.[23] The other bodies concerned with training were the Medical Advisory Committee of the faculty and the Joint Committee of Higher Training of Anaesthetists. By 1985, the National Training Committee would have trained 65 anaesthetists to consultant standard. The numbers sitting the examinations had increased substantially with approximately 400 candidates sitting the Primary examination twice yearly. In view of these large numbers, the introduction of a cut-off mark in the MCQ exam would have to be considered. The faculty was keen that it be recognised as the training body for the specialty by the Postgraduate Medical and Dental Board and by the Medical Council. The board agreed to award a medal in honour of Dr Edmund Delaney, former board member, who had died in 1979. The medal was presented by the dean at the AGM in May to Dr

Jennings, a registrar at the Mater Misericordiae Hospital, Dublin.

1981

The Annual Scientific Meeting was held in the RCSI on Saturday 16 May. The theme was 'Obstetric and neonatal problems.[24]

- Dr James 'Alfie' Moore (Belfast), 'The antacid controversy'
- Dr Jeffrey Selwyn Crawford (Birmingham), 'Maternal awareness versus neonatal depression'
- Dr Maldwyn Morgan (London), 'Pulmonary complications'
- Prof. J. Bonnar (Dublin), 'Coagulation defects'
- Prof. Kieran O'Driscoll (Dublin), 'Obstetric analgesia, is it as simple as it seems'?
- Prof. Sol M. Schnider (San Francisco), 'Indications for regional anaesthesia'
- Prof. G.A. Gregory (San Francisco), 'Immediate care of the neonate'

The AGM was held on Friday 15 May and was followed by the sixth Kirkpatrick Lecture given by Prof. Cecil Gray, CBE. The lecture title was 'On reflection – a possible solution to Ludovic's dilemma'. Dr Charles O'Hagan won the Delaney Medal.

The medical school at the Royal College of Surgeons in Ireland proposed the establishment of a chair of anaesthesia with undergraduate teaching at RCSI and clinical commitments to the new Beaumont Hospital. The dean, Dr McCarthy, along with Drs Riordan and Woodcock, met the registrar of RCSI, Mr Grace, and Mr Alan Browne to consider the structuring of the professorial position at RCSI/Beaumont. It was agreed that it would be funded by the college, the faculty and Jervis Street/ Richmond/Beaumont Hospitals. RCSI also agreed to the 'Faculty of Anaesthetists Johnston and Johnston Library' being housed within the college.

An international conference of English-speaking faculties and boards of anaesthesia took place in London. Arising from the discussions on training, the faculty was pleased to receive notification from Dr E.S. Siker of the American Board of Anesthesiology that 'Holders of the Fellowship certificate … would be allowed to enter the A.B.A. [American Board of Anesthesiology] examination system on successfully completing one year of clinical anaesthesia training in an accredited programme'

The honorary treasurer presented the accounts for 1980. Income was

£90,817 and expenditure £95,742, resulting in a deficit of £4,925. The board had been informed that a new accounting system had been implemented by RCSI that charged the faculty 5 per cent of the overall college expenditure and this had led to the financial deficit. The possibility of holding meetings outside RCSI was discussed as a means of reducing costs. It was felt that the faculty should be financially independent of the college. The dean, McCarthy, proposed that the college should continue to retain the examination fees and should use these monies to cover the room rental and secretarial costs of the faculty. All other monies (e.g. faculty subscriptions) should be kept by the faculty in a separate account.[25]

The board received further correspondence from the Conjoint Board (RCP & SI) requesting the restoration of the DA examination. Difficulties in recruiting trainee anaesthetists were discussed and the conclusion reached was that this was due to the heavy workload in anaesthesia. The trainee/consultant ratio was 0.42/1 whereas it was 1.38/1 in other specialties.

1982

Dean Dr Gerald Black, 1982–5

The AGM of the faculty took place in the college (RCSI) at 5.30 p.m. on Friday 15 May and was followed by the Harry O'Flanagan Lecture which was delivered by Prof. Eric Nilsson from the University of Lund in Sweden. His talk was titled 'Swedish Anaesthesia: looking back-wards to plan the future'

The Annual Scientific Meeting took place on the following day, Saturday 16 May. The theme was 'Anaesthetic update 1982'.

- Dr Anthony Gilbertson (Liverpool), 'Practical measurements in respiratory failure'
- Dr Keith Sykes (Oxford), 'New methods of respiratory support in acute lung disease'
- Dr Warren M. Zapol (Boston), 'Pathophysiology of adult respiratory distress Syndrome'
- Dr Myles MacEvilly (Dublin), 'Substance p and other neurotransmitters'
- Dr David W. Barron (Belfast), 'Post-operative pain relief using epidural and intrathecal opioids'
- Dr Daniel C. Moore (Seattle), 'Post-operative pain relief using local nerve blocks'

Board of Faculty of Anaesthetists, RCSI, 1985. Front row (left to right): Declan Tyrrell, Kevin Moore, Robin King, Gerry Black (Dean), Denis Moriarty, Padraic Keane, Lorna Browne. Back row (left to right): Rory O'Brien, John Cooper, Myles MacEvilly, Sam Kielty, Seamus Harte, Aidan Kennedy, David Hogan, Morrell Lyons, Richard Clarke. Courtesy of Bobby Studio.

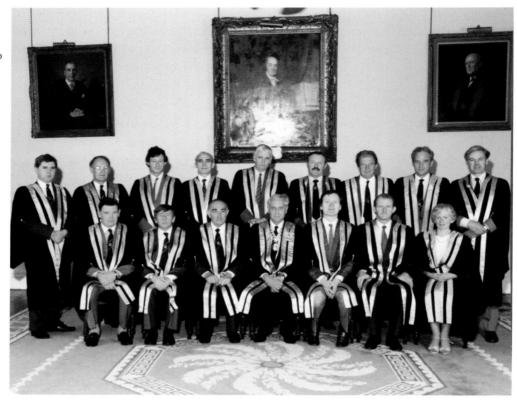

An honorary fellowship was conferred on Prof. Tess O'Rourke Brophy OBE from the Royal Brisbane Hospital, University of Queensland, Australia (she was the first and only woman to receive the honorary fellowship of the faculty). Her citation was read by Black.

The financial relationship between the faculty and the college was discussed again. Keane stated that the long-term objective should be complete control of the finances by the board. The faculty wished to have its own bank account and it was agreed that this would be discussed with the council of the college. Moriarty went to Kuwait to examine in the Primary FFARCS with examiners from the English faculty.

1983

The Annual Scientific Meeting took place on Saturday 21 May; the theme for the conference was 'Cardiovascular problems in anaesthesia and intensive care'.

- Dr Margaret Branthwaite (London), 'Recent advances in cardiac assessment'

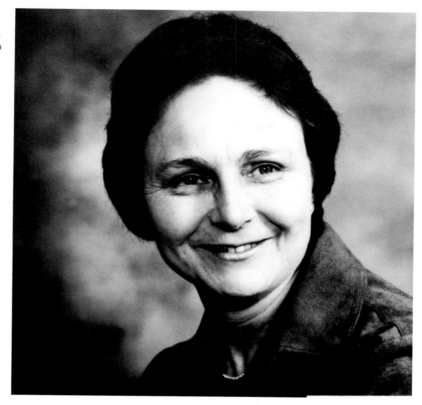

Tess Rita O'Rourke Brophy, the only woman to be conferred with an Honorary Fellowship of the Faculty of Anaesthetists, RCSI. May 1982. Courtesy of the Royal College of Surgeons in Ireland.

- Dr Róisin MacSullivan (Dublin), 'Myocardial ischaemia during anaesthesia'
- Dr Samuel M. Lyons (Belfast), 'Anaesthetic management for the high-risk cardiac patient'
- Dr Ian Carson (Belfast), 'Inotropic drugs'
- Dr Pierre Foëx (Oxford), 'Cardiovascular effects of inhalational anaesthetics'
- Dr John Horgan (Dublin), 'Management of cardiac dysrhythmias'

The annual dinner was held in the RCSI banqueting hall on the Saturday night and was attended by the Minister for Health, Mr Barry Desmond.

A special dinner was held in September to mark the retirement of Gilmartin from his professorship at the Royal College of Surgeons in Ireland. It was decided that a lecture would be inaugurated in his honour. The second Critikon Lecture took place in December 1983 and was given by Prof. Olof Norland from the Karolinska Institute in Stockholm.

As a result of the dispute over finances between the faculty and the college, a new agreement was reached in March 1983. It was agreed that the faculty would have complete control of its finances with a separate faculty account and its own independent accountant. The honorary treasurer would have the right to scrutinise all expenses incurred in using the RCSI facilities for courses, meetings, exams and dinners prior to payment. He or she would receive monthly statements of the faculty account and there would be closer communication between the RCSI accountant and the faculty. Discussions took place in June between representatives of the board of the faculty, the boards of the Richmond and Jervis Street Hospitals and Comhairle regarding the structure of the appointment of a chair in anaesthesia. It was agreed that there should be six teaching and five service sessions.[26]

1984

The year 1984 was both the 25th anniversary of the foundation of the faculty and the bicentenary of the Royal College of Surgeons in Ireland. The Delaney Medal competition took place in March and was won by Dr Terence McMurray. The Annual Scientific Meeting was held over two days for the first time.
The title of the conference was 'Twenty-five years on'.

Scientific Programme:
- Dr B.R. Brown Jr., 'Metabolism of volatile anaesthetics'
- Prof. Richard S.J. Clarke, 'Alternatives to thiopentone over 25 years'
- Dr Joel Kaplan, 'Cardiovascular monitoring'
- Dr William S. Wren, 'Anaesthesia for surgery of the larynx'
- Dr Hugh Raftery, 'Problems in pain management'
- Dr Gordon Jackson Rees, 'Paediatric anaesthesia'
- Dr Joel Kaplan, 'Drug therapy in the patient with cardiac disease'
- Dr S.A. Feldman, 'Advances in neuromuscular block'
- Dr B.R. Brown Jr. 'Management of anaesthesia in patients with liver disease'
  Honorary fellowships were conferred on Prof. Guy Vourc'h and Dr Gordon Jackson Rees at the faculty annual dinner. Coleman read the citation for Vourc'h, describing how he had commenced his medical studies in 1936 but shortly after, these were interrupted by World War Two. He fought in the French army but when France was invaded, he fled with a number of companions in an open boat. After drifting for ten days at sea, he was rescued and then joined the Inter Allied Commandos. He received the British Military Cross for bravery. He is credited with reforming French anaesthesia after the war. Moore read the citation for Dr Gordon Jackson Rees, the renowned

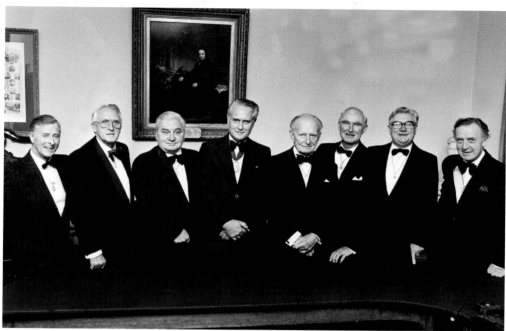

Eight Deans. (Left to right) John R. McCarthy, Harold Love, Joe Woodcock, Gerry Black, Tommy Gilmartin, Ray Davys, John Dundee, William Wren. Courtesy of Bobby Studio.

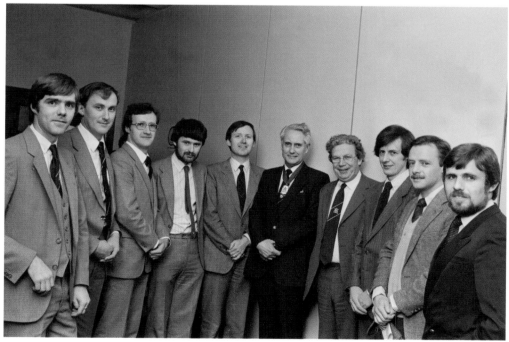

Delaney Medal competition 1984. (Left to right) David O'Toole, Rodney Meeke, Dermot Murphy, Ken Lowry, Denis Moriarty, Gerry Black (Dean), David Hogan, Declan Warde, Gerry Dorrian, Terry McMurray. Courtesy of Bobby Studio.

paediatric anaesthetist. The first Tess Brophy Prizes for the candidate with the highest mark in the Final FFARCSI examination were awarded to Dr Douglas Gilroy from Belfast and Dr W.C. Ho from Merseyside.

In May 1984, the dispute over finances between the faculty and RCSI seemed to be resolved, with the college revoking its authority over the faculty's accounts. Keane and Moriarty opened the Faculty's own account in December.

A total of 386 candidates sat the Primary examination in 1984, 353 presented for the Final fellowship. It was decided that the fellowship examination would, in future, consist of three parts: Part 1 to be an examination on the basic principles and practice of anaesthesia, Part 2 on advanced pharmacology and physiology and Part 3 as previously with the addition of clinical measurement. The new exam would be held for the first time in spring 1986.[27]

The Medical Advisory Committee was chaired by Dr K.P. Moore and met twice during the year. The Winter Faculty Lecture took place in December and was delivered by Prof. Temmerman from Brussels. The final Kirkpatrick Lecture was given in 1984 by Dr Peter Froggatt, titled 'MacDonnell father and son'. It was replaced one year later by the Gilmartin Lecture.

1985
Dean Dr Padraic W. Keane, 1985–8

The dean, Black, visited Damman in Saudi Arabia in January 1985 and inspected the King Fahad Hospital for the purpose of recognition for the requirements of the FFARCSI examination. He provided a satisfactory report and felt that it would be feasible to have the FFARCSI examination held there. The fourth Delaney Medal competition took place in March and the winner was Dr John Boylan.

The Annual Scientific Meeting took place over two days in May. Speakers included Drs Lorna Browne, Anthony Cunningham and Denis Moriarty (all from Dublin), Dr E. McAteer (Belfast), Dr J.H. Donegan (San Francisco) and Prof. H. Turndorf (New York). An honorary fellowship was conferred on Dr J.F. Nunn prior to the annual dinner. The first Gilmartin Lecture, entitled 'From small beginnings', was given by Dundee on the Friday evening of the scientific meeting. The autumn faculty meeting took place in September and featured four speakers, Drs Enda Shanahan and Dermot Phelan from Dublin, Dr Johnson (Belfast) and Dr Comer (Galway). The Winter Faculty Lecture in December was given by Dr Joseph Stoddart of Newcastle-upon-Tyne on 'The treatment of chest injuries'.

On 27 September 1985, Dr Thomas B. Boulton, president of the Association of Anaesthetists of Great Britain and Ireland presented the John Snow Medal to Gilmartin. The medal is normally presented in London but Boulton travelled to Dublin on this occasion, as Gilmartin was unable to travel.

The post of professor of anaesthesia at RCSI was advertised in December 1984, interviews were held in March and Anthony Cunningham was appointed in October 1985. The faculty undertook to make a financial contribution for the first year.

There were 70 training posts in the General Professional Training Programme and 17 posts at Higher Professional Training. Declan Tyrrell circulated details of a proposed Diploma in Intensive Care. It was felt that 12 months' training would be required before candidates could sit the examination.[28]

Another working party was set up between the board of faculty and RCSI Council. Its terms of reference were to explore the relationship between the two bodies, to look at similar arrangements internationally and to make recommendations to the board as to how to implement change. The faculty representatives were Keane (dean), Moriarty (vice dean), Cooper (hon. treasurer), Hogan (hon. secretary), Black and K.P. Moore. RCSI was represented by Mr Victor Lane (president), Mr R.A.E. Magee (vice president), Mr Frank Duff, Mr J.M. McAuliffe Curtin, Mr Stanley McCollum and Prof. Eoin O'Malley.

1986

The Delaney Medal competition was held on 7 March with five papers presented. Dr Frank McDonnell was the winner. The new three-part fellowship examination commenced in April 1986 and the board expressed its thanks to Drs Declan Tyrrell (chairman, Examinations), McCarthy (Part 1), Morrell Lyons (Part 2) and Robin King (Part 3) for progressing its implementation. The Department of Anaesthesia, RCSI was formally established in April when Anthony Cunningham assumed the position of first full-time professor in the specialty in the Republic of Ireland. Dr David O'Toole was subsequently appointed as lecturer and Drs Edward Gallagher, James Gardiner, Anthony Healy and Declan Warde as clinical lecturers.

On 3 April, Prof. Michael Cousins of the Flinders Medical Centre, Adelaide, Australia read a paper entitled 'Opiate pharmacokinetics, a basis for advances in treatment of cancer pain'. The Western Anaesthetic Symposium took place on 5 April with Prof. Cedric Prys-Roberts from Bristol as the visiting speaker.

The themes of the Annual Scientific Meeting in May were anaesthetic aspects of computers, adverse drug reactions and neuromuscular blocking drugs. Speakers included Prof. W.C. Bowman, Prof. Donald Campbell, Dr Michael J.

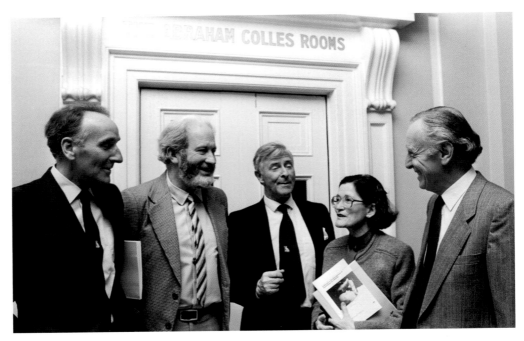

Cousins, Prof. J. Forrest, Drs Michael Slazenger, Rajinder Mirakhur, Gavin Kenny, William Wren, Aidan Synnott and McCann.[29] The second Gilmartin Lecture was given by Sir Gordon Robson but Gilmartin himself was unable to attend because of ill-health.

As a result of the joint working party negotiations, agreement was finally reached in June 1986 on future relations between the board of faculty and RCSI Council. The faculty would henceforth assume independent control of its financial affairs and accounts but these would be audited annually by RCSI. The conference of examiners and the conferring of fellowships of the Faculty of Anaesthetists, RCSI would be conducted solely by the dean and officers of the faculty (i.e. there would no longer be a requirement for the presence of the president or vice president of RCSI).[30]

Prof. Thomas J. Gilmartin, the first dean of the faculty, died on 22 June 1986.

The autumn faculty meeting was held in Cork for the first time. The speakers were Drs Charlie O'Hagan, John D. McAdoo, William P. Blunnie and Peter M. Crean. The meeting was organised by Drs Rory O'Brien and John Cahill. Prof. Anthony Cunningham gave his inaugural lecture in the RCSI on 6 November.

The Winter Faculty Lecture was held on 12 December and was given by

Prof. Lawrence Saidman; its title was 'Clinically important research published in anesthesiology in 1986'.

Des Riordan reported on the progress of the anaesthetic training course in Tanzania which he considered was fulfilling an important role; he recommended that the faculty should continue its support. It was being led by Eugene Egan who had agreed to continue in the role for a further three years.

1987

Dr Eugene Egan from the Christian Medical Centre, Kilimanjaro, Tanzania gave a lecture on 7 January titled 'Ex Africa semper aliquid novi'. The Delaney Medal competition took place on 6 March and the prize was awarded to Dr Noel Flynn for his contribution 'The effect of local anaesthetics on epinephrine absorption following rectal mucosal infiltration'.

The Annual Scientific Meeting took place on 15 and 16 May. The speakers and subjects on Friday 15 May were:

- Dr B.L. Grundy, 'Full heads and full stomachs'
- Dr D. I.Foulkes, 'Transferring critically ill patients'
- Dr P.S. Sebal, 'Sufentanil'

and on the following day:

- Dr John Donohue, 'Renal failure'
- Dr Joseph A. Tracey, 'Renal transplantation'
- Dr B.L. Grundy, 'Intraoperative monitoring of sensory evoked potentials'
- Dr P.S. Sebel, 'Assessment of depth of anaesthesia'
- Dr John Crowe, 'Liver failure and the anaesthetist'
- Dr Pat Doherty, 'Monitoring in paediatric anaesthesia'

Prof. Edmond (Ted) Eger was conferred with an honorary fellowship at the meeting and delivered the Gilmartin Lecture.[31] The autumn faculty meeting took place in September in the Europa Hotel in Belfast and the speakers were Drs O'Brien (Cork), Aidan Sharkey (Ballinasloe), Lesley Fox (Dublin) and Terence McMurray (Belfast). The board agreed to move to a new room in the college which would be known as the dean/committee room and would be exclusively for the use of the faculty.

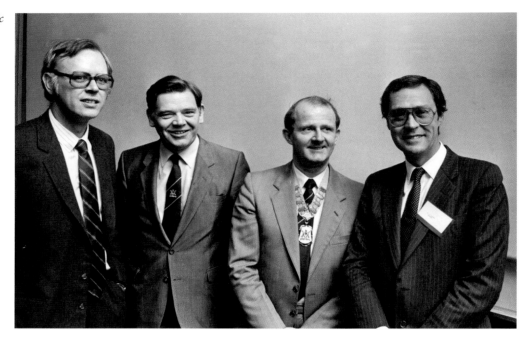

1988
Dean Dr Denis C. Moriarty, 1988–91
In March 1988, a full memorandum of agreement was reached between RCSI and the faculty which replaced that of 1982.

It was agreed that as regards income, the faculty would have:

(1) Annual subscription from the fellows
(2) Dividends and bank interest
(3) Profits (losses) from scientific symposia
(4) Profits (losses) from courses for the Primary and Final fellowship exams
(5) Other income including from suppliers of equipment and drug companies

The faculty would be liable for its expenditure for:

1 Travelling expenses
2 Subscription to the *Journal of the Irish Colleges of Physicians and Surgeons* (*JICPS*)
3 Printing, stationary, postage, telephone and electricity
4 Expenses for the dean and board members, entertainment costs

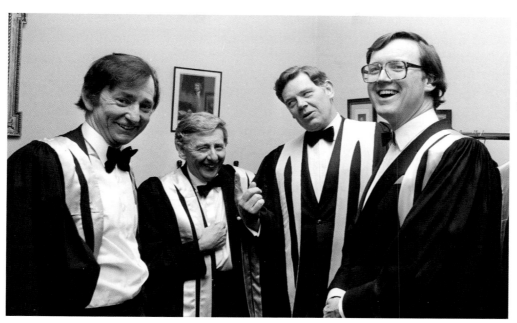

(Left to right)
Des Riordan,
Kevin Moore,
Declan Tyrrell,
Denis Moriarty.
Courtesy of
Bobby Studio.

5 Insurance and auditors fees
6 Contribution towards the academic department

In addition, RCSI would charge the faculty for the use of their facilities for courses, seminars and symposia at one third the commercial rate. It would also be billed for the salary of a full-time secretary. The board of faculty agreed to notify the college of any significant acquisitions or disposal of assets while faculty accounts could in future be audited by the college auditors.[32]

The Delaney Medal competition took place on 3 March and was won by Dr Kieran Crowley. The Annual Scientific Meeting took place on Friday 13 and Saturday 14 May 1988. The speakers were Drs G. Parkes (Addenbrookes), M. Rogers (Johns Hopkins), R.M. Jones (Guy's), Ephraim S. Siker (Mercy, Pittsburgh), Dermot Phelan (Mater, Dublin) and Mr Brian Lane (Beaumont).

Dr Ephraim S. Siker, professor of anaesthetics, University of Pittsburgh, gave the fourth Gilmartin Lecture, 'A measure of vigilance', and was conferred with an honorary fellowship. His citation was given by Richard Clarke. The speakers at the autumn faculty meeting held on 30 September were Prof. Mapleson on 'Efficacy of oxygen masks', Dr Pat Doherty on 'Pulse oximetry' and Dr Aidan Synnott on 'Lung volumes and cardiac output in critically ill patients'. The Winter Faculty Lecture was given by Prof. J.G. Jones who spoke on 'Brain function in anaesthetised patients'.

A committee was set up to coordinate and promote training in intensive care in Ireland. It consisted of two anaesthetists, two surgeons and two physicians. Moriarty and Keane were nominated from the faculty.

Abbott donated an endowment of £3,000 p.a. and the Education Committee felt that this should be used to fund suitable projects. It was decided that those candidates seeking funds from the endowment should submit their research proposal specifying how the funds would be used.

Clarke was appointed as professor of anaesthetics and head of department at Queen's University Belfast following the retirement of Dundee. Moriarty, Keane and Clarke were nominated to the UEMS.

1989

At the board meeting in March, the dean reported on his visit to the new College of Anaesthetists in London and this led to a discussion on future relations with that college, the parity of the exams and the idea of an independent Irish College of Anaesthetists. Three options were proposed at the June meeting : (1) to become a college within a college, (2) to be integrated with 'London', (3) or to become an independent college. A legal opinion given by Dermot Gleeson, senior counsel, stated that RCSI did not have the constitutional right to create a college within a college as this would need an act of the Oireachtas. Some board members felt that the faculty should disaffiliate itself from RCSI. It was agreed that the most realistic option was to maintain the status quo for the moment.

The Annual Scientific Meeting was held in May and the theme was 'The control of pain'. The main speakers were Drs K. Budd, J.A. Moore, C. Wells, W. Blunnie, E. Charlton and Prof. T. Murphy. The theme of the autumn faculty meeting was 'The role of the doctor within hospital management'. The speakers were F. Scott-Lennon, Ann Naylor and L. Flanagan. The Critikon Lecture took place in December and was given by Prof. Jean Louis Vincent who spoke on 'Modern management of heart failure in an I.C.U. setting'.

The dean (Moriarty) and Carson visited Riyadh in Saudi Arabia. It was agreed to hold a Part 1 course there in 1990 followed by the Part 1 examination later in the year. They hoped to hold the Part 2 course and examination at a later date. The Standing Committee in Ireland of the AAGBI produced a booklet 'Anaesthesia in Ireland – the provision of a safe service' which was circulated to all practising anaesthetists.

1990

Cunningham and Clarke gave the first overseas course for the Primary fellowship examination in Riyadh, Kingdom of Saudi Arabia and the board subsequently ratified an agreement to run these courses for three years. The College of Anaesthetists in London was not happy with the faculty running exams in Riyadh as it was already doing so. The dean, Carson and McCarthy held the Part 1 examination in Riyadh in September and this was the first occasion on which the faculty had held an exam outside Ireland.

At the instigation of Dr Dermot Phelan, a joint meeting of the Faculty of Anaesthetists, RCSI and the Intensive Care Society was held in RCPI in March. A working party was convened to examine the feasibility of setting up a diploma in critical care with Dr Gerry Fitzpatrick as convenor.

The Annual Scientific Meeting was held in May on the theme 'Anaesthesia in the '90s'. The main speakers were Prof. Seraj (Saudi Arabia), Prof. T. Healy (UK), Prof. James Bovill (Netherlands), Prof. Bendixen (USA), Dr J.P. Howard Fee (Belfast) and Dr Alan J. McShane (Dublin). Prof. Michael Rosen, the first president of the Royal College of Anaesthetists, was conferred with an honorary fellowship at the meeting and his citation was delivered by John Cooper.

The balance sheet for the ASM showed a healthy profit of £6,971. Prof. Anthony Clare, medical director of St Patrick's Hospital Dublin gave the Gilmartin Lecture. It was decided to award the Abbott endowment to six different projects with each one receiving IR £500. Dr Hussein Nagi won the Delaney Medal. The theme for the autumn faculty meeting was 'Anaesthesia in peripheral hospitals and the speakers were Drs Ann Elizabeth Bourke, P.J. Breen and D. Donnelly. Keane gave a talk at the winter faculty meeting: 'In search of the magic bullet'.

1991

Dean Dr Richard J. Clarke, 1991–4

The board held a meeting in March which was attended by the RCSI accountant. It was felt that the financial agreement between the faculty and the college had not been adhered to and that in future, there should be better communication from RCSI. The faculty accounts were noted as being in a healthy state with over £90,000 in Banque National de Paris (BNP), over £20,000 in investments and £8,000 in the current account. At a later meeting, the honorary treasurer, Gallagher, pointed out that difficulties in collecting annual subscriptions from fellows were due to a failure to process credit card payments and also problems with direct debits. This explained the dramatic reduction in subscription income in 1989/90. A report of the meeting between the faculty and the London college was circulated by Cooper. This led to a wide-ranging discussion on the options open to the faculty. Could they become a faculty of the London college? Would a referendum of all fellows be needed? It was decided to continue discussions with London. Cooper suggested that the faculty should start up a sink fund with a view to buying their own building.

The Annual Scientific Meeting took place on Friday/Saturday 17/18 May after which an honorary fellowship was conferred on Dr Alan Sessler from the Mayo Clinic, Rochester, Minnesota, USA. The Gilmartin Lecture was delivered by Mr Peter Sutherland, former attorney general and European commissioner. His talk was titled 'Europe 1992'. The autumn faculty meeting in October was held in conjunction with the South of Ireland Association of Anaesthetists at the Silver Springs Hotel in Cork. Speakers included Drs Declan O'Keefe (Dublin), Neil McDonald (Dublin), Robert Taylor (Belfast) and Prof. William Shoemaker (Los Angeles) who spoke on 'Augmentation of cardiac output in sepsis'. Prof. Henrik Kehlet delivered the Winter Faculty Lecture, entitled 'Postoperative pain, status and perspectives'. There were three recipients of the Abbott research grants, Drs William Blunnie, James M. Murray and Gerry Fitzpatrick. The Delaney Medal competition was won by Dr Tom Ryan for his paper 'The role of transoesophageal echocardiography during major vascular surgery'.

Prof. Clarke was invited to take over the deanship from Dr Moriarty at the September board meeting. There were new regulations for the Fellowship of the Faculty of Anaesthetists, RCSI (FFARCSI). It was agreed that there would be reciprocity between the FFARCSI and the fellowship of the College of Anaesthetists (in London) in both Part 1 and Part 2 of the respective exams. Candidates who had obtained the European Diploma in Anaesthesiology were exempt from Part 1. The Part 1 revision courses were organised by Dr Rory Dwyer, the Part 2 course was coordinated by Dr Liam McCaughey and the Part 3 by Dr Róisin MacSullivan. Discussions continued on the development of a diploma in intensive care. Dr K.P. Moore, chairman of the Medical Advisory Committee, informed the board that there were currently 23 SRs in post in Ireland

1992

A joint meeting of the Faculty of Anaesthetists, RCSI and the Intensive Care Society of Ireland was held in March. Speakers included Drs Conor Burke, Tess

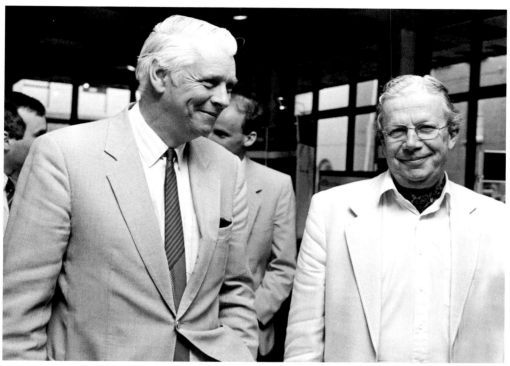

Gallagher and Prof. R.A. Little. The Annual Scientific Meeting took place as usual over the weekend of 15 and 16 May. The main theme was 'Anaesthesia in the elderly'. Speakers and topics included:

- Dr Deirdre McMahon, 'Physiological adaption in a microgravity environment'
- Dr Anthony P. Rubin, 'Development of an acute pain service'
- Prof. John P. Kampine, 'Anaesthesia and the control of breathing'
- Dr Máire McCarroll, 'Difficult airways workshop'
- Dr D.G. Seymour, 'Pre-op states and outcomes in geriatric surgery'
- Prof. Kevin O'Malley, 'Medication in the elderly'
- Dr John P. Alexander, 'Intensive care in the elderly'
- Dr Rory Dwyer, 'Altered anaesthetic requirements in the elderly'
- Prof. John P. Kampine, 'Is there increased anaesthetic risk in the elderly'?

The eighth Gilmartin Lecture was delivered by Dr Maurice Hayes, formerly Ombudsman, Northern Ireland, with the title 'Subsidiarity breeds consent'.

The Autumn Faculty Lecture was given by Dr Felicity Reynolds titled 'Maternal mortality: Anaesthesia in perspective' and was part of a joint meeting in September between the faculty and the Obstetric Anaesthetists Association (OAA). The meeting was followed by a state reception in Dublin Castle.

The winter meeting was held jointly between RCSI and the Faculty on 13 and 14 November. The speakers for the faculty were Drs Ken Lowry who spoke on 'Treatment of sepsis', Robert Taylor on 'Management of the critically burned patient' and Kate Flynn on 'Enteral and parenteral nutrition'. Prof. Runciman from the Royal Adelaide Hospital in Australia gave the Winter Faculty Lecture on 'Cost benefit analysis'.

The winners of the Abbott research grants were Drs David Hill (Belfast), T.H. Boyd (Belfast), Kevin Carson (Dublin), Grainne Nicholson (Dublin) and Paul McDonagh (Dublin). The Delaney Medal was won by Dr Frank Chambers (Galway).

The Part 1 course in Riyadh was given by Henry Craig and Joseph Tracey while that for Part 2 was provided by Howard Fee and Prof. Hall. Richard S.J. Clarke, David Hogan and Aidan Sharkey were examiners in the faculty exams held in Riyadh in September. Liam McCaughey and Róisin MacSullivan were extern examiners at the MMed (Anaesth) examination in Kuala Lumpur in November.

Cunningham circulated a report from the Liaison Committee (between the faculty and the Royal College of Anaesthetists). Prof. Spence, President of the Royal College of Anaesthetists, had informed the Liaison group that if the Irish faculty was to integrate with the college, the faculty members on the college board would be co-opted members only and would have no voting rights on the council. There was a wide-ranging discussion at the board meeting and the consensus view was that the proposals on offer from the English college were disappointing.

1993

The Delaney Medal competition was held on Friday 5 March. Papers were presented by Drs John R. Darling (Belfast), Éamon McCoy (Belfast), David Hill (Ballymena), Deirdre McCoy (Dublin) and Ann Taylor (Dublin). The winner was David Hill from the Waveney Hospital in Ballymena.

The Annual Scientific Meeting was held on 21 and 22 May. The theme was 'Children and anaesthesia'. Speakers and themes included:

- Mrs Patricia Donnelly, 'Psychological preparation of children for surgery'
- Dr Declan Warde, 'Premedication and induction in children'

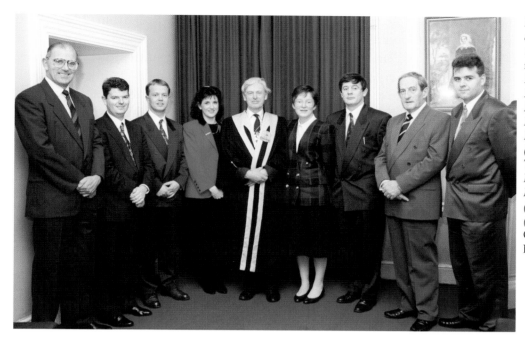

Delaney Medal competition 1993. (Left to right) Keith Lewis (Janssen), David Hill, Eamon McCoy, Deirdre McCoy, Richard Clarke (Dean), Ann Taylor, John Robert Darling, Michael Doherty (Janssen), (unidentified). Courtesy of Bobby Studio.

- Prof. Ronald Miller, 'Muscle relaxants in critical care'
- Dr Peter Crean, 'Management of post-op pain in children'
- Prof. David Hatch, 'Paediatric respiratory physiology'
- Dr Tess Gallagher, 'Management of acute major trauma in children'
- Dr Frances O'Donovan, 'Transport of the critically ill child'

Dr Máire McCarroll coordinated a cardiopulmonary resuscitation workshop.

The seventh Gilmartin Lecture, 'Works of art of medical interest in the National Gallery', was delivered by Mr John Gilmartin, son of the late Prof. Gilmartin. An honorary fellowship was conferred on Ronald Miller from the University of California, San Francisco, and editor of the textbook *Miller's Anaesthesia*.[34]

A joint meeting was held in March between the faculty and the Intensive Care Society of Ireland; the speakers were Drs E. Carton, R. Hone and F. Green. The autumn faculty meeting was held in September at the Royal Dublin Society (RDS) in conjunction with the meeting of the European Society of Regional Anaesthesia; it was organised by Dr James Gardiner and opened by Mary Robinson, President of Ireland. Prof. Philip Bromage gave the Autumn Faculty Lecture titled 'Pain management – masked mischief'. The Winter Faculty Lecture took place in December and was delivered by Prof. Pierre Foëx from Oxford who spoke on 'Silent myocardial ischaemia: a factor of risk'

Seamus Hart, chairman of the Examination Committee, presented new regulations regarding examiners. All anaesthetist examiners would have to be consultants of at least three years' standing in active practice in a substantive post in Ireland or the UK and involved in training anaesthetists. The faculty provided extern examiners in 1993 in Riyadh, London and the University of the West Indies.

The board of faculty also received a document entitled 'Amalgamation of the Royal College of Anaesthetists (RCoA) and the Faculty of Anaesthetists, RCSI' from the Liaison Group working party. It recommended that the faculty take one of three decisions:

1   To accept the amalgamation proposals as they stood
2   To reject the proposals outright and suspend discussions
3   To pursue a number of amendments in negotiation with the RCoA.

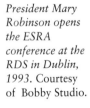

President Mary Robinson opens the ESRA conference at the RDS in Dublin, 1993. Courtesy of Bobby Studio.

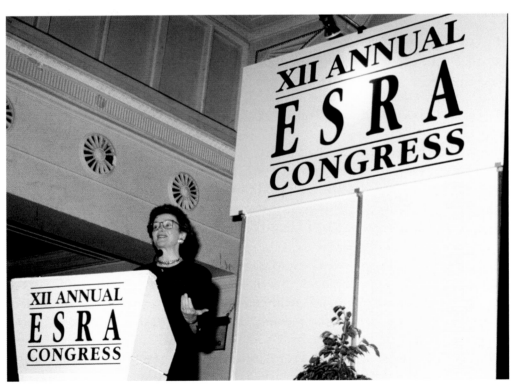

The honorary secretary circulated the report and the recommendations from the Liaison Committee at the March board meeting. It was decided that the proposals from the Royal College were unsatisfactory but it was agreed to keep the lines of communication open. Further meetings took place later between the Liaison Group and Prof. Spence who stated that there would be no financial aid forthcoming and he indicated that there was a time limit on the discussions.

The board received a request from Comhairle on the provision of adolescent and paediatric anaesthetic services. A draft document prepared by MacSullivan and Cunningham was accepted by the board in response to this request.

Cooper highlighted a number of grievances with regard to the financial affairs of the faculty. At a meeting with RCSI in September, the faculty outlined its long-term aspiration to acquire independent headquarters. RCSI pointed out that it hoped to obtain independent degree-conferring status, reiterated the benefits to the faculty of being part of the college and its wish to maintain a cordial relationship. The faculty decided to seek a legal opinion from Mr Dermot Gleeson, senior counsel: (1) to ascertain the status of the faculty within RCSI, (2) to explore the possibility of acquiring a headquarters outside RCSI, and (3) to examine the ability of the faculty to continue the FFA within RCSI. Whereas the board felt that an independent college was not yet realistic, it decided to study the feasibility of purchasing a faculty headquarters. Cooper, Blunnie and Fitzgerald were asked to prepare a feasibility report. The faculty had assets of approximately £250,000 available if it decided to purchase premises.

The interim arrangements for the Conjoint Diploma in Intensive Care Medicine were presented to the board. The diploma could only be awarded to candidates already successful at the fellowship or membership examinations of the Colleges of Surgeons, Physicians or of the Faculty of Anaesthetists, RCSI. There would be an obligatory six months' training period in a recognised intensive care unit. The working party was composed of Gerry Fitzpatrick as chairman, Maura Hainsworth (Faculty), Brian Keogh (RCPI), Gavin Lavery (Intensive Care Society of Ireland) and David Bouchier-Hayes (RCSI). Phelan reported that at the Board of Intensive Care Medicine meeting in November, it had been decided to proceed with the Diploma in Intensive Care Medicine and it was hoped that the first examination would be held at the end of 1994.

The honorary secretary outlined the problems encountered in conducting the elections for the board as being due to deficiencies in the college database of fellows 'in good standing'. The cost of a new computer, server and software that would be needed to rectify the problem would be over £7,000.

An extraordinary general meeting was held on 10 September to discuss the amalgamation proposals vis-à-vis the Royal College of Anaesthetists and to present the board's position. There were heated exchanges and spirited discussion about recent elections to the board of faculty as there was a perceived imbalance in regional representation. As a result of these discussions, new regulations were presented extending the franchise for board elections to 'fellows in good standing' resident overseas. The new regulations also stipulated that fellows in default of their annual subscription would not have the right to nominate candidates nor be permitted to vote.

1994
Dean Dr John Cooper, 1994–7

Mr Dermot O'Flynn, President of RCSI, stated that the council of the college would support the faculty in its wish to purchase a headquarters. It was decided that Blunnie, Cooper and Fitzgerald would draw up a 'Headquarters Finance Programme' in conjunction with Crann Peter & Co., accountants/auditors. Their financial report was presented at an Extraordinary Board Meeting held on 10 April and made a number of recommendations. These included: (1) clarification of the legal/affiliation position with the RCSI, (2) a more consistent method of recording the financial affairs of the faculty, and (3) to establish the precise number of subscription-paying fellows. The honorary treasurer was to obtain a breakdown of examination income/expenditure from RCSI, which was an ongoing bone of contention. It was decided to appoint a membership secretary to audit the faculty database of fellows, to correspond with them and to invoice them for their annual subscription.

The Delaney Medal competition was held on Friday 4 March in the Albert Lecture Theatre, RCSI. Seventeen papers had been submitted of which eight were chosen for presentation. The final eight were presented by Drs David Green, Nuala Cregg, Marie Doyle, James Lyons, Grainne Nicholson, Eleanor O'Leary, Donal Buggy and T.J. Tinder. The medal was awarded to Donal Buggy.

The Annual Scientific Meeting took place on 21 and 22 May. The format was changed with panel discussions/case presentations and free paper sessions on Friday morning followed by lectures in the afternoon. The conferring ceremony took place later in the afternoon followed by the Gilmartin Lecture entitled 'Egyptian medicine' which was given by Prof. John Nunn. On the Saturday, there were refresher courses and workshops.

The autumn faculty meeting was held in the Ulster Folk Museum in Belfast in September. Drs Kevin Milligan spoke on 'Intrathecal clonidine in orthopaedics', Joseph Lee on 'Cerebral blood flow', Jeanne Moriarty on 'Day case anaesthesia' and David O'Flaherty on 'Ambulatory epidurals'. The Winter Faculty Lecture in December was given by Prof. Sir Donald Campbell, titled 'The typhoon of change'.

The Calman Report from the UK and the Tierney Report – 'Medical manpower in acute hospitals – a discussion document' – were presented at the May meeting of the board. The Tierney Report covered the general issues of trainee numbers, the consultant/trainee ratio, specialty training, continuing medical education and certificates of completion of specialist training. The Medical Advisory Committee chairman, MacSullivan, proposed a number of changes in response to the Tierney Report, including the identification of training posts, each post to be numbered with a letter indicating the training programme with which it was associated (e.g. S=southern region, W=western region etc), identification of non-training posts, centralised application for general professional training and recognition of the subspecialties of ICU and pain within anaesthesia. Phelan reported for the Board of Intensive Care Medicine on training developments and recognition of ICUs for training.

At the September board meeting, John Cooper took over as dean from Prof. Richard Clarke. The honorary secretary then presented a draft document, 'A memorandum and articles of association', which proposed incorporating the faculty as a company, the 'Faculty of Anaesthetists, R.C.S.I.'. This was a complex legal affair and required a number of actions to be taken:

(a) Preparation of a draft memorandum and articles of association
(b) Submission of the draft memorandum and articles of association to RCSI council for approval
(c) Submission of the draft memorandum and articles of association to the fellows of the faculty for approval
(d) Acquisition of a licence from the Minister for Industry and Commerce
(e) Execution of the memorandum and articles of association by seven board members
(f) Lodgement of documentation in the Companies Office

Cooper indicated that having had meetings with the RCSI Council and legal representatives, they agreed that they would facilitate the incorporation of the Faculty of Anaesthetists, RCSI.[35]

The board responded to a query from Comhairle on subspecialty recognition

273

by stating that there were four categories of consultant anaesthetist: (1) consultant anaesthetist, (2) consultant anaesthetist/specialist in intensive care medicine, (3) consultant anaesthetist with special interest in intensive care medicine, and (4) consultant anaesthetist with a special interest in pain medicine.

1995

A joint overseas meeting with the Royal College of Surgeons in Ireland took place in Bahrain on 13 March with workshops on trauma (Eleanor O'Leary) and cardiac disease (Róisin MacSullivan and Inder Bali). The Delaney Medal competition also took place in March. John Sear, reader in anaesthesia at Oxford, was the extern judge and the medal was awarded to Dr Jennifer Porter.

The Annual Scientific Meeting on 19 and 20 May covered a number of different topics. The Friday programme commenced with 'Controversies/ Debates', which included 'Rationing ICU services' and 'The pill and orthopaedics'. The afternoon session was on 'Total intravenous anaesthesia'. The Saturday workshop was on 'Regional anaesthesia' and the Saturday refresher course covered 'Newer inotropic agents', 'Neonatal emergencies' and 'The epidural space revisited'. An honorary fellowship was conferred on Prof. David Morrell, University of Witwatersrand, South Africa. Fellowships by election were conferred on Dr Angela Enright, the first female president of the Canadian Anaesthetists Society, and on Dr Richard Seed, from Riyadh. The eleventh Gilmartin Lecture was given by Prof. Seamus Heaney, Boylston Professor, Harvard University, entitled 'The operation of poetry'.

The autumn faculty meeting on 'Contemporary trends in obstetrical anaesthesia' was held in the Rotunda Hospital in September and was followed by the Autumn Lecture delivered by Dr Anthony Rubin from Charing Cross Hospital on 'Anaesthesia for ophthalmic surgery'. The Winter Faculty Lecture took place in December and was given by Dr Maldwyn Morgan from the Hammersmith Hospital, London, who spoke on 'How to get a paper published'.

The Medical Council informed the board of the proposal to establish a register of medical specialists and requested that the faculty clarify the criteria required of a person completing specialist training in Ireland. The 'criteria for inclusion on the specialist register' agreed by the faculty were: (1) a primary medical qualification, (2) possession of a specialist qualification by examination in anaesthesia which is recognised as equivalent to the FFARCSI, and (3) to have completed a structured training programme comparable to that of the possessors of the Certificate of Completion of Specialist Training.

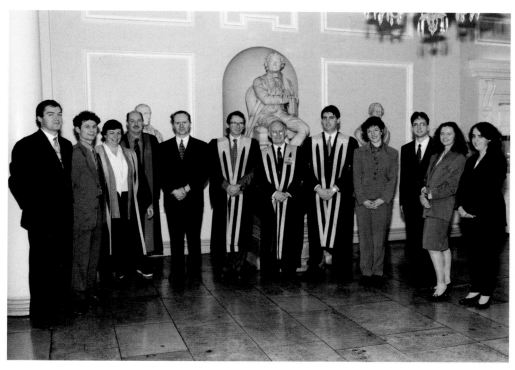

Delaney Medal competition 1996. (Left to right) Dermot Kelly, Jimmy Lyons, Carlos McDowell, Nigel Webster, John Browne, Liam McCaughey, John Cooper (Dean), Frank Chambers, (Unidentified), David O'Gorman, Nuala Cregg, Fidelma Kirby. Courtesy of Bobby Studio.

Arising from this, the board established a Credentials Committee to consider requests for inclusion on the specialist register.[36] The board adopted new training requirements for the specialty; basic specialist training would be for two years, followed by senior (specialist) training of four years' duration. Fee informed the board that the examination for the fellowship would revert to a two-part exam, commencing in September 1996. It was also proposed that an Objective Structured Clinical Examination (OSCE) would be introduced into the Part 1 examination. There was controversy over the decision to reduce the training requirement for the Final fellowship examination from 36 months to 30 months and the effect this had on reciprocity with other colleges. A new three-year contract was agreed with the Riyadh armed forces hospital with the faculty providing courses and examinations until 1997.

An extraordinary general meeting of the faculty was held on Friday 8 September at which the Memorandum and Articles of Association – Incorporation of a Company – were presented and approved by the fellows of the faculty. On 12 October 1995, the Council of RCSI approved the Memorandum and Articles of Association submitted by the faculty and also approved the licence agreement between RCSI and the faculty. At the board meeting in December, the Memorandum and Articles were signed by the seven founder board members who then became the directors of the new company. The seven founding members were:

- Dr John Cooper, Dean
- Prof. Anthony J. Cunningham, Honorary Secretary
- Dr William P. Blunnie, Honorary Treasurer
- Prof. J.P. Howard Fee, Chairman Examination Committee
- Dr G. Carlos McDowell, Chairman Education Committee
- Dr Róisín MacSullivan, Chairman Medical Advisory Committee
- Dr William McCaughey
-

Mr Philip Curtis recorded the signing ceremony for the faculty archives. Copies of the Memorandum and Articles of Association were forwarded to the Department of Enterprise and Employment and another copy was lodged in the company's office.

1996
The Delaney Medal competition was held on 1 March and was won by Dr Fidelma Kirby for her paper 'Permissive hypercapnic ventilation'. The event was facilitated by Janssen-Cilag. The Annual Scientific Meeting took place on Friday 17 and Saturday 18 May. Speakers on the Friday included Drs Gavin Lavery (Belfast), Kate Flynn (Dublin), Patrick Benson (Dublin), Declan Warde (Dublin), John Cahill (Cork), Prof. John Kampine (USA) and Mike Harmer (UK). The Saturday morning refresher course included:

- Prof. John Kampine (USA), 'Risks in anaesthesia for the hypertensive patient'
- Dr Mary Bowen (Dublin), 'Update on eclampsia'
- Dr Brian Kavanagh (Canada), 'Acute respiratory failure'
- Dr Niall Hughes (Dublin), 'Carotid endartectomy'
- Dr Michael Harmer (Wales), 'Post-operative nausea and vomiting'

Other speakers on Saturday were Drs John McAdoo (Cork), Tom Schnittger (Dublin), Kevin McKeating (Dublin), James Murray (Belfast) and Peter Farling (Belfast). An honorary fellowship was conferred on Prof. John William Hall, professor of physiology at UCC and the 12th Gilmartin Lecture was delivered by Prof. Mary McAleese, professor of law at Queen's University Belfast.

The autumn faculty meeting took place in September. The speakers were Drs Robert Darling (Belfast), Gary McCleane (Craigavon), Michael Carey (Dublin) and Gerry Coughlan (Galway). The Winter Faculty Lecture was given by Dr Sheila Watts, entitled 'Clinical guidelines'.

The inaugural meeting of the company limited by guarantee, the 'Faculty of Anaesthetists, R.C.S.I.' took place on 21 June 1996 in the dean's room, RCSI. The registered office of the new company was Messrs Hayes and Sons, solicitors, 15 St Stephen's Green, North, Dublin 2. Blunnie opened a bank account in the name of the new company.

Prof. Fee outlined new guidelines for the appointment of examiners. A mock OSCE exam was held in September. It was decided to use trained actors for the OSCE and Mr Fintan Foy of the RCSI examination office stated that this would cost approximately £800 per examination. Overseas examinations were again held in Riyadh.

A register of medical specialists was to commence in January 1997. The board wrote to the Medical Council requesting that the specialty should be called 'Anaesthesia' and not 'Anaesthetics' and asked that both pain management and intensive care medicine should be included under the specialty.[37] It was noted that the board of the faculty should be the recognised body for training. The new Primary examination took place in October and McCaughey presented the results. The overall pass rate was 36 per cent although the new OSCE had a pass rate of 86 per cent.

1997

Dean Dr William P. Blunnie, 1997–8

Prof. Peter Hutton (Birmingham) was extern adjudicator at the annual Delaney Medal competition which was won by Dr C. Renfrew for his paper titled 'A new method of carbon dioxide absorption for low-flow anaesthesia'. The Annual Scientific Meeting took place on Friday and Saturday, 16 and 17 May, followed by the 38th anniversary dinner on the Saturday night. Prof. Cedric Prys-Roberts was conferred with an honorary fellowship, and Hainsworth read his citation. The 13th Gilmartin Lecture 'The University Bill 1996' was given by Dr Art Cosgrove, president of University College Dublin. The Abbott endowments for 1997 were awarded to five candidates, Drs Áine Ní Chonchubhair, Kai Rabenstein, Jacinta McGinley, Harry Frizelle and Geraldine O'Leary. The autumn meeting was held in conjunction with the Royal Victoria Eye and Ear Hospital in September and Prof. Kathy McGoldrick delivered the Autumn Faculty Lecture.

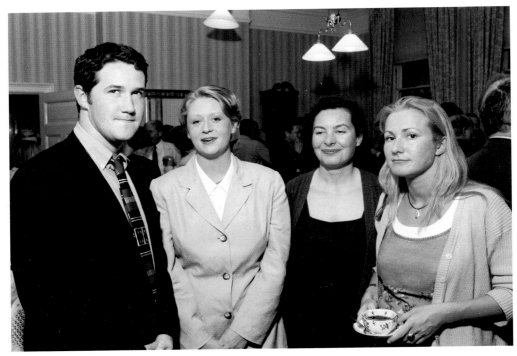

Prof. James Eisenkraft, Mount Sinai Medical Centre, New York delivered the Winter Faculty Lecture on 'Complications of anaesthesia delivery systems'.

The board instituted a new training committee commencing on 1 January 1997. Membership included representatives from the board, the Association of Anaesthetists of Great Britain and Ireland, the Department of Health, the Royal College of Anaesthetists, hospitals, pain management and intensive care medicine and a non-consultant hospital doctor (NCHD). The function of the committee would include establishing the required number of specialist registrars and making recommendations to the board regarding inclusion on the specialist register.[38]

The Medical Council had established the Register of Medical Specialists and the faculty was recognised as the authority to assess the anaesthetic training of applicants for the Certificate of Completion of Specialist Training (CCST). The Training Committee would supervise the programme and issue these certificates. Its inaugural meeting took place in August and was attended by Dr W. MacRae representing the Royal College of Anaesthetists (RCoA). The committee decided that logbooks would be mandatory for both Basic Specialty and specialist registrar (SpR) trainees and it was agreed that a research period of up to six months would be recognised for training. There were 209 approved training posts in anaesthesia with 45 unapproved posts and there were 29 SpR posts but the dean, Blunnie, felt that the establishment of the latter should be 80 to meet future needs.

Moriarty and Fee had meetings with Queen's University Belfast investigating the possibility of instituting a simulator centre for the teaching of anaesthesia. A committee was set up by the board to oversee the acquisition of a simulator.

The dean informed the board at the September meeting that he had written to Prof. Kevin O'Malley, registrar at RCSI, regarding changing the title from the 'Faculty of Anaesthetists, R.C.S.I.' to the 'College of Anaesthetists, R.C.S.I.'. This change in title was accepted by RCSI later in the year. Cooper then welcomed Mr Peter McLean, President of RCSI to the meeting before handing over the chain of office to the incoming dean, William Blunnie. The new dean informed the board that on 4 July 1997, the faculty had been granted charitable status by the Revenue Commissioners and now had its own seal.

Cunningham produced a document on 'Criteria for Hospital Educational Approval' including references to intensive care medicine and pain management. This was approved and circulated to regional training committees. MacSullivan presented a report, 'Feasibility study projection re purchasing premises for the Faculty of Anaesthetists', in which it was stated that at least 7,000 square feet would be needed. A number of auctioneers had been retained in the search for suitable premises. The chairman of the Credentials Committee, Fitzgerald, reported that the Medical Council had changed the nomenclature in that it would now maintain a 'Register of Medical Specialists' and would issue a 'Certificate of Specialist Doctor'.

Further discussions took place regarding accreditation and training in intensive care medicine. Correspondence was tabled from Dr Declan O'Keeffe on the development of a training programme and diploma in pain management.

1998

Dr W. MacRae of Edinburgh, past president of the Association of Anaesthetists of Great Britain and Ireland, was conferred with an honorary fellowship at the Annual Scientific Meeting. The Gilmartin Lecture was given by Ms Pauline Marrinan Quinn, entitled 'What is an ombudsman?'

The following amendments to the Articles of Association of the Faculty of Anaesthetists, RCSI were agreed by the fellows of the faculty at the AGM held on Saturday 16 May 1998:

(a) To change the name 'Faculty of Anaesthetists' to 'College of Anaesthetists'

(b) To substitute 'Board of the Faculty' with 'Council of the College'
(c) To replace 'Dean of Faculty' with 'President of the College'
(d) To replace 'Vice-Dean' with 'Vice-President'
(e) To insert 'Intensive Care Medicine' and 'Pain Management' as faculties

Phelan, chairman of the Finance and General Purposes Committee, reported that all investments held by RCSI on behalf of the faculty would be transferred to faculty accounts. This figure was approximately £145,000. The faculty (later the college) would be registered for PAYE and PRSI and would employ its own staff. MacSullivan presented an outline guide, 'College of Anaesthetists proposed premises – Draft Budgetary outline'. It was agreed that space would be needed to hold the Delaney Medal competition as well as the autumn and winter meetings. Phelan reported back from the Board of Intensive Care Medicine that the first Diploma in Intensive Care (DIBICM) examination had taken place on Wednesday 10 June 1998 at St Vincent's Hospital. There were 11 candidates of whom nine were successful.

The board discussed a memorandum from the Department of Health on a proposed sub-consultant grade. There was unequivocal rejection of this concept by the board members. It was agreed that Basic Specialist Training would be run at regional level under the supervision of the Training Committee but the SpR rotation would be a national scheme with trainees being rotated throughout the country. Cooper, past dean, agreed to be the convenor of a meeting of interested parties to establish a diploma in pain management under the auspices of the faculty. The dean reported that he and MacSullivan, Phelan, Howe, Cooper and Moriarty were continuing to examine various properties throughout the city as potential premises for the faculty/college.

Prof. Mary McAleese, President of Ireland, was conferred with an honorary fellowship by William Blunnie, first president of the College of Anaesthetists of Ireland, on 23 September 1998. This is now taken as the foundation day of the college.[39]

The motto for the coat of arms, 'Salus dum vigilamus', was agreed with the deputy herald following a meeting with Blunnie and Phelan. Pat Fitzgerald also had an input into the design. The college was granted its coat of arms by the Heraldic Office in December 1999. The specialty had finally become independent, 151 years after MacDonnell gave the first anaesthetic in Ireland. A short time later, in 2000, the new college would finally leave RCSI to move to its own premises at 22 Merrion Square.

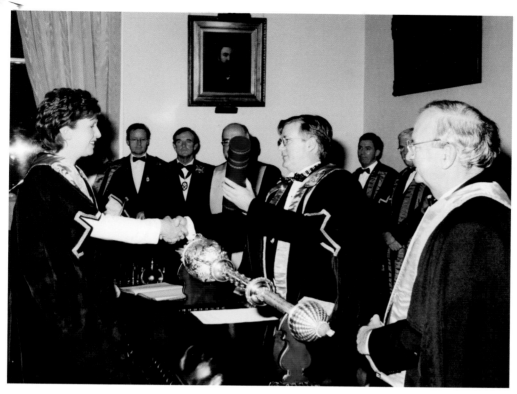

President Mary McAleese is conferred as the first Honorary Fellow of the College of Anaesthetists of Ireland by William Blunnie on 23 September 1998.
Courtesy of Bobby Studio.

References

1   Faculty of Anaesthetists, RCSI, Minute Book 2, 1970–4, p. 10.
2   *Ibid.*, p. 11.
3   *Ibid.*, p. 9.
4   *Ibid.*, p. 36.
5   *Ibid.*, p. 30.
6   *Ibid.*, p. 34.
7   *Ibid.*, p.39.
8   *Ibid.*, p. 47.
9   Richmond C. 'Bjorn Ibsen', *British Medical Journal*, 2007, 335, p. 674.
10   Faculty of Anaesthetists, RCSI, Book 2, 1970–4, p. 74.
11   *Ibid.*, p. 89.
12   *Ibid.*, pp. 94–5.
13   *Ibid.*, p. 96.
14   Faculty of Anaesthetists, RCSI, Minute Book 3, pp. 303–4.
15   *Ibid.*, p. 331.
16   *Ibid.*, p. 346.
17   *Ibid.*, p. 348.
18   *Ibid.*, pp. 414, 419.
19   *Ibid.*, p. 410.

20 Spence A.A., Editorial. 'European Academy of Anaesthesiology' *British Journal of Anaesthesia*, 1978, 50, pp. 1171–2.

21 Faculty of Anaesthetists, RCSI, Minute Book 3, p. 447.

22 *Ibid.* p. 459.

23 *Ibid.*, p. 506.

24 *Ibid.*, p. 513.

25 *Ibid.*, p. 523.

26 Faculty of Anaesthetists, RCSI, Minute Book 4, p. 569.

27 Faculty of Anaesthetists, Extracts from annual report, RCSI (1983–4).

28 *Ibid.* (1984/1985).

29 Faculty of Anaesthetists, Minute Book 4, p. 635.

30 *Ibid.*, p. 653.

31 *Ibid.*, p. 657.

32 Minutes of the Board of the Faculty, meeting 11 March 1988, p. 4.

33 Minutes of the Board of the Faculty, 17 May 1991, Book 4, p. 1.

34 *Ibid.*, Board meeting, September 1992, p. 5.

35 *Ibid.*, Board meeting, September 1994.

36 *Ibid.*, Board minutes, 1995.

37 *Ibid.*, Board minutes, December 1996, p. 2.

38 *Ibid.*, Board minute, March 1997, p. 3.

39 *Ibid.*, Board minutes, May 1998.

Chapter 20

The Western Anaesthetic Symposium (1979)*

John Cahill

The Western Anaesthetic Symposium is the flagship of academic anaesthetic meetings in the west of Ireland, the first of which was held in spring 1979 at University College Galway (UCG). It quickly became established as an annual event in the anaesthetic calendar.

Galway, the 'City of the Tribes', with its unique history and charm, had much to offer as a venue for the launch of a new anaesthetic meeting but its distance from other major cities, Dublin, Belfast and Cork, could well have been a disadvantage. The reverse, in fact, turned out to be the case as the meeting quickly gained a reputation not just for the excellence of the academic programmes but for the accompanying hospitality and the unique settings in some of the most beautiful locations in the west of Ireland.

While the organisation of such academic events requires a team effort, one name, that of Padraic Keane, is synonymous with this particular one, and rightly so.

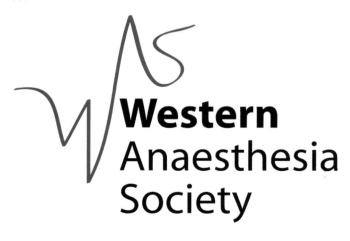

The Western Anaesthesia Symposium and the Western Anaesthesia Society

Padraic Keane was born in Oranmore, a short distance from Galway city. He graduated MB BCh BAO from UCG in 1960 and trained in anaesthesia at the Manchester Royal Infirmary (UK), Galway Regional Hospital (now University College Hospital Galway) and at the University of Boston, Massachusetts. He returned to his native city in 1970 to take up an appointment as consultant anaesthetist with responsibility for anaesthetic services at Galway Regional Hospital.

Despite the heavy clinical workload and the energy expended in developing the anaesthetic department, Padraic Keane understood the need for a regional anaesthetic forum, and in 1979, with the help of likeminded colleagues, his aspiration became a reality. The first meetings were held at UCG or at Galway Regional Hospital but very soon the meeting venues reflected the beauty and charm of Connemara and beyond. Arguably the most notable of these was Ballynahinch Castle. This sixteenth-century castle set on the banks of the Ballynahinch salmon river has been the home of the O'Flaherty Chieftains, the legendary renegade princess Grace O'Malley, Richard Martin MP (also known as Humanity Dick in recognition of his work as an animal rights campaigner or Trigger Dick because of his feats as a duellist!!) and the Maharajah Ranjitsinji. Tucked away in exquisite surroundings, delegates, their spouses, invited speakers and trade exhibitors all experienced the hospitality and warm welcome that characterised Padraic Keane and his wife Bernie. Trainees were especially welcome and the Registrars' Prize competition was an essential part of the meeting. The event, which quickly became known as 'the Galway Meeting' was hugely successful and acted as a perfect counterpoint to the Annual Scientific Meeting of the (then) Faculty of Anaesthetists, RCSI in Dublin.

From the outset, the list of speakers had an international flavour, with renowned clinicians from North America, Britain and mainland Europe contributing to the programme. This, of course, proved to be a great boost in establishing the symposium on a firm footing and was due in no small part to Padraic Keane's personal charm, communication skills and the many contacts that he had built up while training overseas. Notwithstanding his ability to attract speakers from abroad, Padraic Keane was always conscious of the expertise and talent to be found on his own doorstep at UCG and from the hospital medical and surgical staff, and there were regular contributions from the Departments of Physiology and Anatomy at UCG and from the Departments of Medicine and Surgery at Galway Regional Hospital.

The educational reach of the symposium was much broader than the weekend of the meeting. Trainees at all levels were encouraged to engage in research projects in the knowledge that the 'Galway Meeting' was a welcoming forum for them to present their work. In 1983, an exchange programme between the Department of Anaesthesia at Galway Regional Hospital and the Department of Anesthesiology at the Milwaukee Medical Centre, Wisconsin was established. It afforded opportunities for scientific research and clinical practice to anaesthetic trainees on both sides of the Atlantic and many research papers arising from the exchange programme have been presented in Galway.

In 2003, the O'Beirne and Costello Gold Medal competitions were established in recognition of Dr Peter O'Beirne (1943–1992) and Dr Joseph Costello (1938–1998). The O'Beirne Medal was awarded for the best oral presentation and the Costello Medal for the best poster. Joseph Costello and Peter O'Beirne were close friends and colleagues of Padraic Keane's at Galway Regional Hospital and had played a major role in establishing the annual symposium.

Serious and intense though the academic sessions at these may have been, they were never bereft of humour or the occasional light-hearted distraction. Padraic Keane's knowledge and love of horseracing was well known and serves as an example of his ability to accommodate diverse subjects to the mutual benefit of all. The usual date of the symposium was in early April, which, of course, coincided with the running of the Aintree Grand National. These two events were never considered in any way incompatible, so that when the need arose, events at Liverpool were simply 'incorporated' as part of the scientific programme by means of a large screen wheeled to the rostrum, the traditional draw for the sweepstake made, while the gravelly tones of (the late) Peter O'Sullevan, 'the voice of racing', described the fortunes and misfortunes of the horses as they negotiated the fences at Aintree. Not surprisingly, the Saturday afternoon session was always well attended and many a guest speaker was surprised and enthralled. The genuine affection and loyalty which Padraic Keane engendered is perhaps best demonstrated by the unique 'record' held by Dr John Cooper (Belfast) of having attended every single Western Anaesthetic Symposium from its inception in 1979 until 2019.

By the time Padraic Keane retired from clinical practice in 2001, the meeting was firmly established as an annual event of the highest academic standard and unique hospitality, and its success was guaranteed by a cohort of young consultants who had been appointed in the intervening years. The number of consultants in the Department of Anaesthesia at University College Hospital, Galway had increased fourfold – the increase in trainee numbers was even greater

– and many of these consultants had completed part of their training in Galway and subsequently taken part in exchange programmes with American universities.

To the fore in this regard was Dr Noel Flynn, who with the help of a small number of committed fellow consultants, ushered the symposium into the new millennium. Flynn is a graduate of UCG and worked as a research fellow under the guidance of Prof. John Kampine at the Milwaukee Medical Centre, Wisconsin. He was appointed as a consultant anaesthetist at University College Hospital, Galway, initially as a locum in 1992 and then permanently in 1994 and he became the driving force behind the meeting when Padraic Keane relinquished the reins.

In 2011, the Western Anaesthesia Society came into being with the Western Anaesthetic Symposium as its Annual Scientific Meeting. The society continues the work of representing the professional, educational and medico-political needs of anaesthetists, intensivists and pain physicians in the west of Ireland.

Chapter 21

The Intensive Care Society of Ireland (1987)*

John Cahill

The Intensive Care Society of Ireland (ICSI) was founded on 20 June 1987 at the Royal College of Surgeons in Ireland (RCSI) following a critical care meeting held earlier that day at the same venue.

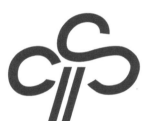

Intensive Care Society of Ireland

The Intensive Care Society of Ireland.

The broad objectives of the new society were to develop a unified approach to the subject of intensive care medicine in Ireland, to develop clinical standards and to establish formal training and education for clinicians wishing to specialise in the discipline. Interim officers were agreed (chairman, vice chairman, honorary secretary, honorary treasurer and trainee representative) and a submission was made to the Healthcare Funding Commission advocating the reorganisation of healthcare provision to accommodate and develop the subspecialty.

The Annual Scientific Meeting of 1988, also held in RCSI, was followed by the first AGM and the officers and council members were formally approved. Dr Dermot Phelan was elected president, Dr Gavin Lavery became vice president, Dr Ron Kirkham was made honorary secretary, and Dr Gerry Fitzpatrick became honorary treasurer. The new council members included Drs Gerry Dorrian, Inder Bali, Carlos McDowell, Prof. Denis Moriarty, Dr Ed Major, president of the

Intensive Care Society, United Kingdom (ICS UK, co-opted), Ms Catherine Guihen, Irish Association of Critical Care Nurses (IACCN) representative and Dr Mary White, trainee representative.

In 1983, ICS (UK) held its Annual Scientific Meeting in Dun Laoghaire on the invitation of the medical faculty of Trinity College. The local organising team was led by Ron Kirkham. Sponsorship by pharmaceutical companies and medical device suppliers was organised, and support also came from members of the Technical Committee of the Electro-Technical Council of Ireland – the body which until 2018, advised the Irish government on standards and regulations for all medical electrical devices. The meeting was a resounding success, with over 400 delegates from Ireland, the UK and further afield attending, making it, at the time, the largest ICU conference held in these islands. The conference concluded with a gala dinner held in the dining hall in Trinity College with entertainment provided by the College Singers.

In 1986, the IACCN was founded in order to promote the art and science of critical care nursing. The association is a not-for-profit organisation representing critical care nurses across Ireland and has a clear vision, mission statement and set of objectives.[1]

Celebrating the 30th anniversary of the ICSI at a joint meeting with the Northern Ireland Intensive Care Society in Belfast in 2017, Dermot Phelan recalled the society's early days and noted what a momentous year 1987 had been – Ireland won the Eurovision song contest, Stephen Roche won the Tour de France, but there was tragedy too with the massacre at the Cenotaph in Enniskillen where 11 people lost their lives.

Reviewing the intensive care landscape in Ireland prior to 1987, Dr Phelan noted that intensive care facilities developed slowly during the 1950s, largely in support of open heart surgery but also certain acute medical conditions such as tetanus and poliomyelitis.[2] Reports of mitral valvotomy and surgery for coarctation of the aorta in Ireland began to appear in the literature in the early 1950s.[3-5] The first mitral valvotomy at the Mater Misericordiae Hospital in Dublin was carried out in 1956 and in order to facilitate the medical and nursing care required, two beds (the forerunners of what would now be termed intensive care beds) were later designated for use by postoperative cardiac surgical patients.

---

*This account is based largely on a presentation made by Dr Dermot Phelan in Belfast on 7 June 2017 to mark the 30th anniversary of the ICSI. It describes some aspects of the history of the ICSI until the early 2000s, when the College of Anaesthetists of Ireland moved into its new home at 22 Merrion Square North, Dublin.

A respiratory failure unit with two beds opened at the Royal Victoria Hospital Belfast in 1961 and by 1971, the unit had expanded to 11 beds.[1]

In the mid- and late-1970s, the Faculty of Anaesthetists, RCSI established three regional anaesthetic training schemes and the National Senior Registrar Training Scheme, and intensive care medicine became part of the syllabus for the Final fellowship examination. As the clinical and teaching demands of the developing specialty increased, individual consultants with a particular interest in this area began to take a leading role and this group of clinicians became the prime movers in establishing an organisation that could promote and advocate on behalf of intensive care medicine. There were practical problems, however. Intensive care sessions were not recognised as part of a consultant's contractual workload and therefore not remunerated, nor was there a mechanism for receiving payment for patients with private health insurance treated in an intensive care unit (ICU). These issues only began to be addressed with the introduction and subsequent refinement of the Consultants' Common Contract, first introduced in 1981, recognition by Comhairle na nOspidéal of the post of consultant anaesthetist with special interest in intensive care in 1995[6] and prolonged negotiations between the Irish Standing Committee of the Association of Anaesthetists of Great Britain and Ireland (AAGBI) and the Voluntary Health Insurance Board (VHI).

From the outset, the newly founded ICSI immediately set about organising a spring meeting, an Annual Scientific Meeting (ASM) in the summer with speakers from renowned ICUs abroad, and an autumn (out-of-town) meeting. There were also twice-yearly refresher courses held in the spring and autumn for those preparing for exams. An advisory committee on training in intensive care medicine was also set up in conjunction with the Faculty of Anaesthetists, RCSI. At the third ICSI Annual Scientific Meeting held in the King's Hall, Belfast, the society crest was agreed following a competition – the winning design was submitted by Dr Colette Pegum, a consultant anaesthetist at the Royal Victoria Eye and Ear Hospital, Dublin. In 1989, ICSI became affiliated to the World Federation of Societies of Intensive and Critical Care Medicine (WFSICCM) and the first ICSI news bulletin appeared in 1990.

Despite early progress, the society experienced a number of practical difficulties, not least of which was the lack of a permanent headquarters. In those early days, 'Head Office' was variously located in the Anaesthetic Department or the intensive care unit at the Mater Misericordiae Hospital (Dublin), or a number of other Dublin addresses, including the College of Anaesthetists of

Ireland and the Royal Academy of Medicine in Ireland.

Venues for business and council meetings of the society also proved a challenge as council members worked at locations all over Ireland. This challenge, however, had a hugely positive effect as it helped to foster the concept of island-wide membership and representation which is now one of the guiding principles of the society. Council meetings were held at the home of Dr Carlos McDowell in Baltray and at the Ballymascanlon House Hotel, both in County Louth. Nowadays mobile phones, the internet and facilities to conference call have made the task of organising council and business meetings infinitely easier. None of these facilities was available in the early days of ICSI, so important meetings almost always had to be face-to-face.

The out-of-town meetings quickly became fixtures in ICSI's calendar and within half a dozen years, the society had visited Castlebar, Craigavon, Ballymena, Belfast, Galway, Kinsale and Waterford. The ICSI meeting in Kilkenny in 1991 included a wide-ranging discussion on the subject of the transport of critically ill patients with contributions from ambulance personnel, ICU nurses and clinicians from a wide range of specialties. The result was the publication in 1994 of the report 'Transport of the Critically Ill'.[7] which was presented to the then Minister for Health, Brendan Howlin TD, and which led directly to the introduction of the Mobile Intensive Care Ambulance Service (MICAS) in 1996.

The 1994 ASM of the society held in Killiney Castle, County Dublin a joint meeting with ICS (UK) and representatives of both societies were invited to Áras an Uachtaráin as guests of Mrs Mary Robinson, President of Ireland.

Also in 1994, the Irish Board of Intensive Care Medicine (IBICM) came into being; it was given the responsibility of organising formal training and accreditation in intensive care. The IBICM was an intercollegiate entity and was set up after extensive discussions between ICSI, the Faculty of Anaesthetists, RCSI, RCSI itself and the Royal College of Physicians of Ireland (RCPI). The first chairman of the new IBICM was Dr Dermot Phelan.

The initial examination for the Diploma of the Irish Board of Intensive Care Medicine (DIBICM), under the Conjoint Board of the Royal College of Physicians of Ireland and the Royal College of Surgeons in Ireland (RCP & SI) was held in 1996. There were five successful candidates.

Since then, the Joint Faculty of Intensive Care Medicine of Ireland (JFICMI) has replaced the IBICM with Brian Marsh as the first dean.[8,9]

Promoting formal training and accreditation in intensive care medicine was one of the first stated objectives of the ICSI, and anaesthesia trainees were quick to acknowledge the importance of the new society in this regard. The first Annual Scientific Meeting of the Anaesthetists in Training in Ireland (ATI), held at University College Cork in October 1987, was devoted to the topic of intensive care with contributions from Dr Dermot Phelan, Dr Declan Warde, Prof. Anthony J. Cunningham and guest lecturer Prof. Hugh Seeley, St George's Hospital, London. Two-month training modules in intensive care medicine were introduced in 1994 by IBICM and by the time the first Diploma in Intensive Care Medicine examination was held in 1996, 13 ICUs, including those in the Royal Victoria Hospital, Belfast and Belfast City Hospital had been accredited for training; six months' training in intensive care was a prerequisite for entering the exam. Over time, training modules in the specialty were made available to postgraduate medical and surgical non-consultant hospital doctors (NCHDs) and in 2011, the option for newly qualified medical graduates to rotate through intensive care during their intern year was introduced and has become extremely popular.

The first Kate Flynn Prize competition was held at the society's 1998 autumn meeting in Galway in commemoration of Dr Kate Flynn whose career as a consultant at Beaumont Hospital was cruelly cut short by her untimely death in 1997. Family members including Kate's father, travelled from Kerry to attend the inaugural medal competition, lending a particular poignancy to the first Kate Flynn Prize presentation. As a trainee, Kate had been a speaker at the first ASM of ICSI and subsequently trained in intensive care medicine in Australia. The winner of the inaugural Kate Flynn Prize was Dr Michael Scully, a trainee anaesthetist at the Mater Misericordiae Hospital, Dublin with a presentation entitled 'Activated Protein C and meningococcal sepsis – do we have the solution?'

Over the years, many other Irish trainees worked in Australia with the result that the development of training in intensive care medicine in Ireland at all levels was hugely influenced by experience gained in, and the continuing link with that country – initially with the Faculty of Anaesthetists of the Royal Australasian College of Surgeons (FARACS) and later by the College of Intensive Care Medicine of Australia and New Zealand (CICM–ANZ). Kate Flynn was an exceptional doctor with a strong personality whose great passion was the welfare of her critical care patients. Hence the decision to hold a premium case report competition to recognise her major contribution to intensive care medicine and to honour her memory.

Dermot Phelan MB FFARCSI, FJFICMI, FCICM (ANZ), Dip Med Management
Dermot Phelan was educated at the Franciscan College, Gormanston and attended medical school at University College Galway graduating MB, BCh, BAO in 1974. He completed his intern year in Queensland, Australia at the Alexandra Hospital, Brisbane. The intern year included a module in anaesthesia and intensive care which was quite novel at the time, and this proved to be the spark that ignited a career-long commitment to intensive care medicine which had an enormous effect on the development of the specialty in Ireland, and on the careers of numerous young trainees.

Dr Dermot Phelan

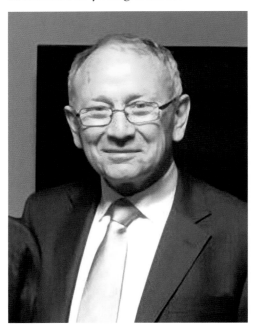

He began training in anaesthesia at the Royal Perth Hospital, Western Australia in 1977 and returned to Ireland in late 1978 to complete anaesthesia training and gained the Fellowship of the Faculty of Anaesthetists, RCSI (FFARCSI) in 1979. He trained in intensive care medicine at the Flinders Medical Centre, Adelaide from 1980 to 1983 and was then appointed as a fellow at the Royal Children's Hospital Melbourne in 1984 before returning to the Mater Misericordiae Hospital, Dublin as a consultant anaesthetist in 1985.

During a career spanning more than 30 years, Dermot Phelan played a leading role in helping to have intensive care medicine in Ireland recognised as a specialty in its own right, and in establishing internationally recognised training rotations, examinations and accreditation for intensive care medicine.

He was instrumental in setting up the Intensive Care Society of Ireland (ICSI) and was its founding president. He was member of Council of the Intensive Care Society (UK) and was the first chairman of the Irish Board of Intensive Care Medicine (IBICM). He was dean of the Joint Faculty of Intensive Care Medicine (JFICMI), chairman of the Management Committee of the Mobile Intensive Care Ambulance Service (MICAS) and specialty editor for the *Irish Journal of Medical Science*.

As a council member of the European Society of Intensive Care Medicine (ESICM), he was chair of Professional Development, served on the Executive and Finance Committees, was editor in chief of Patient-centred Acute Care Training (PACT), the ESICM Multidisciplinary Distance Learning Programme for Intensive Care Doctors, and chair of the European Diploma in Intensive Care Medicine.

During the critical period between 1995 and 2001, when the Faculty of Anaesthetists was preparing to become an independent college, Dermot Phelan was a member of the board of faculty and later a member of the council for the new college, serving as vice president, treasurer, chairman of the Examination & Accreditation Committees and as an examiner in the fellowship exam.

In 2006, he was awarded the President's Medal of the College of Anaesthetists of Ireland for services to the faculty and college and for his distinguished contribution to the development of anaesthesia and intensive care medicine in Ireland. He retired from full-time clinical practice in 2015 but continues to contribute to the work of the JFICMI.

Presidents of the Intensive Care Society of Ireland	Year elected
Dr Dermot Phelan	1987
Dr Gavin Lavery	1990
Dr Gerry Fitzpatrick	1992
Dr Jeanne Moriarty	1994
Dr Ken Lowry	1996
Dr Kieran Crowley	1998

References

1 Irish Association of Critical Care Nurses, 'Vision, Mission, Aims & Objectives', available at iaccn.ie (accessed 30 June 2021).
2 Dundee J.W., 'The last of the fifty – a time for change', *Ulster Medical Journal*, 1986, 55, pp. 15–22.
3 O'Farrell T.P, Brennan P., Mulcahy R., et al., 'The surgery of mitral stenosis', *Irish Journal of Medical Science*, 1951, 26, pp. 193–210.
4 O'Connell T.C.J. and Mulcahy R., 'Emergency mitral valvotomy at full term. A report of a case', *British Medical Journal*, 1955, 1, pp. 1191–2.
5 Gearty G.F., 'Some Highlights of the Half Century', The Irish Cardiac Society 1949–1999, available at https://www.irishcardiacsociety.com/pages/page_box_contents.asp?pageid=

879&navcatid=293 (accessed 30 June 2021).

6   'Comhairle na nOspidéal seventh report: August 1992 to June 1995 Appendix C', available at http://hdl.handle.net/10147/82116 (accessed 30 June 2021).

7   'Report on Transport of the Critically Ill', Intensive Care Society of Ireland, 1994.

8   'Memorandum and Articles of Association, Joint Faculty of Intensive Care Medicine of Ireland', available at https://jficmi.anaesthesia.ie/wp-ontent/uploads/2019/06/JFICMI-MaAA-2019.pdf (accessed 30 June 2021).

9   'New legal/financial (governance) status for Joint Faculty', available at https://jficmi.anaesthesia.ie/news/new-legal-financial-governance-status-for-joint-faculty/ (accessed 30 June 2021).

Chapter 22

The Development of Academic Departments

Joseph Tracey

The first professor of anaesthesia anywhere in the world was Dr Ralph Milton Waters at the University of Wisconsin who was appointed to the Medical Faculty in 1927 and became full professor in 1933. He stated that his intentions were four-fold: to provide the best service to patients, to teach anaesthesia to medical students, to train postgraduate doctors in administering anaesthetics and to carry out research.[1] The first chair to be endowed was the Henry Isaiah Dorr chair of research and teaching in anaesthetics and anaesthesia at Harvard University, Boston in 1917 but the post wasn't filled until 1941 when Henry Beecher was appointed.[2] As an aside, Ed Lowenstein has claimed that Isaiah Dorr himself was the first person to hold the title of professor of anaesthesia when, in 1889, he was appointed as professor of dentistry, anaesthetics and anaesthesia at the Philadelphia Dental College.[3]

In 1936, it was proposed that the University of Oxford should develop a postgraduate medical school with chairs in medicine, surgery, obstetrics and gynaecology. Lord Nuffield offered to endow these to the sum of £1.25 million. In a casual conversation at Huntercombe Golf Club, he told some of his medical acquaintances about the proposed endowment. Among the group was an anaesthetist, Dr Robert Reynolds Macintosh, who is reported to have replied jokingly that anaesthesia had been forgotten yet again. As a result of this, Nuffield decided that there should be a chair in anaesthetics and that he wished Macintosh (who had given him an anaesthetic previously) to be the Nuffield Professor. The academic establishment at Oxford was initially opposed to the appointment of a chair in the specialty, believing that a readership would suffice but Nuffield prevailed and increased his endowment to £2m to achieve his aim.[4] Macintosh took up the appointment in February 1937 becoming the first professor of anaesthesia in Europe.[5]

Robert Reynolds Macintosh. Courtesy of the Royal College of Surgeons in Ireland.

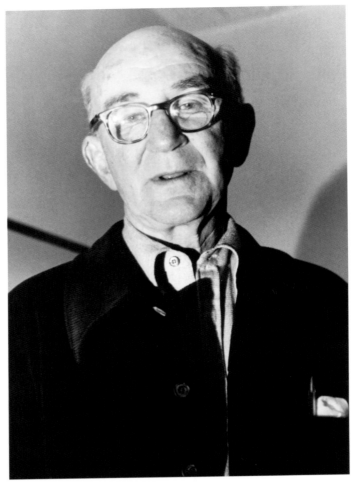

The establishment of other chairs throughout Britain followed, with the appointment of Dr Edgar Alexander Pask in Newcastle (1949), Dr William Woolf Mushin in Cardiff in 1953 (conferred honorary FFARCSI in 1964) and Dr T. Cecil Gray in Liverpool in 1959 (conferred honorary FFARCSI in 1962).[5] Macintosh was conferred with an honorary FFARCSI in 1964.

Queen's University Belfast

The first university department of anaesthetics in Ireland was established at Queen's University Belfast in 1958 when Dr John Wharry Dundee was appointed as head of department and senior lecturer. He had been a senior lecturer in Liverpool prior to his appointment to Belfast. The new post was jointly funded

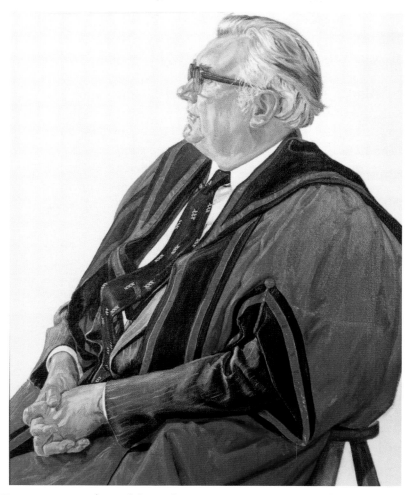

by the Department of Health and Queen's University and was allocated four rooms at the new Institute of Clinical Science – these were used for research and teaching. Dundee was subsequently promoted to full professor in 1964 , the first professor of anaesthetics to be appointed in Ireland. He was dean of the Faculty of Anaesthetists, RCSI from 1970–3. He retired from clinical practice in 1987 and was awarded the OBE two years later.

Dr Richard Samuel Jessop Clarke was appointed senior lecturer in 1965, as reader in 1972 and received his personal chair in 1980. He became head of department with a substantive chair when he replaced Dundee in 1988. He was dean of the Faculty of Anaesthetists, RCSI from 1991–4. He retired in 1994.

James (Alfie) Moore was an obstetric anaesthetist at the Jubilee Hospital on the Belfast City Hospital campus. He had qualified from Queen's University Belfast (QUB) in 1952, received his FFARCS in 1957, his MD in 1961 and a PhD in 1974. He was a research fellow at the Mercy Hospital, Pittsburgh and senior tutor in the Department of Anaesthesia, Royal Victoria Hospital (RVH). He was involved in a number of research projects with Dundee; some would say that he was his right hand man and a key person in the early days of the Academic Department at QUB. He received a personal chair around 1990. He published widely in the field of obstetrics, particularly on pain relief in labour. Later he participated in benzodiazepine studies with Dundee as well as research on the use of histamine (H2) receptor antagonists in the prevention of Mendelson's syndrome. He was a member of the Board of the Faculty of Anaesthetists, RCSI for many years, was an examiner in pharmacology in the Primary exam and also examined in the Final fellowship.

Dr James Gamble was appointed senior lecturer in 1980 and was succeeded by Dr John Patrick Howard Fee as senior lecturer in 1981. Fee was subsequently appointed professor and head of department in 1995 following the retirement of Richard Clarke. He retired in 2009. Dr Rajinder Mirakhur became senior lecturer in 1990 and was appointed to a personal chair in 1996.[5,6]

Trinity College Dublin

The first academic anaesthetic post in Ireland was filled by Thomas Percy Claude Kirkpatrick, visiting physician at Dr Steevens' Hospital, Dublin who was appointed lecturer in anaesthetics at Trinity College Dublin (TCD) in 1910. He held the position until 1948 when he was replaced by Dr Victor McCormick, who would later be a member of the first board and vice dean of the Faculty of Anaesthetists, RCSI. He was succeeded in turn by Dr Edmund Delaney and then by Dr Ron Kirkham who was appointed in 1980. Dr Gerard Fitzpatrick was appointed lecturer in 1993 and became associate professor of anaesthesia in 2012.

Royal College of Surgeons in Ireland

In 1964, the Council of the Royal College of Surgeons in Ireland appointed Dr Thomas J. Gilmartin as lecturer in anaesthetics to its medical school, initially for a period of five years. He became associate professor in 1965. This was the first such academic post in anaesthetics in the Republic of Ireland.[7] Prof. Gilmartin retired in 1983.

In 1984, at the instigation of Dr Joseph Woodcock and Dr Des Riordan of

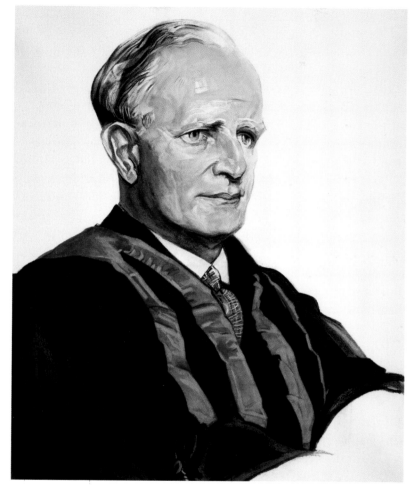

Thomas James Gilmartin. Portrait by Carey Clarke copied from the original pastel by Sean Keating.

the Charitable Infirmary, Jervis Street, an agreement was reached between the hospital, the Faculty of Anaesthetists, RCSI and the Council of RCSI to fund a full chair in anaesthetics. Prof. Anthony J. Cunningham was appointed in October 1985 and took up the post on 1 April 1986. The chair was based in RCSI with clinical attachments initially at the Charitable Infirmary, Jervis Street, and the Richmond Hospital both in Dublin. The two hospitals amalgamated on a single site as Beaumont Hospital in 1987. Dr David O'Toole was appointed as first lecturer and Ms Patricia Casey as research assistant.[8]

National University of Ireland

The west of Ireland soon followed suit with the appointment in 1989 of Dr

Padraic Keane (then chairman of the Department of Anaesthetics at Galway Regional Hospital), as the Critikon/Johnson and Johnson Professor of Anaesthetics. This was the first chair in anaesthesia in the National University of Ireland (NUI) and the first at University College Galway (UCG).

Dr Denis Moriarty was appointed lecturer in anaesthesia at University College Dublin (UCD) in December 1986, the first such academic post in the specialty at the college. He became UCD's first professor of anaesthesia (with a clinical commitment to the Mater Misericordiae Hospital) in January 1991. The post was funded for specific academic sessions as well as having funding (from both public and private sources) for a tutor/lecturer. Moriarty retired in 2006.[9]

Meanwhile, in Munster, Drs Seamus Hart, John McAdoo and Rory O'Brien applied pressure on University College Cork (UCC) for the establishment of an academic department of anaesthesia. The members of the Department of Anaesthesia at Cork University Hospital covenanted personal funds to the university to establish the financial basis necessary to kick-start the establishment of such a post and as a result, Dr George Shorten was appointed as first professor of anaesthesia and intensive care medicine at UCC in 1997.

Professorial appointments in Ireland until 1998

1964   Prof. John W. Dundee, Queen's University Belfast (QUB), first Professor of Anaesthesia in Ireland

1965   Prof. Thomas J. Gilmartin, Associate Professor (RCSI)

1986   Prof. Anthony J. Cunningham (RCSI)

1988   Prof. Richard S.J. Clarke (QUB) (Personal Chair in 1980)

1989   Prof. Padraic Keane, Critikon/Johnson and Johnson Chair (UCG, NUI)

1990s   Prof. James 'Alfie' Moore (QUB), Personal Chair

1991   Prof. Denis Moriarty, University College Dublin (UCD, NUI)

1995   Prof. P.J. Howard Fee (QUB)

1996   Prof. Rajinder Mirakhur (QUB), Personal Chair

1997   Prof. George Shorten, University College Cork (UCC, NUI)

References

1 Waters R.M., 'Pioneering in anesthesiology', *Anaesthesia*, 1949, 4, pp. 125-30.

2 Gravenstein J.S. and Beecher H.K., 'The introduction of anesthesia into the university', *Anesthesiology*, 1998, 88, pp. 245–53.

3 Lowenstein E., Dorr H.I., et al., 'Henry Isaiah Dorr was the first person to hold the title professor of anaesthesia', *Anesthesiology*, 2000, 93, p. 1160.

4 Sykes K. and Bunker J., *Anaesthesia and the practice of medicine. Historical perspectives*,

London: Royal Society of Medicine Press, 2008, pp. 70–1.

5   Nunn J.F., 'Development of academic anaesthesia in the UK up to the end of 1998', *British Journal of Anaesthesia*, 1999, 83, pp. 916-32.

6   Clarke R., *The Royal Victoria Hospital Belfast: A history, 1797–1997*, Belfast: Blackstaff Press, 1997, pp. 210–11.

7   Council RCSI, Minutes Book, available from Heritage Centre, RCSI, File RCSI/COU/28 (1938–1960).

8   RCSI Annual Report, 1986, pp. 14–15, available from Heritage Centre, RCSI.

9   Personal communication from Prof. D. Moriarty.

Chapter 23

The House at 22 Merrion Square

Joseph Tracey

The College of Anaesthesiologists of Ireland is located in a fine Georgian building at 22 Merrion Square, Dublin and has been based there since the year 2000. The house is over 250 years old and has an interesting history. In the 1700s, the most fashionable part of Dublin lay to the north of the river Liffey where Luke Gardiner had developed places such as Mountjoy Square, Rutland Square and Sackville Mall (now O'Connell Street). The land south of the river was mainly slob- and farmland and had not yet been developed. In 1713, Dublin Corporation leased Sir John Rogerson the farm rights to 133 acres of this

22 Merrion Square. Photographs by the author (left) and Bobby Studio (right).

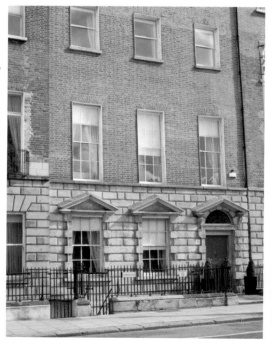 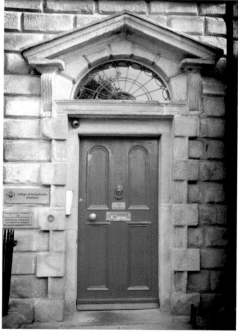

slobland so that he could reclaim it. Rogerson built a long stone quay along the south bank of the river and as a result, the land was no longer liable to flooding. The Fitzwilliam family, which had become established in the area in the thirteenth century, had steadily expanded their holding so that 500 years later they owned 1,377 acres on the southeast side of the river, a massive landbank that would be worth billions of euro today.[1] Their estate included three of the radial routes out of Dublin, the old Artichoke Road, Baggot Street and Leeson Street[2] and extended from west of Trinity College southwards between Donnybrook Road and the coast as far as their family seat at Merrion Castle on Mount Merrion in Blackrock.

In 1745, James Fitzgerald, the Earl of Kildare, had a town house built facing down Molesworth Street and just east of where Merrion Square would eventually be located. When a friend observed to the Earl that the site was a bit remote, Fitzgerald had declared, 'They will follow me wherever I go'.[3] He predicted that if he moved to the southside of the city, the aristocracy would follow him, abandoning the then fashionable northside areas such as Rutland Square and Henrietta Street. The house, which was styled like a ducal palace, was designed by Richard Castle (also known as Richard Cassels) who had also designed the Fitzgeralds' country home, Carton House, outside Maynooth. This palace, which was initially known as Kildare House was subsequently renamed Leinster House

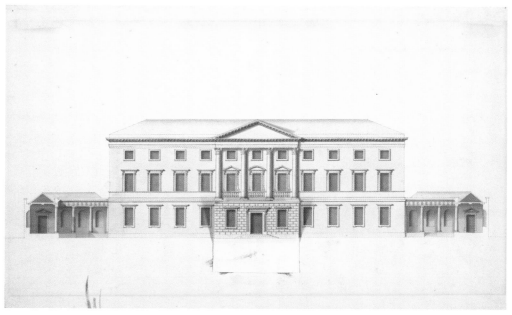

Drawings of the façade of Leinster House by Richard Castle (Cassells). Courtesy of the Irish Architectural Archive.

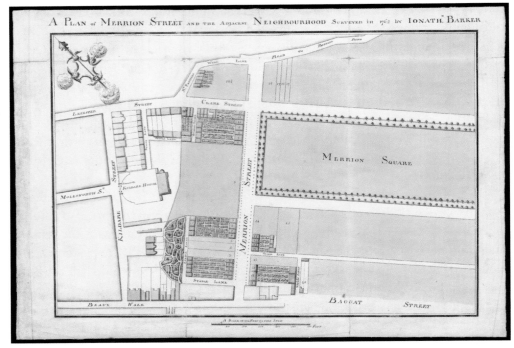

in 1766, when Fitzgerald became the first Duke of Leinster. This 'elevation' of
the Fitzgeralds made the southside of the river even more fashionable. The house
was sold in 1815 and was subsequently occupied by the Royal Dublin Society
for over a century before becoming the home of Oireachtas Éireann in 1922.

The 7th Viscount Richard Fitzwilliam saw the move of the aristocracy to
the southside that had been predicted and realised the potential for development
of the family's estate. He appointed his younger brother William to oversee this
development which began with the building of Merrion Street in 1758 alongside
Kildare House. The street included Mornington House where Arthur Wellesley,
Duke of Wellington, was born in 1769. The Fitzwilliams approached John Ensor
to design a square to the east of Merrion Street and this can be seen in the
drawings by Barker from 1762 and 1764 which show the layouts of the plots
around the square.

They soon realised that they were sitting on a veritable goldmine. In a letter
which William wrote to his brother the Viscount he stated, 'I think the present
building madness can never hold but however keep it up for our own sakes as long
as possible'.[1] They decided to sell the lots in groups of two or three but insisted
that the houses be of good quality 'be good and substantial, three stories and a

304

half above the cellar, with a front area of eight feet and a flagged pavement'.[4] They insisted on an unbroken terrace except for one carriage archway at the centre of the north side allowing access to the mews. The first lots were all bought by groups of tradesmen, carpenters, plumbers, plasterers and master builders all working for each other in a form of barter. The Fitzwilliams offered these developers discounted rates if they used the granite from their own quarries in the Dublin mountains and also on their bricks which were made in their brickfields.[5] In total, 92 houses were built with the initial development being on the north side which is where number 22 is located. Standard houses were sold in 1760 at a price of £1,500. The north side is unusual in that most of the houses, including number 22, have granite rustication on the hall/ground floor. This rustication 'lends a sense of strength and solidity to the structure'.[1] This feature is not seen on the other sides of the square as the Fitzwilliam quarries at Ticknock were flooded in 1779 and so cheap granite was no longer available to the developers. As a streetscape, Merrion Square is unrivalled in Dublin with its long regular row of eighteenth-century brick and granite fronted terraces rising above the plantings of the park in the centre. A contemporary account referred to how 'Most of the houses on the north were constructed of stone as far as the first floor which gives them an air of magnificence inferior to nothing of the kind, if we except Bath'.[6]

The garden in the centre of the square was for the private use of the residents only and they would have been key-holders. A characteristic of the Georgian garden-square was that there should be an uninterrupted promenade along the boundary railings and this walkway around the periphery has been reinstated with the recent redevelopment of the square by Dublin City Council. In Merrion Square park, the footpath on the north side was wider than that on the south as this was the more popular side on which to stroll. This was because the north side was sunnier with the paths on the south side shadowed by the buildings which were quite elevated above the level of the park: 'The footway on the North side is in summer evenings the resort of all that is elegant and fashionable in the vicinity'.[6] The original gardens were lightly planted leaving wide open spaces so that 'looking from their windows [residents] may not long at a time lose sight of their children'.[7] It was only later that the Victorians started to plant trees around the periphery of the park obscuring the view into the gardens. The Georgians also felt that their new houses should be seen from the park as part of the landscape/cityscape. The recent changes to the landscaping in Merrion Square park reflect the original Georgian concept of more open spaces and less dense planting.[7] In 1789, Antrim House was built by Denzille Holles, Earl of Clare, to a design by John Ensor. This was the biggest house on the square with an 82-foot frontage which closed off the vista of the Georgian mile. Holles' name has been perpetuated in Holles Street, Clare Street and Denzille Lane; the lane runs behind the houses on the north side of the square.

In 1791, the residents obtained an act of parliament allowing them to enclose the square with an iron railing and in 1792 the Rutland Memorial was erected at the western end of the park; it is situated across the street from the National Gallery of Ireland (built in 1854). By 1794, the plantings in the gardens were completed and the iron railings had been erected.

In 1816, Fitzwilliam died and left his estate to George Augustus Herbert, 11th Earl of Pembroke. Thus the Fitzwilliam Estate became the Pembroke Estate. The names Fitzwilliam and Pembroke are still commonly seen in south County Dublin in place names such as Fitzwilliam Square, Merrion Road and Pembroke Road.

Numbers 20 and 21 Merrion Square were built as a pair by Francis Ryan, a plasterer and by Thomas Sherwood, a plumber, and construction started in 1764. They bought the lots together and then took one house each with Sherwood taking number 21.[8] This then became number 22 in 1845 when a narrow house was built (now number 13) in the carriage arch half way down the terrace.[8] Construction on numbers 20 and 21 had reached roof level by February 1768. A large group of tradesmen was busy completing the chimneys when the rear stack collapsed killing seven men and injuring five others:

> A very unfortunate accident happened last week by two houses number 21 and 22 Merrion Square he (Mr. Lacy) was building for Ryan and Sherwood, for as they were stopping the chimneys, the rere of them fell down, by which there were seven men killed and five wounded. This was supposed by some owing to the great fall of snow we had here of late that prevented the works cementing and by others to bad materials – if the latter be the case, Lacy must have a great deal to answer for and i think that it must be a reproach to him all his life

stated a letter from Elizabeth Fagan .[9]

Number 22 stands out in the terrace because 'a most unusual stone detail to the structural openings is to be seen in a house built by T. Sherwood, No 22, Merrion Square North. The stone pediment detail appears above each ground floor windows and also above the entrance door'.[10]

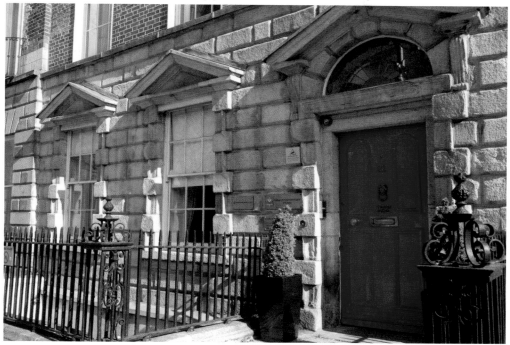

Facade of 22 Merrion Square showing stone pediment detail and granite rustication. Photograph by the author.

It was also noted that 'No 22 is exceptional in having moulded and quoined architraves and pediments to the door and windows ... standard 1760s' joinery and cast cornices inside.'[8]

Residents at 21/22 Merrion Square in the eighteenth, nineteenth and twentieth centuries are listed below:

1798	Mrs Stopford[11]
1830	Mr James Lalor[12]
1834–40	Miss Lucretia Taylor[13]
1841	Vacant
1842–3	Major William Stewart[14]
1843–50	Andrew Geraghty, solicitor (1845 the number changes to 22)
1851–3	J.C. Egan, FRCSI
1854–72	William Gibson, Taxing Master
1872–84	Mrs O'Connor
1890–1901	Samuel R. Mason, FRCSI
1902–8	Mrs Mason

1909–25	Dr Edward Emanuel Lennon
1935–55	Dr D. O'Brien, LDS
1963	T.C. O'Mahoney, solicitors
1996–2000	Slatterys PR/ Mr Ray Moran/ Mr Shea O'Flanagan
2000	College of Anaesthetists

The houses in Merrion Square were mainly owned in the eighteenth century by the nobility and by members of the Irish parliament. Following the Act of Union of 1801, the aristocracy moved to London to be near the Parliament at Westminster. As a result, in the nineteenth century, the majority were occupied by wealthy merchants, doctors or solicitors[15] and number 22 was no different.

The earliest resident listed in the Irish Georgian Society records is a Mrs Stopford who was living there in 1798. The National Archives of Ireland hold correspondence dated 1830 from Mr James Lalor[12] at 21 Merrion Square (in the letter he proposes to the government the purchasing and draining of bogs as a form of employment for the poor). All the subsequent residents are listed in *Thom's Directory*[13] which was first published in 1834. Miss Lucretia Taylor lived there from 1834 to 1840. The only possible reference to her is that there was a school at 18 Wicklow Street owned by a lady of that name. Major William Stewart[14] who lived there from 1842–3 was a former commander of the Donegal Regiment and also a former chief police magistrate for County Limerick. There are numerous references to Andrew Geraghty (1843–50) in the papers of the time as his practice seemed mainly to involve conveyancing.

Dr John C. Egan
Dr John Cruise Egan acquired his Licence in Midwifery from the Dublin Lying-in Hospital (now the Rotunda) in 1840, qualified LRCSI in 1841, received his MD from Glasgow the following year and obtained his FRCSI in 1845. He lived at number 22 from 1851 to 1853 and worked at the Westmoreland Lock Hospital. He published a number of papers: 'The diagnosis and treatment of Syphilitic disease' in the *Dublin Medical and Quarterly Journal*, 'Syphilis contracted by nursed children' in the *Dublin Medical Press*, and 'Gonorrhoea in the female' in *The Lancet*.[16] He was a member of the Council of the Surgical Society of Ireland and also of the Dublin Natural History Society.

The Gibson family
William Gibson, who lived in the house from 1854 until his death in 1872, was

the son of John Gibson, a United Irishman who had taken part in the 1798 Rising in Cavan. William was a solicitor and subsequently taxing master at the Court of Chancery. He was evidently well off as there are records in the Registry of Deeds that show that he was capable of making large loans of 700 pounds to a William Rathborne in 1850 and then a mortgage (on several properties in Meath and Merrion Square) of 1000 pounds to his son Gorges [sic] Rathborne ten years later in 1860. He was married to Louisa Grant and had six children.

Edward Gibson was their third child and was born in 1837. He graduated first place and gold medallist, BA from Trinity College Dublin (TCD) in 1858. He became a barrister in 1860, received his MA in 1861 and an honorary LLD from Trinity in 1881. He became a King's Inn bencher and then Queen's counsel in 1872. He was elected to Westminster representing Dublin University as a Conservative member of parliament (MP) from 1875 to 1881 and was attorney general from 1887–80. Finally, he was made Lord Chancellor in 1885 and became a peer in the same year, becoming the 1st Lord Ashbourne. In the same year, he drafted the Purchase of Land (Ireland) Act which created a fund that allowed tenants to buy the land they rented and pay the loan back over a number of years. This became known as the Ashbourne Act.[17] He was married to Frances Colles, granddaughter of the surgeon Abraham Colles, and they had eight children, four boys and four girls. One of their daughters, Violet Gibson, gained notoriety for her attempted assassination of Benito Mussolini in 1926. This story is recounted in *The woman who shot Mussolini* by Frances Saunders.[18] Number 22 passed out of the family on the death of William Gibson in 1872 . Edward himself had a house in Fitzwilliam Square for a number of years but moved back to Merrion Square in 1897 into number 12, which is probably the house described in Saunders' book.[13]

Samuel Roberts Mason

Mason lived in the house from 1890–1901. He was born in York Street, Dublin on 5 November 1852. He was educated at the Academic Institute, Harcourt Street and later attended the Ledwich School of Medicine in Peter Street, Trinity College Dublin and Mercer's Hospital. He received an Arts degree from the University of Dublin in 1873 and his MB in 1874, FRCSI in 1879 and MD in 1883. He was a fellow of the Royal Academy of Medicine in Ireland and a member of the Court of Examiners, RCSI. He was elected master at the Coombe Lying-in Hospital in December 1883 and was appointed lecturer in midwifery and on 'the diseases peculiar to women' to the Ledwich School in 1877. In 1893, he became professor of midwifery at RCSI and held this office until 1899 when he resigned.

He married Mary Elizabeth, eldest daughter of J. Shine from Limerick, in 1882. His only child was killed in an accident in 1895 when he was just eight years old. Dr Mason himself died a few years later on 9 January 1901.[19] His widow stayed on in the house until 1908.

Edward Emanuel Lennon

Lennon lived in the house from 1909–25. Originally from Newcastle House in Enfield, County Meath, in his youth he had travelled to America to earn his fortune. When he had earned enough money, he returned to Dublin and decided to study medicine. He was a student at the Royal College of Surgeons in Ireland and at the Meath Hospital where he qualified LRCSI in 1882, LRCPI in 1883

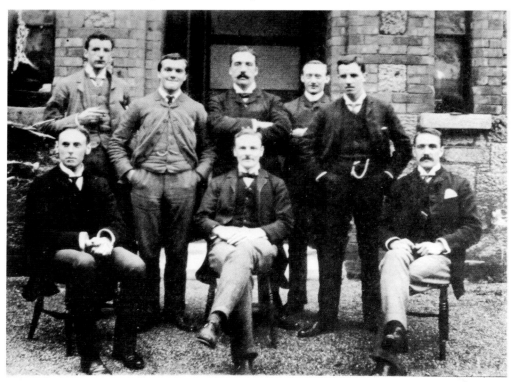

Dr Edward E. Lennon (seated front left) in a photo of Meath Hospital staff, 1887. Reproduced from Ormsby L.H. History of the Meath Hospital and County Dublin Infirmary, Fannin, 1892.

WILFRED WYNNE,
Ex-Resident and Clinical Clerk.

JOHN A. BURLAND,
Ex-Resident.

JOHN RYAN,
Ex-Resident and Clinical Clerk.

ANDREW McFARLAND,
Ex-Resident and Clinical Clerk. H. HILDIGE,
Ex-Resident and Clinical Clerk.

EDWARD E. LENNON,
Senior Assistant Physician.

FRANK PORTER NEWELL,
House Surgeon.

JAMES CRAIG, M.B.,
Junior Assistant Physician.

and became MRCPI in 1890 and FRCPI in 1892. He was appointed senior clinical assistant at the Meath Hospital in August 1886 and physician to the hospital in 1893, a position he held until his death in 1940. He married Eileen Mary Cole Metge from Navan in 1908, one year before he moved to number 22 Merrion Square. They had two children, Maeve and Edward. 'He is described as a handsome man, very gregarious and often found at social gatherings. When he entered the wards, the nurses' hearts were "all a flutter"'.[20] He was a fellow of the Royal Academy of Medicine in Ireland, Censor in RCPI and a demonstrator in anatomy at the Carmichael College, Dublin.[21] He is seated front left in the photograph of the Meath Hospital staff from 1887. When he left the house in 1925, he moved around the corner to number 38. He finally moved back to the family home at Newcastle House in 1936.

Dr Donough O'Brien, LDS

O'Brien lived in the house with his family from 1935–55 and this was the last family to live there. He had his dental practice in the house but also let consulting rooms. A number of prominent doctors of the time had their rooms there, including Mr Tom O'Neill (MB BCh BAO 1935, FRCS 1941) who was a surgeon

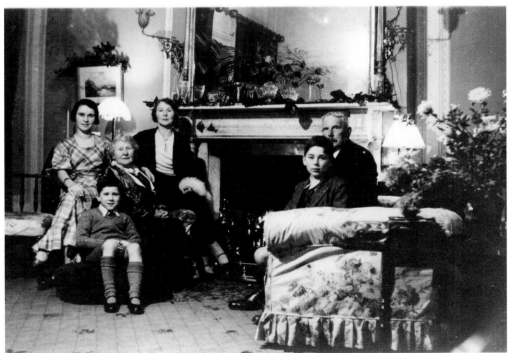

Photograph taken in the front drawing room (now the Board Room) of 22 Merrion Square by Dr Donough O'Brien, Christmas 1935. (Left to right) Oona O'Brien, Ronan O'Brien, their grandmother Louisa Hardy, Mrs Ida O'Brien, Declan O'Brien and Oswald Hardy. Courtesy of Oliver O'Brien.

in Sir Patrick Dun's hospital, and Dr Charles Herbert McMahon MB BCh BAO 1932, FRCPI 1939) a physician, also at Sir Patrick Dun's.

Dr Robert Emmet Davitt who was a visiting physician and anaesthetist at the Charitable Infirmary in Jervis Street also had rooms in the house. He was a son of Michael Davitt, founder of the Land League, a Home Rule politician and member of parliament (1892–9). In 1932, Davitt gave the only anaesthetic ever administered in the house when he anaesthetised Ronan O'Brien, a child aged four years, for the removal of a lump in his neck. The operation took place in

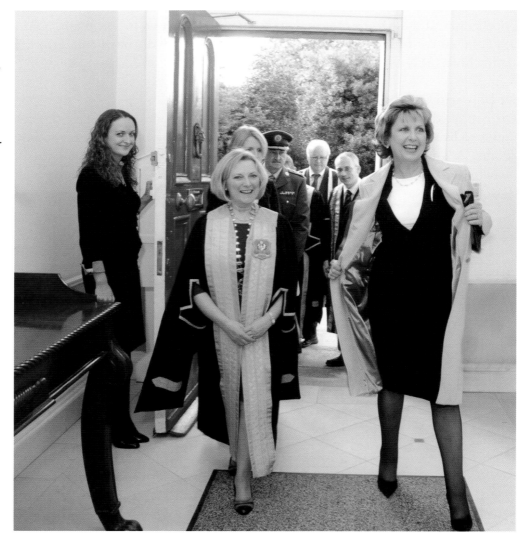

President Mary McAleese with Jeanne Moriarty at 22 Merrion Square after its refurbishment, 2010. Courtesy of Bobby Studio.

one of the bedrooms on the top floor of the house and the surgeon was Oliver St John Gogarty, ear, nose and throat surgeon and poet (personal account from Mr Oliver O'Brien). Dr Davitt was subsequently elected to Dáil Éireann as a Cumann Na nGaedheal TD from 1933–5.

* * *

The house was occupied after 1955 by a number of different businesses and was no longer used as medical consulting rooms. The College of Anaesthetists of Ireland purchased the building in the year 2000 at a cost of €3.6 million and it has been the home of the specialty ever since. The vendors were two well-known Dublin surgeons but they had not used the building in their clinical practice. It was completely refurbished in the early years of the millennium under the supervision of the conservation architect Roisin Hanley and was formally re-opened by President Mary McAleese in October 2010. The specialty finally had a home of its own, 151 years after MacDonnell first used ether for surgery in January 1847.

References

1   Casey C., *The Eighteenth-Century Dublin Town House*, Dublin: Four Courts Press, 2010, pp. 97–9.
2   McCullough N., *Dublin an Urban History*, Dublin: Anne Street Press in conjunction with Lilliput Press, 2007, p. 129.
3   Craig M., *Dublin 1660–1860: The shaping of a city*, Dublin: Liberties Press, 2006, p. 159.
4   Matthews N., 'The development of Merrion Square', vol. 1. (unpublished master's thesis for Urban and Building Conservation (MUBC), UCD, 1997, p. 29.
5   Casey, *Dublin Town House*, p. 100.
6   *The Georgian Society Records of Eighteenth Century Domestic Architecture and Decoration in Dublin*, vol. IV, Shannon: Irish University Press, 1969, pp. 69–70.
7   Merrion Square conservation plan, Howley Hayes Architects, 2014, pp. 6–7.
8   Casey C., *The Buildings of Ireland. Dublin*, New Haven and London: Yale University Press, 2005, pp. 582–3.
9   Matthews N., 'Merrion Square' in M. Clark and A. Smeaton (eds.) *The Georgian Squares of Dublin. An Architectural History*, Dublin: Dublin City Council, 2006, pp. 60–1.
10 *Ibid.*, p. 65.
11 *Georgian Society Records*, vol. IV, p. 80.
12 National Archives of Ireland, CSO/RP/SC/1830/1347.
13 *Thom's Directory*, 1834–1900.
14 National Archives of Ireland, CSO/RP/SC/1821/1350.
15 Meenan F.O.C., 'The Georgian squares of Dublin and their doctors', *Irish Journal of Medical Science*, April 1966, 484, pp. 149–54.

16 'John Cruise Egan', *Medical Directory*, 1861, p. 881.

17 Maume P. '*Gibson, Edward*' in *Dictionary of Irish Biography*, vol. 4 Gaffkin–J., Cambridge: Cambridge University Press, 2009, pp. 66–8.

18 Saunders F.S., *The Woman Who Shot Mussolini*, London: Faber and Faber, 2010.

19 Cameron C.A., *History of the Royal College of Surgeons in Ireland, and of the Irish Schools of Medicine: Including a Medical Bibliography and a Medical Biography*, Dublin: Fannin, 1916, p. 629.

20 Turner J., *The Murphys of Rathcore Rectory*, Victoria: Friesen Press, 2020, pp. 109–10.

21 Ormsby L.H., *Medical history of the Meath Hospital and County Dublin Infirmary, from its foundation in 1753 down to the present time*, Dublin: Fannin and Co., 1888, p. 251.

PART III

Chapter 24

Biographies

SECTION 1
Deans of the Faculty of Anaesthetists, Royal College of Surgeons in Ireland

1960–4	Thomas J. Gilmartin
1964–7	Joseph A. Woodcock
1967–70	G. Raymond Davys
1970–3	John W. Dundee
1973–6	William S. Wren
1976–9	S. Harold Love
1979–82	John R. McCarthy
1982–5	Gerald W. Black
1985–8	Padraic W. Keane
1988–91	Denis C. Moriarty
1991–4	Richard S. Clarke
1994–7	John Cooper
1997–8	William P. Blunnie

Thomas James Gilmartin (1905–1986)
LRCP & SI LM DA FFARCS FFARCSI FRCSI (Hon)THOMAS 'TOMMY'

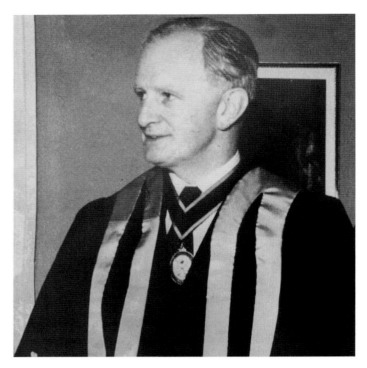

GILMARTIN was born in Ballymote, County Sligo in 1905, the son of James Gilmartin JP and his wife Rita Coghlan. His mother died from puerperal fever shortly after his birth. He was educated initially by the Sisters of Saint Louis at Kiltimagh, County Mayo then at Summerhill College, Sligo and subsequently Belvedere College, Dublin. He attended medical school at the Royal College of Surgeons in Ireland and graduated LRCP & SI in 1929. He then trained in anaesthetics in Birkenhead General Hospital, the Royal Southern Hospital in Liverpool and St Mary's Hospital, Paddington, London. He returned to Dublin in 1931, where he was appointed as assistant anaesthetist in Mercer's Hospital under the supervision of Dr P. Gaffney before returning to London for a further year. On this occasion he worked at the Hammersmith Hospital where he gained experience with Boyle's apparatus. He obtained the DA in 1937. He became visiting anaesthetist to Mercer's Hospital in 1946 and was also visiting anaesthetist to the Dublin Skin and Cancer Hospital (Hume Street) and the Dublin Dental Hospital (both of which would have been within walking distance of Mercer's) as well as Peamount Sanatorium. Gilmartin is credited with introducing curare into anaesthetic practice in Ireland in 1945. He is reputed to have acquired a sample of the drug which was brought to Ireland from North America by the boyfriend of a staff nurse in the operating theatre of Mercer's Hospital.

Gilmartin was involved in the development of the Diploma in Anaesthetics (DA) in Ireland which was a conjoint examination of both the Royal College of Physicians of Ireland and the Royal College of Surgeons in Ireland. The first examination was held in 1942 and he himself received the Irish DA in 1943.[1]

In 1945, he applied to the Royal Academy of Medicine in Ireland (RAMI) to form a Section of Anaesthetics. The Academy agreed to the addition of a new section provided that a committee of at least 12 anaesthetists could be formed. This committee was duly convened with Dr Thomas Percy C. Kirkpatrick as president and Tommy Gilmartin as secretary. The inaugural meeting was held in 1946 to commemorate the centenary of the discovery of anaesthesia. The main speaker was Dr Ivan Magill who delivered a lecture on 'Current topics in anaesthetics'. Dr Gilmartin subsequently held the position of president of the section.

In 1949, he was a foundation fellow of the new Faculty of Anaesthetists of the Royal College of Surgeons of England and was granted the FFARCS by election. In 1950, he was chairman of a committee of the Irish Medical Association that produced a seminal 'Report on the Anaesthetic Services in Ireland'. This led to better recognition of the role of the specialty in the health service and to better working conditions and remuneration for anaesthetists.

In 1959, he was a founding member and first dean (1960–4) of the newly formed Faculty of Anaesthetists, RCSI and was a foundation fellow (FFARCSI 1960). Whereas it had been stipulated in the standing orders of the faculty that the role of dean should be for three years only, it was decided by the board of the faculty to grant Dr Gilmartin an extra year at the end of his term as a 'lap of honour' in appreciation of the role he had played in its foundation.

He was a member of the Council of the Association of Anaesthetists of Great Britain and Ireland (AAGBI) and subsequently vice president (1973–5). He was awarded the John Snow Silver Medal by AAGBI in 1985 and his citation was read by Dr Bill Wren. In 1964, the Council of the Royal College of Surgeons in Ireland (RCSI) appointed him as lecturer in anaesthetics for a period of five years and in 1965 he was made an associate professor of anaesthetics at College. This was the first anaesthetic professorship of any kind in the Republic of Ireland and was a significant step for the specialty. It came a year after the appointment of John Dundee as professor of anaesthetics at Queen's University Belfast. Gilmartin received an honorary fellowship of the Royal College of Surgeons in Ireland (FRCSI) in 1974, and remains the only anaesthetist in Ireland to have been awarded this accolade. His citation was given by the well-known surgeon and past-president of RCSI Mr Terence Millin.[2] He was elected as an honorary member of the Société Française d'Anesthésie et de Réanimation (SFAR) (French Society of Anaesthesia) in 1976 and a foundation academician of the European Academy of Anaesthesiologists in September 1978.

The author (J.T.) was a first-year senior house officer (SHO) in anaesthetics in Mercer's Hospital in 1977 and worked under his supervision. Dr Gilmartin was in his seventies and coming towards the end of his career. He was polite and reserved but keen to demonstrate how to use some of the older types of anaesthetics such as trichloroethylene and methoxyflurane (halothane was the most commonly used potent inhalational agent at that time). He had particular expertise in dental anaesthesia and was, at one time, president of the Association of Dental Anaesthetists. He was deeply involved in the Royal College of Surgeons in Ireland, was president of their graduates' association in 1960 and was elected president of the 'Bi' (a student society, the 'Biological Society' run jointly by RCSI and RCPI) at RCSI in 1980. He retired from anaesthetics and from Mercer's Hospital on its closure in 1983.[3]

Tommy Gilmartin married Peggy Maiben in 1936 and they lived in a fine Georgian house at number 32 Baggot Street, Dublin. He was a member of Portmarnock Golf Club and of the Royal Irish Yacht Club. They had one son, John, who was a well-known art historian.

The Gilmartin Lecture was inaugurated in his honour in 1985 with the first lecturer being Prof. John Dundee. The second lecture was delivered on 16 May 1986 by Sir Gordon Robson but unfortunately Prof. Gilmartin was unable to attend as he was ill. He died shortly afterwards on 22 June 1986.[4]

In 2019, his son John left a bequest to the College of Anaesthesiologists of Ireland of a portrait of Prof. Gilmartin by Carey Clarke, copied from an original pastel by Seán Keating, and it now hangs in the boardroom at 22 Merrion Square.

JT

References

1   Andrews H., 'Gilmartin, Thomas James' in *Dictionary of Irish Biography*, vol. 4, Gaffikin–

J., Cambridge: Cambridge University Press, 2009, pp. 98–9.

2   Millin T., 'Citation on behalf of Thomas James Gilmartin', *Anaesthesia*, 1974, 31, pp. 647–8.

3   Tracey J.A., 'Dr Thomas James Gilmartin', available at https://www.rcoa.ac.uk/dr-thomas-james-gilmartin (accessed 6 January 2021).

4   Lectures given by Drs David Wilkinson and Des Riordan, and personal recollections.

Joseph 'Joe' Augustine Woodcock (1919–1997)
LRCP & SI DA FFARCSI FFARCS (Hon)

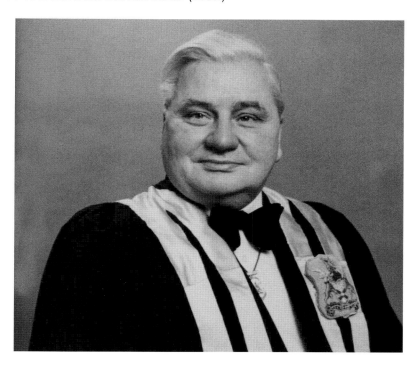

JOE WOODCOCK was born in Dublin on 1 May 1919. His father, Samuel Woodcock, had a grocery store on Thomas Street and his mother was Annie (*née* Mooney). The family lived on Brighton Road in Rathgar. He was educated at Blackrock College, boarding there from 1932 until 1936. He then changed school to St Mary's, Rathmines to sit the Matriculation examination before studying medicine at the Royal College of Surgeons in Ireland. He graduated LRCP & SI in 1944.[1]

Joe started his internship in the Charitable Infirmary, Jervis Street, Dublin in 1944 and subsequently became the anaesthetic senior house officer there. He

321

passed the Diploma in Anaesthetics examination in 1946 and was appointed visiting anaesthetist to the Charitable Infirmary in August of that year on the resignation of Dr Nagle. He remained in post for the next 40 years. He was a progressive consultant and was the lead in a number of significant developments at the hospital. He was the first anaesthetist to be chairman of the Medical Board, instigated the development of the intensive care unit and of a freestanding surgical day care unit and was also responsible for the introduction of a recovery room. Joe was the co-founder of the first dialysis unit in Ireland along with Dr Gerry Doyle, Prof. William O'Dwyer and Dr Michael Carmody.[2] The main instigator for this development was the hospital gynaecologist, Dr Arthur P. Barry, who wanted a treatment for young women who were developing renal failure from post-partum haemorrhage. The group went to Leeds to purchase a dialysis machine and brought it back to Ireland where it was left to Dr Woodcock to assemble it. Initially, dialysis was only carried out during the night and the members of the group each took turns in dialysing the patients. The service commenced in 1958.

In the 1950s barbiturates were among the commonest poisons taken as a deliberate overdose; the recommended treatment at the time was supportive care and dialysis. Consequently the Charitable Infirmary, Jervis Street began to receive a number of additional referrals for dialysis treatment for these patients. Because of this, Dr Woodcock found himself providing advice over the phone on the management of poisoned patients. At this time, he was the honorary secretary of the board set up by the Royal College of Surgeons in Ireland to advise on the formation of the new Faculty of Anaesthetists, RCSI. On one of his trips to London to liaise with the Faculty of Anaesthetists of the Royal College of Surgeons of England he went to visit the newly opened poisons unit at Guy's Hospital where he met its director, Dr Roy Goulding. As a result of the information and support he received from Guy's, he decided to develop a similar unit in Ireland. With the support of the Department of Health and the Irish Medical Association, he founded the National Poisons Information Centre at the Charitable Infirmary, Jervis Street in June 1966. Over 50 years later, the centre (now based at Beaumont Hospital) still provides advice to emergency care departments and other doctors on the management of poisoned patients. It also provides advice to the general public.[3]

The first meeting of the Board of the Faculty of Anaesthetists, RCSI took place on 15 December 1959. Dr Woodcock was a member and was elected honorary secretary. He was a foundation fellow of the new faculty (FFARCSI 1960) and was elected dean in 1964, a post he held for three years. He was elected a fellow of the

Faculty of Anaesthetists of the Royal College of Surgeons of England in 1965 and was a foundation academician of the European Academy of Anaesthesiology in 1978.

In 1985, Dr Des Riordan and Dr Woodcock approached the faculty for their support in funding a new chair in anaesthesia. They then successfully negotiated with the Royal College of Surgeons of Ireland who agreed to replace the post at RCSI (which had become vacant on the retirement of Prof. Gilmartin) with a full-time professorship in anaesthesia. The appointment was based initially at the Charitable Infirmary, Jervis Street with some sessions at the Richmond Hospital and later transferred to Beaumont Hospital following the amalgamation of the Richmond and Jervis Street Hospitals in 1987. This was the first full-time chair in anaesthesia in the Republic of Ireland.

Dr Woodcock was a superb organiser and this is evident from the number of developments he implemented in Jervis Street. He was also one of the prime movers in the organisation required to bring about the new faculty of anaesthetists and all the correspondence from the Advisory Committee in 1959 is from his home in Rathgar, Dublin. He retired from clinical practice in 1985 and was proud to say that he was replaced by the newly appointed professor of anaesthesia, Dr Anthony Cunningham.

Personal life

Dr Woodcock was first married to Mrs May Cullen, a widow who had one daughter, Mary. Following the death of his wife, he married again, this time to Mrs Inagh Gibson. He lived in a beautiful 'upside-down' bungalow on Zion Road, Rathgar and regularly invited all the anaesthetic staff for dinner. When one of these guests said how impressed they were with his culinary abilities, he confessed that he had a cook who came round when he entertained. He was a keen shot (with the shotgun) and was very involved with the Irish Clay Pigeon Shooting Association (ICPSA). He was club secretary for many years and the Joe Woodcock Trophy is still awarded at the annual international 'down-the-line' shooting competition hosted by the ICPSA. He was a member of the Slane Castle shooting syndicate and shot there every Saturday during the shooting season. There was always a chance of being handed a brace of pheasants on a Monday morning with instructions to hang them for a few days before putting them in the pot. He was a founder of the Rathgar Credit Union and continued to be involved with it during his retirement.

He died in August 1997.

JT

References

1 Information from Clare Foley, Archivist, Blackrock College, Dublin.
2 Beaumont Kidney Centre, available at Beaumont.ie/kidneycentre-aboutus-department history (accessed 24 August 2021).
3 Tracey J.A., 'Department of Anaesthetics' in E. O'Brien (ed.), *The Charitable Infirmary 1718–1987. A farewell tribute*, Dublin: Anniversary Press, 1987, p. 130.

Geoffrey Raymond Davys (1919–2012)
MB BCh BAO DA FFARCSI FFARCS (Hon)

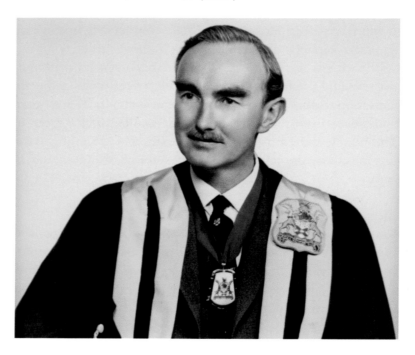

GEOFFREY RAYMOND 'RAY' DAVYS was born in Dublin on 21 April 1919 to James Davys, a bank manager, and his wife Emily (*née* Egan). After completing his secondary school education at Clongowes Wood College, County Kildare he studied medicine in University College Dublin graduating MB BCh BAO in 1941. During his student years, he supplemented his spending money by performing in drama productions broadcast on the national radio station, Radio Éireann. He worked for six months as a house physician and house surgeon in the original St Vincent's Hospital on St Stephen's Green in the city, following which he moved to England. After spending one year in Darlington, County Durham in casualty and orthopaedic house officer posts, he travelled south to Greenwich, London for further experience. He joined the Royal Air Force Medical Service in 1944 and served in the UK, France, Belgium and Germany, attaining the rank of War Substantive Flight Lieutenant.[1] Returning in 1947 to Dublin and St Vincent's Hospital (where he was to spend the rest of his working life, initially as assistant and later as a consultant anaesthetist), Ray Davys soon passed the examination for the Diploma in Anaesthetics of the Conjoint Board of the Royal College of Physicians of Ireland and the Royal College of Surgeons in Ireland (DA [RCP&SI]). Prior to and following the 1970 relocation of St Vincent's to Elm Park, Dublin, he played a major role in the planning and further development of the new hospital's intensive care unit (ICU); in addition, he attended Cherry Orchard Fever Hospital for many years, caring for poliomyelitis survivors who required long-term (sometimes permanent) iron lung or cuirass ventilation. He was also a visiting anaesthetist to the National Children's Hospital, Harcourt Street.

A foundation fellow of the Faculty of Anaesthetists, RCSI, Ray served on the faculty board from its inception on 12 December 1959. At the first board meeting, the Fellowship Election Committee, which subsequently adjudicated on applications for election to fellowship without examination, was formed. He was a member from the outset, and for many years afterwards. He acted as the chairman of the faculty's Finance and General Purposes Committee, sat on the Medical Advisory and also the Education and Examinations Committees and was honorary secretary to the board. He was elected as the third dean in 1967, fulfilling the role with distinction until 1970. Quite remarkably, in over 15 years of board membership, he was absent for just three meetings. In 2010, by which time the Faculty of Anaesthetists, RCSI had become the College of Anaesthetists of Ireland, he was awarded the College Medal in recognition of his outstanding service to the specialty of anaesthesia over many years.

Ray was active in the Dublin Anaesthetists Travelling Club and contributed to the medical literature until shortly before his retirement in 1985, writing on such subjects as cardiac arrest, postanaesthesia vomiting and fibreoptic bronchoscopy in the ICU.[2,3] He enjoyed sailing and walking, had a wide circle of friends, and was an entertaining and engaging raconteur.[4] Pre-deceased in 2004 by Marie-Patricia (*née* White), his wife of over half a century, he died in the hospital which he had served with loyalty and distinction for almost 40 years, and where he was affectionately known by generations of anaesthesia trainees as the 'Wing Commander', on 26 December 2012.

DW

References

1   'G.R. Davys', available at forces-war-records.co.uk/records/6427807/war-substantive-flight-lieutenant-g-r-davys-royal-air-force-medical-branch/ (accessed 13 February 2021).

2   Davys R. and Gallagher E., 'Postanaesthetic vomiting: A trial of cyclizine tartrate', *Journal of the Irish Medical Association*, 1957, 40, pp. 84–5.

3   Gibney R.T., Brennan N.J., Davys R. and Fitzgerald M.X., 'Fibreoptic bronchoscopy in the intensive care unit', *Irish Journal of Medical Science*, 1984, 153, pp. 416–20.

4   O'Farrell N., 'Obituary. Raymond Davys', *British Medical Journal*, 2013, 347, f4474.

JOHN WHARRY DUNDEE (1921–1991)
OBE MD PhD FFARCS FFARCSI FRCP

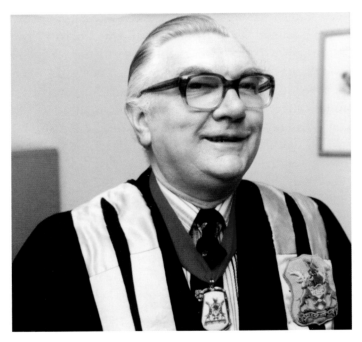

Born on 8 November 1921 to William Dundee, a farmer, and his wife Matilda ('Tilly', *née* McRoberts) at Ballynure, near Larne, County Antrim, JOHN DUNDEE received his secondary education in Ballyclare High School. Having studied medicine at Queen's University Belfast (QUB), he graduated MB BCh BAO in 1946. His early appointments were as house physician, house surgeon and resident anaesthetist at the City and County Hospital, Londonderry where he met his future wife Sarah (Sally) Houston.[1] Within two years of becoming a doctor, he had successfully passed the examination for the DA (RCP & SI).

Anaesthesia in the early years after World War Two was experiencing rapid growth following the introduction of thiopentone and the muscle relaxant curare. Liverpool, where the legendary T. Cecil Gray had been appointed reader in anaesthesia in 1947, was at the centre of new ideas, particularly in anaesthetic pharmacology. Dundee moved to the city for further training and with the exception of a one-year sabbatical during which he worked as a research fellow with Robert Dripps and Henry Price at the University of Pennsylvania, Philadelphia, USA, he spent most of the next decade there, his first position being as resident anaesthetist at the Walton Hospital, Fazakerley. From the outset, he demonstrated extraordinary energy and initiative where both clinical work and academic research were concerned. He was appointed lecturer in anaesthesia at the University of Liverpool in 1950 and, two years later, consultant anaesthetist to the Walton and United Liverpool Hospitals. During his time in the city, he obtained an MD from QUB for his thesis on 'Sensitivity to and detoxification of thiopentone' (for which he did all his own analytical work in the laboratory while simultaneously working in a busy clinical post) and a PhD from the University of Liverpool on 'Thiopentone and other thiobarbiturates'. He was also involved with studies on curare, a major interest of Gray's, and in early work on hypothermia for neurosurgical anaesthesia.[1,2] He was elected to Fellowship of the Faculty of Anaesthetists of the Royal College of Surgeons of England (FFARCS) in 1953.

John Dundee returned to Belfast in 1958, when he was appointed to a joint consultant/senior lecturer in anaesthetics post at the Royal Victoria Hospital (RVH) and QUB. He set about building up the department, initiating a range of postgraduate activities some years before the introduction of organised training schemes in any part of Ireland. These included teaching for trainees preparing for the FFARCS examinations and continuing education for consultants which incorporated regular clinical meetings. He also began an extensive programme of clinical research, at first continuing his own work on thiopentone but gradually covering other intravenous induction agents, most of the opioids, phenothiazines and anti-emetics as well as anticholinergic drugs, muscle relaxants and inhalational anaesthetics.[1] His efforts ultimately led to him producing approximately 600 scientific papers in 30 years and supervising 50 theses for higher degrees. Apart from published papers, his work was summarised in his four textbooks on intravenous anaesthetic agents and one on clinical anaesthetic pharmacology.[3]

One less well-known aspect of Dundee's contribution to anaesthesia is the keen interest that he had in the management of chronic pain. In about 1952, while in Liverpool, he assumed the running of a pain clinic started by Cecil Gray four years earlier.[4] He continued working in that area in Belfast until an enthusiastic colleague relieved him of the responsibility. Similarly, he was, along with Dr Robert 'Bob' Gray, a major force behind the establishment of an intensive care unit, the first in Northern Ireland, at the Royal Victoria Hospital. He was appointed as first professor of anaesthetics at Queen's in 1964, a post he held until his retirement in 1987.

John Dundee, a foundation fellow, served on the Board of the Faculty of Anaesthetists, RCSI from its first meeting on 12 December 1959. He was immediately nominated to sit on the Education Committee, of which he was chairman for many years, and played a leading role in the development of both the Primary and Final FFARCSI examinations, in each of which he became a regular examiner. He worked also on the Finance and General Purposes Committees. His tireless efforts were recognised when he was elected dean, the first from Northern Ireland, in 1970. While Thomas Gilmartin is rightly perceived as having been the moving spirit in establishing the faculty, it is largely thanks to Dundee's contribution that it was seen as an all-Ireland body from the outset.[1] By the time of his retirement from the board in 1979, he had served for an unbroken 20 years since its inauguration. In 1985, he returned to deliver the inaugural Gilmartin Lecture, titled 'From Small Beginnings'. He had become a Fellow of the Royal College of Physicians (FRCP) during the previous year and was president of the Royal Academy of Medicine in Ireland from 1989 to 1991.

His work in Ireland does not appear to have hindered his involvement with various UK committees. He was elected to the Council of the Association of Anaesthetists of Great Britain and Ireland and the Board of the Faculty of Anaesthetists of the Royal College of Surgeons of England, and served as president of the Section of Anaesthetics, Royal Society of Medicine (1979–80). He also sat on the Committee on Safety of Medicines and was associate editor of the *British Journal of Anaesthesia*.

After retirement, Dundee's interest having been stimulated on a visit to China, he turned to studying alternative medicine, and in particular, the use of acupuncture as an anti-emetic during cancer chemotherapy. Outside work, he was a fine musician and played in a dance band that entertained troops during World War Two. He subsequently became skilled as a church organist and in later life, played the instrument at church services and also sang in the choir at

Windsor Presbyterian Church, Belfast. He was president (1985–7) of the Christian Medical Fellowship of the United Kingdom and Ireland.

John Wharry Dundee, who had been made an Officer of the Order of the British Empire (OBE) in the 1989 New Year's Honours List for his services to medicine in Northern Ireland, died suddenly just three weeks after the passing of his wife Sally, on 1 December 1991.

DW

References

1 Clarke R.S.J., 'John Wharry Dundee', available at history.rcplondon.ac.uk/inspiring-physicians/john-wharry-dundee (accessed 13 February 2021).
2 Clarke R.S.J., 'Obituary. JW Dundee', *British Medical Journal*, 1992, 304, p. 710.
3 Palmer R., Wildsmith T., 'Dr John Wharry Dundee', available at rcoa.ac.uk/dr-john-wharry-dundee (accessed 13 February 2021).
4 'John Dundee', available at peoplepill.com/people/john-dundee (accessed 13 February 2021).

William 'Bill' S. Wren (1929–2006)
MB BCh BAO DA FFARCSI FFARCS

WILLIAM STEPHEN WREN was born on 21 July 1929 in Dun Laoghaire, County Dublin. Educated by the Christian Brothers, he subsequently studied medicine at University College Dublin, graduating in 1952. As with many other newly-qualified Irish doctors of the time, he immediately went to England to work. Within a year, he began training in anaesthesia, working at the Whittington Hospital, Whipps Cross and the Royal Postgraduate Medical School at the Hammersmith Hospital, both in Greater London. It was at the latter that his interest in the specialty became a lifelong commitment, a decision which was to have a profound effect on its development in Ireland.

Bill Wren returned to Ireland in 1956 to take up a consultant anaesthetist post in Sligo. Soon afterwards, he moved to the newly-opened Our Lady's Hospital for Sick Children in Crumlin, Dublin. It was (and remains) the largest paediatric hospital in the country and much of the children's surgery which had previously taken place in general hospitals was carried out there. In the early 1970s, the programme for paediatric cardiac surgery was successfully launched. In parallel with the rapid evolution of surgical services, Wren developed the fledgling but expanding Anaesthetic Department and the associated subspecialty of paediatric intensive care with vision, drive and unbending commitment; traits which were

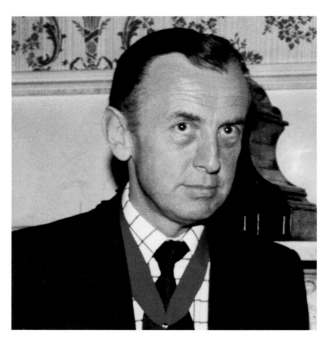

ultimately to benefit the teaching and practice of anaesthesia in all parts of Ireland. Later in his Our Lady's career, he directed his attention to anaesthetic research and was lead investigator of several published trials which explored the effects of both old and new inhalational anaesthetic agents in children.[1–3]

The Faculty of Anaesthetists, RCSI had been inaugurated in 1960; Wren was aware of the critical importance of the new body and despite his exceptionally heavy clinical workload, soon became involved in its affairs. He was first elected to the board of faculty in 1968, and served until 1982, both as secretary and then as dean from 1973 until 1976. From this vantage point, he saw the need for a formal anaesthetic training programme in Ireland. In 1972, with characteristic directness and determination, he launched the Eastern Regional Training Scheme, a general professional programme based in the Dublin teaching hospitals with Our Lady's at its hub, which was overseen by a subcommittee of the faculty, the Medical Advisory Committee. Wren prompted and encouraged colleagues in other parts of the country to develop similar programmes with the result that the Southern and Western schemes, based in Cork and Galway, were developed subsequently. Shortly afterwards, the National Senior Registrar Scheme was launched, once again with him as chairman and the principal driving force and also acting as vice chairman of the Joint Committee for Higher Training in Anaesthesia. The concept of a regulated rotational training programme involving the teaching hospitals was well ahead of thinking at the time in many other medical specialties in Ireland and later formed the model on which a number of other schemes were based.

Wren was a long-time member of the Association of Anaesthetists of Great Britain and Ireland (AAGBI) and was elected to council on two occasions, firstly in 1971 and again 12 years later. He was a member of the Advisory Council, and served as vice president (1976–8) and acted in 1977 as the organising chairman for the Annual Scientific Meeting of the association which was held in Dublin and was a joint meeting with La Société Française d'Anesthésie et d'Analgésie et d'Réanimation (SFAAR) the French Society of Anaesthesia, Analgesia and Intensive Care.

In 1997, in recognition of his contribution over the years, he was awarded the distinction of being elected to AAGBI honorary membership. In 1985, he took on the responsibility of coordinating the joint meeting of the Association of Paediatric Anaesthetists of Great Britain and Ireland and the Section of Anesthesiology of the American Academy of Pediatrics, also held in Dublin.

Recognition of Bill Wren's organisational expertise was not confined to Britain and Ireland. His involvement in anaesthetic affairs at European level was considerable and he contributed to a number of European Congresses of Anaesthesiology between 1970 and 1986, by way of presenting scientific papers or as organising chairman of paediatric anaesthesia sessions, and often both. He was an invited or guest speaker at meetings of national societies in over a dozen major European cities, and was founding honorary secretary of the European Academy of Anaesthesiology, serving on its Senate from 1979–84. In North America, he was visiting professor or guest lecturer at many prestigious institutions including the University of Arizona, the Johns Hopkins School of Medicine, and hospitals for children in Boston, Montreal and Toronto. Back in Ireland, he was honoured in a unique manner in 1988 when he was invited by the Minister for Health, Dr Rory O'Hanlon, to become medical advisor to the Department of Health. This appointment represented an enormous compliment to the man himself and by extension to the specialty in which he worked.

William Stephen Wren retired from clinical practice in 1994 after 37 years as consultant anaesthetist at Our Lady's Hospital for Sick Children. During that time, his contribution not just to paediatric anaesthesia but also to the training of Irish anaesthetists was outstanding. He was an inspirational teacher and motivator who represented his specialty with distinction. He died in Dublin in August 2006.

JC

References

1 Wren W.S., McShane A.J., McCarthy J.G., Lamont B.J., Casey W.F. and Hannon V.M., 'Isoflurane in paediatric anaesthesia', *Anaesthesia*, 1985, 40, pp. 315–23.
2 Wren W.S., Synnott A. and O'Griofa P., 'Effects of nitrous oxide on the respiratory pattern of spontaneously breathing children', *British Journal of Anaesthesia*, 1986, 56, pp. 274–9.
3 Wren W.S., Allen P., Synnott A., O'Keeffe D. and O'Griofa P., 'Effects of halothane, isoflurane and enflurane on ventilation in children', *British Journal of Anaesthesia*, 1987, 9, pp. 399–409.

Samuel Harold Swan Love (1920–2010)
MD DA FFARCS FFARCSI

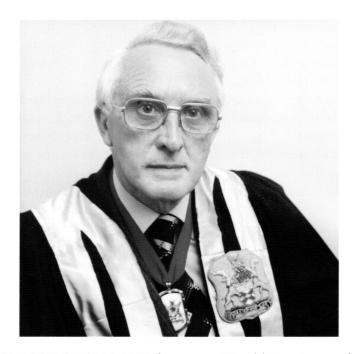

SAMUEL HAROLD SWAN LOVE (known as Harold Love), one of the first Irish anaesthetists to specialise exclusively in the management of children, was born at 365 Ormeau Road, Belfast on 30 July 1920 to Andrew Love, a draper, and his wife Lizzie (*née* Simpson), a former milliner. He attended Bangor Grammar School following which he entered the medical school of Queen's University Belfast (QUB), graduating MB, BCh, BAO in 1945. After time spent in house officer posts at the Royal Victoria Hospital (RVH) in the city, he moved to England where he worked initially as resident anaesthetist and later as anaesthetic registrar at Darlington Memorial Hospital in County Durham. He obtained the DA (RCP & SI) in 1949, was awarded a doctorate in medicine (MD) by QUB in 1952 and went on to become a Fellow of the Faculty of Anaesthetists of the Royal College of Surgeons of England (FFARCS) in 1953. He obtained the DA (RCP & SI) in 1949, was awarded a doctorate in medicine (MD) by QUB in 1952 and became a fellow by election of the Faculty of Anaesthetists of the Royal College of Surgeons of England (FFARCS) in 1953.. Having previously served as senior registrar in anaesthetics, he was appointed consultant anaesthetist to the Royal Victoria Hospital and the Royal Belfast Hospital for Sick Children (RBHSC) in 1954.

Harold Love was a highly skilled clinician with a special interest in paediatric cardiac anaesthesia and intensive care and also a dedicated teacher, who gave many years of loyal and devoted service to the hospitals in which he worked. A popular father figure in the latter part of his career, he commanded great respect among his professional colleagues, both at home and abroad, and his warm personality was reflected in his close relationships with them.[1] He was a regular contributor to the anaesthetic literature; his published papers included a number on various aspects of anaesthetic pharmacology and both intermittent positive pressure ventilation and dental anaesthesia in children.[2,3]

A founder member of the Association of Paediatric Anaesthetists of Great Britain and Ireland (APAGBI) in 1973, he served as the third president and the first based outside England, from 1979–82. In recognition of his contributions to paediatric anaesthesia and to APAGBI itself, he was awarded honorary life membership in 1988. He was also a founder member of the European Academy of Anaesthesiology.

Harold, a foundation fellow, was a member of the Board of the Faculty of Anaesthetists, RCSI from its first meeting on 12 December 1959. He was soon nominated to and sat for a number of years on the Election Committee which filled the important role of making recommendations to the board as to which candidates for election to foundation fellowship or fellowship of the faculty without examination should be approved. He later worked on the Finance and General Purposes Committee and subsequently had a major input into the faculty examinations, serving as both a member and chairman of the Education and Examinations Committee for some years and also contributing his services as examiner in the Final fellowship from 1965 until shortly after his retirement from clinical practice in 1984. He became vice dean in 1974, and two years later, had the signal honour of being the first dean to be elected unopposed, serving from

1976–9. In the words of Dr John R. McCarthy, his immediate successor in that position, he not only worked hard on behalf of the faculty, but also graced the office with dignity, and had the wisdom to 'save us from our own folly' – this latter comment was made in reference to a potentially damaging decision initially taken by the board but subsequently reversed following mature reflection on the part of the dean and an emergency meeting convened by him.

Harold Love's flair for administration was widely recognised and following his retirement from clinical practice in 1984, he was appointed part-time medical administrator of the Royal Group of Hospitals in Belfast (1984–7). He became honorary archivist to RBHSC in 1991 and subsequently wrote an excellent history of the hospital.[4] He was also able to spend more time pursuing his love of golf on the world-famous links of Royal County Down Golf Club. He had a deep Christian faith and remained active in his church throughout his life. He died on 19 December 2010.

DW

References

1   Black G., 'Obituary. Samuel Harold Swann Love', available at www.apagbi.org.uk/about-us/council/newsletter (accessed 14 February 2021).
2   Love S.H.S., 'The complications of dental anaesthesia', *British Journal of Anaesthesia*, 1968, 40, pp. 188–96.
3   Love S.H.S. and McC Reid M., 'Intermittent positive pressure ventilation in infants and children: The longterm effects in 74 survivors', *Anaesthesia*, 1976, 31, pp. 374–9.
4   Love H., *The Royal Belfast Hospital for Sick Children: A History 1948–1998*, Belfast: Blackstaff Press, 1998.

John R. McCarthy (1928–2021)
MB BCh BAO DA FFARCSI FRCPI FFARCS (Hon)

DR JOHN R. MCCARTHY (or John R. as he was widely known) was born in Dublin on 23 July 1928 and lived initially on Raglan Road and then Herbert Park in Donnybrook. He was educated at St Xavier's School nearby at 58 Morehampton Road. This is described as being a school for the sons of Catholic gentlemen and existed from 1933–61.[1] He attended medical school at University College Dublin graduating in 1951. He spent his clinical years as a medical student at the Mater Misericordiae Hospital, Dublin and he remembers his first time assisting at an operation. The procedure was cataract surgery under general anaesthesia, the surgeon was in his eighties and John R. had to hold a torch

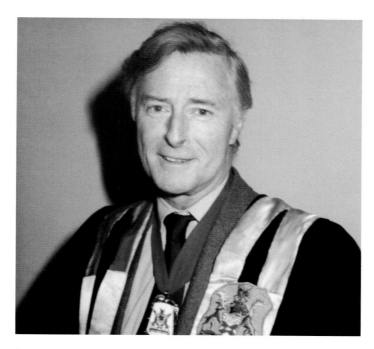

focused on the patient's eye for the duration of the operation.

Following his internship at the Mater, he went to London where he initially worked in internal medicine but soon realised that career prospects were limited and changed to a career in anaesthesia.

After a number of years in London, he returned to the Mater Misericordiae Hospital in Dublin where he spent three years as an anaesthetic registrar and sat the Conjoint Diploma in Anaesthetics examination in 1953 – it was the only anaesthetic qualification in Ireland at the time. John held consultant posts initially at Our Lady's Hospital for Sick Children in Crumlin as well as in the National Maternity Hospital, Holles Street before also being offered a post in the Mater which he accepted on 1 January 1957. Whilst a consultant, he passed his Membership examination of the Royal College of Physicians of Ireland (MRCPI) in 1957 and was made a fellow of that college (FRCPI) in 1979. He continued to work in all three hospitals for a some time but after seven years ceased working at Our Lady's Hospital for Sick Children.

John was involved in the first cardiac surgical procedure in the Mater Hospital which was a mitral valvotomy performed by Prof. Eoin O'Malley in 1961. Subsequently, he continued his involvement with cardiac surgery and was the anaesthetist in the first cases in which cardiopulmonary bypass was used in the Mater in the early 1970s. He received his Fellowship of the Faculty of Anaesthetists, RCSI (FFARCSI) in 1962 . He was a member of the board of the faculty for a number of years before being appointed dean from 1979–82. During his time as dean, the first steps were taken by the faculty towards independence from RCSI. The financial arrangements with RCSI were questioned and new arrangements were proposed which would give the faculty more financial independence. At that time, he was conferred as a Fellow of the Faculty of Anaesthetists , Royal College of Surgeons (FFARCS) in England.

He retired from the Mater in 1994 at the age of 66 years but continued to work in private practice at the Bon Secours Hospital in Glasnevin and at the Mater Private Hospital. He finally retired from clinical practice at the age of 80.

He was married to Patricia (*née* Boylan) and had four children and six grandchildren. He was a keen golfer and was a member at both Milltown Golf Club in Dublin and Rosses Point Golf Club in Sligo. He also enjoyed playing bridge and doing the crossword. He was proud of the fact that he won a trophy at bridge in his 90s. He died on 24 September 2021.

This biography is based on an interview with Dr McCarthy in 2019.

JT

References
1   Doran B.M., *Donnybrook: a History*, Dublin: The History Press Ireland, 2014, p. 59.

Gerald 'Gerry' Wilson Black (1925–2019)
MD PhD FFARCS FFARCSI FRCPI

GERALD WILSON BLACK, known as Gerry, was born in Belfast in1925 and received his early education at Inchmarlo Preparatory School, followed by The Royal Belfast Academical Institution. After graduating from Queen's University Belfast (QUB) in 1949 and initial anaesthesia training in his native city, he worked as a research fellow in the Department of Anesthesiology, University of Pennsylvania, USA. He was appointed as consultant paediatric anaesthetist to both the Royal Belfast Hospital for Sick Children (RBHSC) and the Royal Victoria Hospital in 1960.

His numerous postgraduate qualifications included the Fellowship of the Faculty of Anaesthetists of the Royal College of Surgeons of England (1955) and doctorates in both medicine (MD) and philosophy (PhD) awarded by QUB in

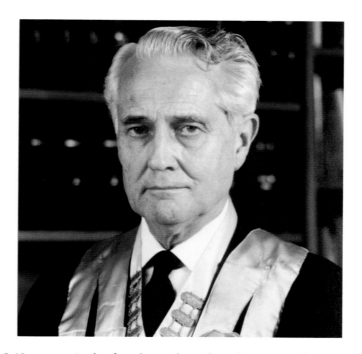

1959 and 1969 respectively, for theses based on his research. He was elected to Fellowship of the Faculty of Anaesthetists, RCSI (FFARCSI) without examination in 1961 and was conferred with that of the Royal College of Physicians of Ireland (FRCPI) in 1974.

Gerry Black had a special interest in the perioperative management of newborn infants and recognising the need for more comprehensive medical and nursing care of this group and also of critically ill older children, he pioneered the development of paediatric intensive care in Northern Ireland. The paediatric intensive care unit at RBHSC, of which he was in administrative charge, was established in 1967 and was one of the first in the United Kingdom.

His research and numerous publications on the action of volatile anaesthetics and, in particular, their sympatho-adrenal, circulatory and metabolic effects established Gerry's international reputation as a leading authority on the subject.[1,2] This aspect of clinical pharmacology, on which his PhD thesis was based, had previously been largely neglected and his work was regularly cited in standard anaesthesia textbooks. He was invited in 1978 by the Medical Research Council (UK) to be co-organiser of a comprehensive clinical trial to investigate the possible adverse effects of halothane and other anaesthetics on the liver with particular reference to the effects of repeat administration. In later years, he was engaged with the study of the effects of volatile anaesthetics in children and also, the interaction of anaesthetics and muscle relaxants.[3] This work was carried out in association with various research fellows, several of whom were subsequently awarded doctorates as a result. In total, he was author or co-author of approximately 50 peer-reviewed journal publications and almost 20 book chapters.

Gerry was totally dedicated to his work and involved in all aspects of hospital life. At different times, he was chairman of the Divisions of Anaesthetics and Paediatrics of the Royal Group of Hospitals and also of the Medical Staff Committee at RBHSC. He served as president of the Northern Ireland Society of Anaesthetists (1979–81) and the Ulster Paediatric Society (1981–2). Outside Northern Ireland, his roles included that of council member (1975–8) and vice president (1981–3) of the Association of Anaesthetists of Great Britain and Ireland, and vice chairman of the Joint Committee for Higher Training of Anaesthetists, Royal College of Surgeons of England (1983–5). He was a founder member of the Association of Paediatric Anaesthetists of Great Britain and Ireland (APAGBI), served as president from 1985 for two years and, in recognition of his outstanding contributions over many years to paediatric anaesthesia in general and to the APAGBI in particular, was awarded honorary life membership in 1995.

Having been an examiner in pharmacology in the Primary fellowship examination for some years beforehand, Gerry was elected to the Board of the Faculty of Anaesthetists, RCSI in 1970. He was immediately appointed to serve on the Education and Examinations Committee, of which he later became chairman, playing a leading role in planning and implementing the introduction of multiple choice questions to faculty examinations. He also sat on the Finance and General Purposes Committee. He became an exchange examiner in clinical measurement for the London faculty's Primary fellowship examination in 1971, and continued to examine in both Dublin and London for many years. Gerry was dean of the Faculty of Anaesthetists, RCSI from 1982–5, having served as vice dean from 1979. He was the Irish faculty's eighth dean and the third from Northern Ireland.

Gerry Black, one of the outstanding anaesthetists of his generation, has been described as a delightful colleague, co-operative and generous, whose wise counsel was often sought. He enjoyed teaching and in 1986, was appointed as honorary lecturer in paediatric anaesthesia, QUB. He encouraged and supported trainees in their career development, inspiring many, and continued to do so until his retirement. Gerry was a private and unassuming man, yet gregarious, with a quick wit and dry sense of humour. He defused many a tense moment in the operating theatre with an amusing comment delivered with perfect timing from the head of the operating table.[4]

Keen on sport, Gerry played rugby and cricket as a schoolboy and was awarded a cricket Blue at Queen's University as a skilful left-arm spin bowler. He travelled widely over the decades, forming many enduring friendships along the way, and was invariably accompanied by his wife Dorothy. He had a great interest in history, maintained his enthusiasm for cricket and rugby throughout his life and on retirement, enjoyed more time on the course of the Royal Belfast Golf Club.[5]

While medicine was an important part of Gerry's life, his wife and two daughters were his priority. He and Dorothy, an ophthalmologist, met at medical school at Queen's. They were very happily married and celebrated their 56th wedding anniversary some months before her death in 2008.

Gerald Wilson Black died in 2019 having led a long and exceptionally productive life.

DW

References

1 Black G.W., 'A review of the pharmacology of halothane', *British Journal of Anaesthesia*, 1965, 37, pp. 688–705.
2 McArdle L., Black G.W., Unni V.K.N., 'Peripheral vascular changes during diethyl ether anaesthesia', *Anaesthesia*, 1968, 23, pp. 203–10. This publication won an award for the best paper submitted to the journal *Anaesthesia* during 1968.
3 Gallagher T.M. and Black G.W., 'Uptake of volatile anaesthetics in children', *Anaesthesia*, 1985, 40, pp. 1073–7.
4 Love H., *The Royal Belfast Hospital for Sick Children: A History 1948–1998*, Belfast: Blackstaff Press, 1998.
5 Coppel D.L., 'Gerald Wilson Black', *British Medical Journal*, 2020, 369, m2425.

Padraic Keane (1936–2016)
MD FFARCS FFARCSI

PADRAIC KEANE was born in Oranmore, a short distance from Galway city. The eldest of three children, he grew up in an atmosphere steeped in sporting endeavour and historical lore, both of which were to have a major influence on his attitudes and achievements as an anaesthetist and administrator.

He was educated at St Mary's College, Galway and graduated MB BCh BAO

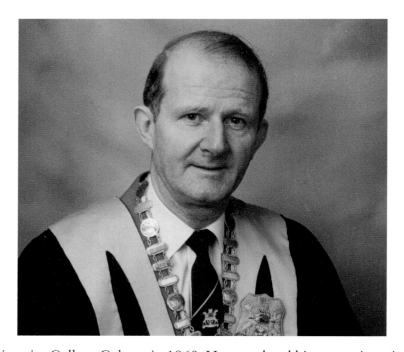

from University College Galway in 1960. He completed his pre-registration house posts at Galway Regional Hospital and Castlebar General Hospital before heading for Manchester to begin training in anaesthesia. Returning to his native city two years later, he continued his training at the Regional Hospital before taking up a fellowship post at the University of Boston, Massachusetts. This period of transatlantic training had an enormous influence on his career, culminating in the award of an MD from University College Galway (UCG) and setting the seeds for the future development of all aspects of the specialty of anaesthesia on a regional and national level.

He returned to Galway in 1970 to take up an appointment as consultant anaesthetist and director of anaesthetic services at Galway Regional Hospital. The hospital was the flagship of the Western Health Board, and under his direction, the anaesthetic department played a leading role in the development of the medical services in the region. A new intensive care unit was opened, and a recompression chamber for the treatment of acute decompression sickness and gas gangrene was installed. Obstetric epidural and acute postoperative pain services were established, and training and education in anaesthesia were reorganised by the establishment of the Western Regional Anaesthetic Training Scheme, and the inclusion of the hospital on the National Senior Registrar Rotation.

In 1979, Padraic Keane was instrumental in establishing the Western Anaesthetic Symposium, an annual scientific meeting in the west of Ireland. The meeting quickly gained great popularity and continues today as one of the stand-out academic meetings in the Irish anaesthetic calendar.

He was elected to the Board of the Faculty of Anaesthetists, RCSI in 1975 and became dean in 1985. His deanship was remarkable for two reasons. Firstly, since the foundation of the faculty in 1960, all deans had been based in either Dublin or Belfast. Padraic Keane was the first exception to this practice. Secondly, he succeeded in disentangling the finances of the Faculty of Anaesthetists, RCSI from those of the Royal College of Surgeons in Ireland (RCSI); this was the first step on the road towards establishing the independent College of Anaesthetists of Ireland. The special working party jointly chaired by the RCSI president (Reginald A.E. Magee) and Dr Keane successfully completed its work in 1987. Thereafter, the annual accounts of the faculty were published separately, in 1991 the first separate conferring ceremony took place, and in 1998 the College of Anaesthetists of Ireland came into being.

A career-long member of the Association of Anaesthetists of Great Britain and Ireland (AAGBI), he initiated discussions in 1987 which led to the establishment of the Standing Committee in Ireland and in 2002, he was made an honorary member of the association.

He was an examiner in the Final medical examination at UCG and the Primary and Final fellowship examinations of the Dublin and London faculties, extern examiner for doctorate degrees at Queen's University Belfast and vice chairman of the Joint Committee for Higher Training of Anaesthetists. In 1983, on the recommendation of the medical faculty in Galway, he became postgraduate coordinator to the Postgraduate Medical and Dental Board which had responsibility for overseeing the development of core courses and examinations for all hospital specialities. In the same year, he established an exchange programme with the Department of Anesthesiology at the Milwaukee Medical Centre, Wisconsin.

Padraic Keane was appointed Critikon/Johnson & Johnson Professor of Anaesthesia at UCG in 1989. He served on the Irish Medical Council, acting as chairman of the Ethics Committee. His particular areas of interest were patient safety, and postoperative pain relief.[1, 2, 3] A witty and engaging lecturer, he spoke on many occasions at regional and national meetings in Ireland and as guest lecturer at prestigious North American institutions including the Brigham and Women's and Beth Israel Hospitals, Boston; he was also visiting professor at

SAFETY AS WE WATCH

Parkland Memorial Hospital, Dallas and the Harvard Medical School.

Padraic Keane was a genuine sports enthusiast. He represented his county at hurling, playing left corner back on the Galway senior hurling team in the early 1960s. At the time, Galway hurlers competed in Munster in the All-Ireland Championship and had to contend with the might of Tipperary and Cork so success proved elusive. The National Hurling League however proved a little more rewarding.[4, 5, 6]

Some years later, realising the pressures athletes are subjected to in the modern era, he convinced the Gaelic Athletic Association (GAA) of the need for a Medical Advisory Committee. Padraic Keane retired from clinical practice in May 2001 after a hectic career spanning more than 30 years. Unassuming, quietly spoken and always approachable, he nevertheless had dynamism, vision and sheer tenacity: he had a significant effect on the development of anaesthesia in Ireland and on the careers of countless of trainees.

JC

References

1 Keane P., 'Anaesthesia in Ireland 1987 – how safe is it!', *Irish Journal of Medical Science*, 1998, 157, p. 51.
2 Colbert S.T., O'Hanlon D.M., McDonnell C., Given F. and Keane P., 'Analgesia in day case breast surgery – the value of preemptive tenoxicam', *Canadian Journal of Anaesthesia*, 1998, 45, pp. 217–22.
3 O'Hanlon D.M., Colbert S.T., Keane W.P. and Given F.H., 'Preemptive bupivacaine offers no advantages to postoperative wound infiltration in analgesia for outpatient breast biopsy', *American Journal of Surgery*, 2000, 180, pp. 29–32.
4 'Galway fight back to draw with Clare', *Irish Independent*, 7 November 1960, p. 17.
5 'Galway never in difficulty', *Irish Press*, 13 March 1961, p. 12.
6 'Tipperary purple patch decisive', *Irish Independent*, 3 July 1961, p. 14.

Denis C. Moriarty (1944–)
MB BCh BAO FFARCSI FFARCS FCPS Malaysia (Hon) FJFICMI

DENIS MORIARTY was born in Dublin on 20 October 1944. His parents were Dr Michael Moriarty (d. 1965) a consultant physician at the Mater Misericordiae Hospital in the city and his wife Catherine (d. 1990), a radiographer. He was educated at the Catholic University School (CUS) on Lower Leeson Street and subsequently studied medicine at University College Dublin (UCD), qualifying MB BCh BAO in 1968. During his internship at the Mater, he attended a lecture given

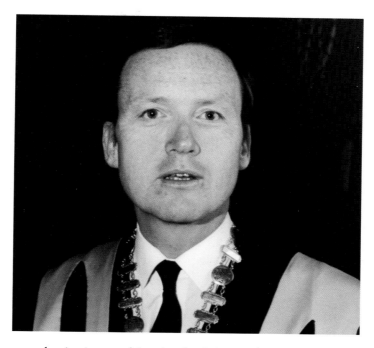

by an Irish anaesthesiogist working in the Mayo Clinic titled 'Anaesthesia, the specialty of the future' and as a result, decided that it was the career for him. He then travelled to the UK for specialty training in anaesthesia. His first post was as a senior house officer (SHO) at the Royal Free Hospital (1970), he was a registrar at University College Hospital (1971) and the Royal Brompton Hospital (1972) and completed his London training as a senior registrar at the Clinical Research Centre in Northwick Park (1973). He received his Fellowship of the Faculty of Anaesthetists, RCSI in 1971 and two years later the FFARCS. In 1974, he was appointed as a consultant anaesthetist at the Royal Brompton Hospital in Chelsea, West London, which specialised in cardiac and pulmonary surgery. Later that year, he moved to the USA to take up a fellowship post in Respiratory Medicine/Intensive Care at the Mayo Clinic in Rochester, Minnesota (1974–6).

He was appointed as a consultant anaesthetist to the Mater Misericordiae Hospital in his native city in 1975 and returned to Ireland to take up the post during the following year. He also attended Our Lady's Hospital for Sick Children in Crumlin (1976–96) one day per week as part of the Paediatric Cardiac Care Team with the noted cardiac surgeon Mr Maurice Neligan. In 1996, he reverted to being full-time at the Mater. His areas of interest were cardiothoracic anaesthesia, intensive care medicine and the advancement of anaesthesia as a major medical specialty.

He was designated lecturer in anaesthesia in December 1986, the first academic post in the specialty at UCD. He was subsequently appointed as the university's first full-time professor of anaesthesia in January 1991. The post was funded for specific academic sessions as well as having a tutor/lecturer post associated with it (paid for by both public and private funds). He was awarded an honorary fellowship of the College of Physicians and Surgeons, Malaysia in 1991.

Prof. Moriarty was very much involved with the Faculty of Anaesthetists, RCSI throughout his career, was a member of the board of the faculty from 1980–92 and was elected dean from 1988–91. He was, again, a member of the board from 1994–8 when the faculty became an independent college and was a member of the council of the college from 1998–2006.

He was an examiner in the fellowship examinations from 1977 until 2015. In 1983, while acting as an exchange examiner with the English faculty in Kuwait, he was approached by two Saudi anaesthetists who were interested in having the Irish equivalent hold their examination in the Kingdom of Saudi Arabia. A few years later, when he was dean of the faculty, he received further enquiries from the Saudi anaesthetists and as a result, he travelled to Riyadh with Dr Ian Carson. It was agreed that the faculty would initially run a Primary fellowship course there and following that, they would hold the Primary examination. The following year, Denis Moriarty, Ian Carson and John R. McCarthy held the first overseas Primary examination in the city. The examinations and annual courses continued in the city for the next 10 years before transferring to Oman.

During his term as dean, Prof. Moriarty continued the process of financial separation of the faculty from RCSI that had been started by his predecessor Prof. Padraic Keane. He reorganised the fellowship examination so that it was more independent of the college by having its own conferring ceremony, and also by running the exams and courses in Saudi Arabia. In the early 1990s, the University of the West Indies (UWI) contacted the faculty requesting an external examiner for their examinations. Prof. Richard Clarke was the first to travel to Jamaica in this role. Prof. Moriarty succeeded him in 1993 and this relationship continued for a number of years with the faculty supporting the UWI in advancing their academic departments as well as providing extern examiners.

Following the foundation of the College of Anaesthetists of Ireland in 1998, Denis continued as a member of council and then as vice president (2004–5) until he retired from the college in 2006.

He was married in 1977 to Dr Fiona Scanlon, who practised as an ophthalmologist. They have four children, three sons and a daughter. One of their sons qualified in medicine and is now a radiologist. He was recently appointed to the Mater, marking a fourth generation of doctors in the family and a third generation of medical consultants at that hospital.

Now retired, Denis spends his time with family, likes to read histories, biographies and books on politics. He is a member of historical societies, the University of the Third Age and organises twice yearly lectures and lunches in the college for the retired fellows group. He also enjoys hill walking and is a member of Milltown Golf Club.

JT

Based on conversations with Prof. Moriarty and information provided by him.

Richard Samuel Jessop Clarke (1929–)
BSc MD PhD FFARCS FFARCSI

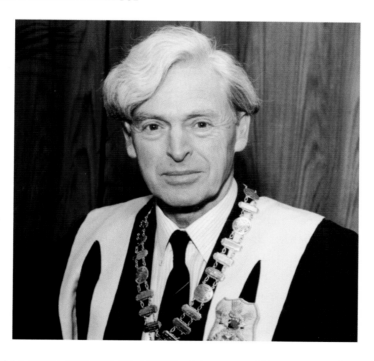

RICHARD SAMUEL JESSOP CLARKE, elder son of Dr Brice Richard Clarke (a noted chest physician) and his wife, Doreen Matilda (*née* Cassidy), was born on 7

July 1929 in Newtownbreda, Belfast.[1,2] Educated at the Royal Belfast Academical Institution and Queen's University Belfast (QUB), he graduated MB BCh BAO in 1954. Four years later he married Elizabeth Kyle ('Kyleen') Colhoun, an occupational therapist from County Londonderry.

His initial medical posts were as a house officer in Belfast City and Musgrave Park Hospitals. He then moved to Oxford, where he first met Kyleen and worked in the Department of Human Anatomy as a member of the scientific staff of the Medical Research Council. He returned to Belfast to commence anaesthesia training, serving in both senior house officer and registrar posts at the Royal Victoria Hospital. Crossing the Irish Sea once more, he became lecturer in physiology and tutor in anaesthesia at St Bartholomew's Hospital and Medical School in London. Back in Belfast again and having spent time as both a senior registrar and senior tutor, he was appointed, in 1965, to the post of consultant/senior lecturer in anaesthetics to the Royal Victoria Hospital and Queen's University.

He was awarded doctorates in medicine (MD) and philosophy (PhD) by QUB in 1958 and 1969 respectively, obtained the Fellowship of the Faculty of Anaesthetists of the Royal College of Surgeons of England (FFARCS) in 1961 and was admitted to Fellowship of the Faculty of Anaesthetists, RCSI (FFARCSI) without examination ten years later.

Richard Clarke was first elected to the Board of the Faculty of Anaesthetists, RCSI in 1981, but his Irish faculty links go back considerably further. He first examined in physiology at the Primary fellowship examination in 1966, and was an exchange examiner in clinical measurement at the London equivalent from 1972 onwards. Upon election to the faculty board, he became a member of the Education and Examinations Committee, which was later divided into two separate components. He continued to serve on both and was chairman of the Education Committee for many years. He was elected vice dean in May 1988 and became dean three years later, serving until 1994.

At the Royal Victoria Hospital, Clarke's clinical work was mainly in cardiac and thoracic anaesthesia, and in intensive care. He has also been a distinguished researcher, with over 200 peer-reviewed publications to his name. His position in Oxford resulted in a number of papers on various aspects of physiology, while after his return to Belfast, he produced a steady stream of anaesthesia-related work, much of it concerned with human pharmacology or metabolism.[3,4] He was awarded a personal professorship in clinical anaesthetics in 1980 and was professor of anaesthetics and head of department at Queen's University from 1988 until his retirement in 1994. He served as president of the Section of Anaesthetics, Royal

Society of Medicine, 1995–6.

Following his retirement, Richard Clarke was appointed honorary archivist to the hospital in which he had worked for so many years. This position gave him access to a large store of material about the institution and its staff, collected over 200 years. In 1997, he produced a major work based on his research, *The Royal Victoria Hospital Belfast: A History 1797–2007*, which has been described as being a masterclass of its kind; it was followed a few years later by a well-received biography of the eminent Belfast surgeon Sir Ian Fraser.[1,5] His magnum opus, however, is undoubtedly *A Directory of Ulster Doctors (who qualified before 1901)*, published in 2013 by the Ulster Historical Foundation, one of many cultural and historical societies in which he has played an active role over the years.[6] The book consists of two volumes containing approximately 1,300 pages, and includes nearly 6,000 names of doctors, practically all accompanied by fascinating biographical information, including details of parentage, birth, marriage and death, and also medical education and subsequent career. It is an invaluable resource for those studying medical or local history, and also for genealogists researching Ulster families. Apart from his medical publications, Richard has had a long involvement in writing on local and family history and has written over 30 books on gravestone inscriptions of Counties Antrim and Down; they constitute a further vast resource that has been salvaged by him for future generations. An erudite man of culture, he has also studied and collected antique sea charts, maps of Ireland and Worcester porcelain and has published extensively on cartographic subjects.

Based telephone conversations with Professor Richard and Mrs Kyleen Clarke.

DW

References

1. Clarke R.S.J., *The Royal Victoria Hospital Belfast: A History 1797–1997*, Belfast: The Blackstaff Press, 1997, p. 152.
2. 'Clarke, Richard Samuel Jessop (Richard)', in B. O'Donnell (ed.), *Irish Surgeons and Surgery in the Twentieth Century*, Dublin: Gill and MacMillan, 2008, p. 601.
3. Clarke R.S.J., Hellon R.F. and Lind A.R., 'The duration of sustained contractions of the human forearm at different muscle temperatures', *Journal of Physiology*, 1958, 143, pp. 454–73.
4. Clarke R.S.J., 'The hyperglycaemic response to different types of surgery and anaesthesia', *British Journal of Anaesthesia*, 1970, 42, pp. 45–53.
5. Clarke R., *A Surgeon's Century: The Life of Sir Ian Fraser*, Belfast: Ulster Historical Foundation, 2004.
6. Clarke R.S.J., *A Directory of Ulster Doctors (who qualified before 1901)*, Belfast: Ulster Historical Foundation, 2013.

John Cooper (1930–)
MB BCh BAO FFARCSI FFARCS
DPMCAI

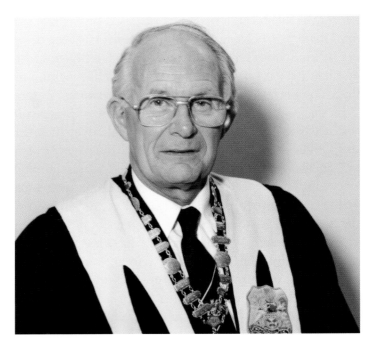

JOHN COOPER was born on 14 October 1930. He entered Queen's University Belfast (QUB) as a medical student in 1949 and graduated MB BCh BAO in 1955. He was a houseman at the Mater Infirmorum Hospital, Belfast and did his postgraduate training at the Mater, the Royal Victoria Hospital and the Royal Belfast Hospital for Sick Children. He received his Fellowship of the Faculty of Anaesthetists, RCSI in 1964 and that of the Faculty of Anaesthetists of the Royal College of Surgeons of England in 1965. In the same year, he was appointed to a consultant post at the Mater Infirmorum Hospital. His areas of interest were intensive care and pain medicine. He was elected to the Board of the Faculty of Anaesthetists, RCSI in 1984 and was subsequently elected dean in 1994, a post he held until 1997. By the time he took over as dean, the faculty had achieved financial independence from RCSI and had started to accrue a capital reserve. Dr Cooper, along with Dr William Blunnie and Dr Pat Fitzgerald, began a search for suitable premises to house the faculty. He received support in this from the then president of RCSI, Mr Dermot O'Flynn who said that the Council of RCSI would assist the faculty in its efforts to acquire its own building. In 1995, in his role as dean, Cooper led the move to incorporate the faculty as a separate company, 'the Faculty of Anaesthetists, RCSI', making it more independent. In the final year of his deanship, the faculty received charitable status.

Following on from his time as dean, he was asked by his successor Blunnie to establish a diploma in pain medicine. He found this to be quite a challenge but he was delighted to be the recipient of the Foundation Diploma in Pain Medicine in 2001. His pioneering work eventually led to the formation of the Faculty of Pain Medicine of the College of Anaesthetists of Ireland in 2008.

Dr Cooper was also actively involved in other areas; he was chairman of the Cardinal Newman Society at Queen's University Belfast from 1961–2 and honorary secretary of the Northern Ireland Society of Anaesthetists, 1975–7. He was a member of the Association of Anaesthetists of Great Britain and Ireland (1970–98) and was elected as an honorary member in 1998. He has been a constant presence and supporter of the Western Anaesthetic Symposium in Galway and has never missed a meeting of this group.

Apart from his role as a consultant anaesthetist, Dr Cooper held a number of senior administrative roles at the Mater Infirmorum Hospital, Belfast. He was general manager of the hospital from 1987–92 when he was appointed chief executive. He realised that the hospital could not continue as a managed hospital of the Eastern Board in Northern Ireland and so led the hospital board in acquiring trust status. He stepped down as chief executive in 1995 and also retired from clinical practice during that year.

However, despite his high-profile career in anaesthesia, Dr Cooper is probably proudest of his sporting achievements, in particular in playing for Queen's in the lead up to the Fitzgibbon Cup (the premier hurling trophy competed for by higher education institutions in Ireland) of 1953. He joined the QUB hurling club in 1950[1] and played with them against University College Cork (UCC) in 1951, and against University College Galway (UCG) in 1952. In 1953, the Fitzgibbon Cup was held in Queen's for just the second time in its history. He played in the semi-final in which QUB defeated UCG. University College Dublin (UCD) defeated Cork in the other semi-final. Dublin were looking for a fourth win in a row which would be a new record. However, the final was deferred because of the Princess Victoria ferry disaster, when the ship, which operated between Larne and Stranraer, sank in the North Channel during a severe storm with the loss of 133 lives. The rescheduled match took place on 26 April 1953 at Corrigan Park in West Belfast and John Cooper was part of the QUB squad but did not play on the day. Queen's won by a single point. It was a significant game in that it was the first GAA match ever to be televised in Ireland (by the new BBC studios which opened that year in Belfast) and it was the first and, to date, the only time that QUB won the Fitzgibbon Cup. This event was commemorated by Comhairle Uladh at Casement Park in 2009 by the awarding of medals to the 'survivors' of the squad. John is proud to have been one of the recipients of this medal.

He is married to Mary (*née* McElroy). His interests are medical education, current affairs, travel, music and gardening.

Based on oral and written information from Dr Cooper.

JT

References

1   Gallagher, C. and Harvey, B., '1953, Annus Mirabilis', available at http //queens.gaa.ie/clubs/hurling/ (accessed 9 August 2021).

William 'Bill' P. Blunnie (1949–)
MB BCh BAO FFARCSI FRCA (Hon) FRCPI (Hon)

DR WILLIAM BLUNNIE was born in 1949 in Kilrush, County Clare where he was educated at the local Christian Brothers school. He studied medicine at University College Galway medical school and graduated MB BCh BAO in January 1974. He interned at Wexford General Hospital and Manorhamilton Hospital before starting his anaesthetic training at the Royal Victoria Hospital, Belfast in 1975. One year later, he became an anaesthetic registrar in Altnagelvin Hospital, Derry; he received his Fellowship of the Faculty of Anaesthetists, RCSI in May 1978. He spent the following two years as tutor/senior registrar (SR) at Queen's University Belfast and the Royal Victoria Hospital. He then rotated overseas taking a post as SR in the Klinicum Statishe in Osnabruck, Germany following which he returned to Ireland in 1981 firstly as SR in the Mater Misericordiae Hospital in Dublin and then back again to the Royal Victoria Hospital.

Bill was appointed as consultant in anaesthesia and intensive care medicine at both the Mater Misericordiae Hospital and the Rotunda Hospital, Dublin, in 1982. He was honorary secretary of the Department of Anaesthesia at the Mater from 1984–8 and subsequently was appointed chairman, a position he held from

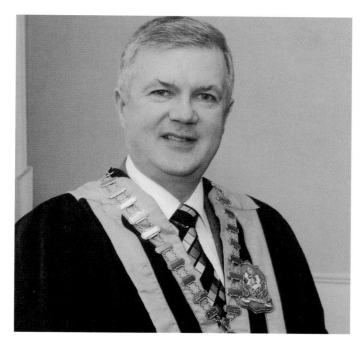

1988 until 1995. He retired from the Mater and the Rotunda in 2012 but continued in private practice at the Mater Private Hospital in Eccles Street, Dublin.

He was a member of the Board of the Faculty of Anaesthetists, RCSI and the Council of the College of Anaesthetists of Ireland consecutively from 1992–2002. During his time on the board/council he served as both a member and as chairman of a large number of different committees (e.g. Education, Examination, Finance, Training etc). He was appointed honorary treasurer in 1992 and dean of the Faculty of Anaesthetists, RCSI in 1997. He was one of the main driving forces in negotiating the separation of the faculty from the Royal College of Surgeons in Ireland and in the formation of the College of Anaesthetists of Ireland (CAI). He was dean of the faculty from 1997–8 and in 1998 became the first president of the new college. Bill continued as CAI president from 1998–2000 and had the honour of conferring its first fellowship on the then president of Ireland, Mary McAleese, on 23 September 1998, a date which is now regarded as the college's foundation day. He himself was conferred with an honorary fellowship by the Royal College of Anaesthetists in December 1998. When he had completed his term as president, he was chairman of the ad hoc house committee set up to purchase a new premises for CAI (1999–2002).

The other committee members were Prof. Denis Moriarty, Prof. Anthony Cunningham, Dr Rory Dwyer and Dr Dermot Phelan. On 25 May 2000, they purchased 22 Merrion Square on behalf of the college as its new headquarters. Following on from that, he was appointed chairman of a project group set up by the college president Dr John McAdoo to renovate the house. It supervised the refurbishment of the house in conjunction with the conservation architect Roisin Hanley and the building firm Clancy Construction. The house was formally opened as the headquarters of the College of Anaesthetists of Ireland by the president of Ireland, Mary McAleese, on 8 October 2010.

Bill was a member of the Irish Medical Council from 1999–2004 representing anaesthesia and radiology, was chairman of the Committee on Medical Ionising Radiation and was a member of the Radiological Protection Institute of Ireland representing the medical profession. He was involved in numerous other groups pertaining to anaesthesia and was convenor of the Irish Standing Committee and council member of the Association of Anaesthetists of Great Britain and Ireland, and also a member of the European Board of Anaesthesiology (EBA UEMS), An Bord Altranais and a founder member of the European Society of Intensive Care Medicine.

He has received recognition internationally for his huge commitment to advancing the specialty. He was conferred with an honorary fellowship by the Royal College of Anaesthetists in 1998, fellowship of the Royal College of Physicians in Ireland in 2008, honorary fellowship of the Romanian and Singapore Societies of Anaesthesia and was elected as an academician of the European Academy of Anaesthesiology. When asked what was his most gratifying achievement in a very busy career, he answered that it was obtaining the Grant of Arms and Badge for the College of Anaesthetists of Ireland. He was adamant, however, in pointing out that this was done in conjunction with his Mater colleague Dr Dermot Phelan and Dr Pat Fitzgerald from Limerick.

Billy retired from clinical practice in 2019. He is married to Monica McMenamin and they have five children. His interests are DIY and travel.

JT

Based on conversations with Dr Blunnie and written information provided by him.

SECTION 2
Professors of Anaesthesia in Ireland (Appointed Pre–1998) Not Already Included in the List of Deans

Anthony J. Cunningham (1947 -)

John P.H. Fee (1947-)

Rajinder K. Mirakhur (1947 -)

George D. Shorten (1961 -)

Anthony J. Cunningham (1947–)
MD FRCP(C) DABA FFARCSI FANZCA FRCPI (Hon) FCMSA (Hon) MSc BA

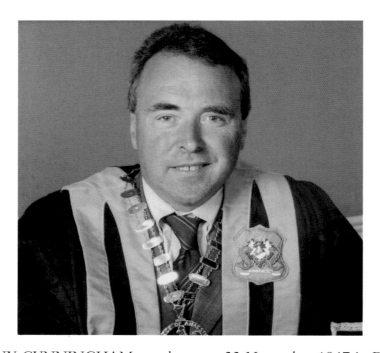

ANTHONY CUNNINGHAM was born on 22 November 1947 in Drogheda, County Louth and went to school at the Dominican College in Newbridge, County Kildare. He studied medicine at University College Galway from 1965–71. Whilst a student, he won a Connaught Minor Rugby medal and was also auditor of the college's Literary and Debating Society in 1968. Following graduation in 1971, he interned at Our Lady of Lourdes Hospital, Drogheda before moving to Canada the following year. He started his training as a resident in internal medicine at the University of Western Ontario in London, Ontario, then moved to a general practice training programme in Brookville, Ontario before starting as an anaesthesia resident at Queen's University, Kingston in the same province. He received the fellowship of the Royal College of Physicians of Canada in 1979. He then did further postgraduate training as fellow in obstetric anaesthesia at the University of Ottawa and subsequently took up a staff position at Ottawa General Hospital as director of the Obstetrical and Pain Service (1979–82).

He returned to Ireland in 1982, initially as consultant anaesthetist at St Vincent's Hospital Dublin. In 1986, he was appointed professor of anaesthesia at the Royal College of Surgeons in Ireland, the first full-time professor of anaesthesia in the Republic of Ireland. His predecessor at RCSI, Prof. Gilmartin had been an associate professor; John Dundee was appointed in 1964 to Queen's University Belfast and was the first professor of anaesthesia in Northern Ireland. His clinical commitments associated with the chair were to the Charitable Infirmary, Jervis Street and the Richmond Hospital, both in Dublin. The two hospitals merged in 1987 to become Beaumont Hospital. After a number of years in Beaumont, he took a sabbatical to go to Yale University School of Medicine in New Haven, Connecticut as a visiting professor (1991–2). This resulted in a number of combined Yale University–Ireland Faculty conferences taking place over the following years. He completed his MD thesis on 'Factors affecting left ventricular performance during abdominal aortic cross-clamping and release' in 1992.

He became involved with the Faculty of Anaesthetists, RCSI soon after returning to Ireland holding multiple sequential roles: honorary secretary (1992–6), chairman of the Final FFARCSI exams (1996–7), chairman of the Education Committee (1997–2000), and finally succeeding Dr William Blunnie on being elected as the second president of the newly formed College of Anaesthetists of Ireland (2000–3). He was coordinator of the MSc programme 'Professionalism in Practice' at the college, as well as being vice president of the European Board of Anaesthesiology and the Irish council representative at the European Society of Anaesthesiologists.

After completing his time at the College of Anaesthetists of Ireland, Prof. Cunningham was elected to the Medical Council and was chairman of its Education and Training Committee from 2006–8. He was a member of the Postgraduate Medical and Dental Board from 2007–8. He has published extensively and is the author of more than 40 review articles and book chapters as well as having presented at meetings and conferences worldwide. In 2021 he published a memoir of his childhood titled *About 1957 – That was When*[1] He even found time late in his career to study for a Bachelor of Arts in Law at the Dublin Institute of Technology, graduating in 2011.

Anthony retired from clinical practice in 2011 to take up the position of foundation dean at Perdana University, Royal College of Surgeons in Ireland School of Medicine, Malaysia, a role he held until 2014. He then returned to Ireland to become the medical director of the Galway Clinic, a private hospital in the west of Ireland.

Anthony was originally married to Bernadette Fitzgerald and they have four children and eight grandchildren. He was married a second time in 2018 to Ann

McGreevy and has three stepchildren from this marriage. He now lives in a bungalow in an idyllic location outside Clonbur, County Galway overlooking Lough Corrib, though he hasn't yet taken up fishing to any great extent. He is a keen tennis player and golfer and has been known to attend the occasional race meeting. His other interests include supporting the County Louth Gaelic football team, Drogheda United Football Club and reading history and politics.

Based on conversations with Prof. Cunningham and written information provided by him.

JT

References
1   Cunningham A.J., *About 1957 – That was When*, Galway: East Rand Publishing, 2021.

John Patrick Howard Fee (1947–)
MD FFARCSI FRCA PhD

HOWARD FEE was born in Belfast on 20 June 1947. His father Charles was a dental surgeon while his mother Violet was an educational psychologist. He attended primary school at Inchmarlo Preparatory School in Belfast and then went to secondary school at the Royal Belfast Academical Institution. From there he enrolled in the medical school at Queen's University Belfast (QUB) in 1966, qualifying MB BCh BAO in 1972. Following his internship at the Lagan Valley Hospital in Lisburn (1972–3) he entered the Northern Ireland Anaesthetic Training Scheme in 1973. He obtained his FFARCSI in 1976 and was subsequently appointed as a consultant anaesthetist at the Mid-Ulster Hospital in Magherafelt, County Londonderry/ Derry. Howard received his MD (honours) from QUB in 1980, was appointed senior lecturer in anaesthetics at the university in 1981 and as a consultant anaesthetist at the Royal Victoria Hospital Belfast at the same time.

In 1986, he took a sabbatical to spend a year as a research fellow at Vanderbilt University and Medical Center in Nashville, Tennessee. He received his FRCA (ad eundem) in 1987 and his PhD in 1990. Howard was appointed professor and head of the Department of Anaesthetics and Intensive Care Medicine at QUB in 1995, a position he held until his retirement in 2009. His research interests were the pharmacology of volatile anaesthetics and benzodiazepines. He has published widely with over 120 research publications

356

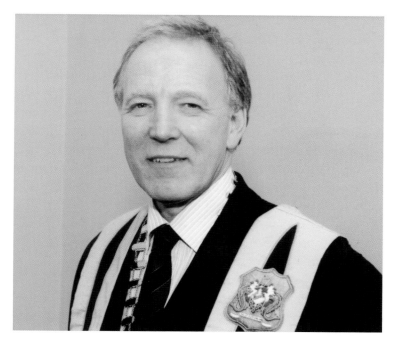

as well as a number of textbooks, *Physiology for Anaesthesiologists* and *Pharmacology for Anaesthesiologists*, both co-authored with James Bovill, as well as *Anaesthetic Physiology and Pharmacology* by William (Liam) McCaughey, Richard S.J. Clarke, William F.M. Wallace and Fee.

He was elected in 1987 as a board member of the Faculty of Anaesthetists, RCSI and served initially until 1997. He was subsequently re-elected as a council member of the College of Anaesthetists of Ireland (CAI) from 1999–2006, was chairman of the Examination Committee and was actively involved along with Dr Liam McCaughey and Dr Joseph Tracey in the development of the Objective Structured Clinical Examination (OSCE) as part of the Primary examination. He was instrumental along with Prof. Anthony Cunningham in developing the overseas Primary examination in Oman. He was elected president of the college from 2003–6. On completing his term as president , he was elected as a council member at the Royal College of Anaesthetists (RCoA) in London from 2007–13.

One of Howard's interests was medical education and he served as a member of the Medline Taskforce on Medical Education in Europe from 2006–7. His involvement in the development of training mannequins and simulators at Queen's lead to the formation of a Queen's University Company, Tru-Corp Ltd. He was a council member of the Anaesthetic Section, the Royal Society of

Medicine from 2000–3 and president of the Ulster Medical Society from 2008–9; his presidential address 'Clouds of unknowing' was a superb synopsis of the history of anaesthesia.

He is married to Eileen and they have one son, Conor, who is a barrister in London. Since his retirement in 2009, Howard has indulged his obsession with Hungary and the Austro-Hungarian Empire. He has been studying the Hungarian language for the last 10 years, initially with teachers in Belfast but now via Skype as his teachers have all returned to Budapest. He visits that city regularly and is also learning German which he finds a little less difficult. His current research interest is Austro-Hungarian postal history and he has exhibited some material in both Dublin and London. His wife Eileen loves ballet, opera and Iceland thus providing Howard with excuses to travel and to indulge these interests.

Finally, when at home in Belfast, he occasionally plays a 'rather fine, listed pipe organ' in his local church.

JT

Based on conversations with Prof. Fee and also written information provided by him.

Rajinder K. Mirakhur (1945–)
MB BS MD FFARCS PhD FFARCSI

RAJINDER MIRAKHUR was born on 14 October 1945 in Srinagar, the northernmost city in India and the capital of the state of Jammu and Kashmir. His father, Mr Prithvi Nath Mirakhur (who died at the age of 103) was an accounts officer in the Jammu and Kashmir administration. His mother Kamla was a home maker. He attended Sri Pratap High School and then Sri Pratap College before studying medicine at the Government Medical College at the Jammu and Kashmir University, Srinagar. After qualifying MB BS in 1966 he did his internship at the Shri Maharaja Hari Singh (SMHS) Hospital in Srinagar before commencing his training in anaesthesia and medicine at the Safdarjung Hospital in New Delhi, India (1967–71). After being conferred MD (Anaesthesia) at the University of Delhi in 1970, he moved to the city of Chandigarh (famous for its architecture and as a planned city by the Swiss architect Corbusier), where he was lecturer and then assistant professor in anaesthesia at the Postgraduate Institute of Medical Education and Research (1971–4). This is one of the highest

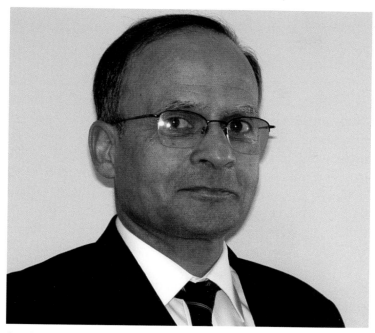

ranked medical colleges in India. He met Prof. John Dundee when the latter was visiting Chandigarh in 1973 and he asked if he could come to Belfast to do some academic work and if possible, a PhD. Although he knew how prolific the Queen's University Department of Anaesthesia was in those days in producing clinical research, he had no idea at the time of the 'troubles' taking place in Northern Ireland. He moved to Ireland in September 1974 to continue his training in Belfast, initially as a senior house officer in the Royal Victoria Hospital, then as registrar, senior registrar, senior tutor and research fellow at Queen's University (1974–80). John Dundee was very supportive, introducing him to several academics in the UK, encouraging him to attend meetings of the Anaesthesia Research Society and the British Pharmacological Society and supporting him in enrolling for his PhD. He was conferred with his Fellowship of the Faculty of Anaesthetists of the Royal College of Surgeons of England (FFARCS) in 1976 and in the following year received his PhD from Queen's University Belfast. He was appointed consultant anaesthetist to the Royal Group in Belfast in 1980 and as senior lecturer, Queen's University and the Royal Hospitals in 1990. He received an ad eundem fellowship of the Faculty of Anaesthetists, RCSI in 1984. He was appointed to a personal chair as professor of anaesthesia, Queen's University Belfast, in 1996, a post he held until his retirement in November 2009.

Rajinder's principal area of interest was undergraduate and postgraduate teaching. He published widely on the physiology and pharmacology of neuromuscular blockade, intravenous and inhalational anaesthetics as well as the pharmacology of anticholinergics. In his clinical practice, he was involved in ophthalmic anaesthesia, orthopaedics and trauma. Although he was an examiner in both the Irish and English faculties and colleges, he was never a member of the Board of the Faculty of Anaesthetists, RCSI or of the Council of the College of Anaesthetists of Ireland. He served on the Council of the Royal College of Anaesthetists, was a member of the Council of the Association of Anaesthetists of Great Britain and Ireland (AAGBI) and was an adviser on overseas doctors' training to the postgraduate dean at QUB.

In 2001, he became the first recipient of AAGBI's Featherstone Award and was conferred with AAGBI honorary membership eight years later. He received the Gold Medal of the Royal College of Anaesthetists, the college's highest honour, in 2011. He has lectured widely and delivered the Winter College Lecture of the College of Anaesthetists of Ireland in 2002 and the Autumn College Lecture in 2010.

He is married to Dr Meenakshi Mirakhur, a neuropathologist at the Royal Victoria Hospital Belfast, now also retired. They have two children, a daughter Dr Anju Mirakhur specialising in respiratory medicine and a son Ajay studying psychiatry and public health. After retirement, he served as the education adviser to the Royal College of Anaesthetists for five years. He is currently a council member of the History of Anaesthesia Society and a member of the Lagan Valley Probus group. He enjoys walking, jogging, generally keeping fit and travel.

JT

Based on written material provided by Prof. Mirakhur.

George D. Shorten (1961–)
MD FFARCSI FRCA DABA PhD DSc (Hon)

GEORGE SHORTEN is a native of Cork city. He was educated at Presentation Brothers College, Cork (PBC) and attended medical school at University College Cork (UCC), graduating MB BCh BAO in 1985. Having completed his intern year at Cork University Hospital, he trained in anaesthesia in Northern Ireland

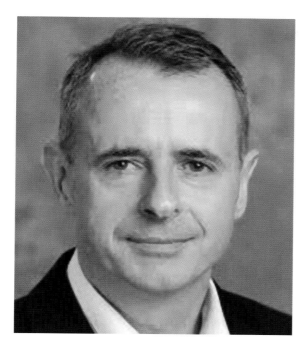

at Craigavon Area Hospital (Portadown), Belfast City Hospital and the Royal Victoria Hospital in Belfast. He obtained the Fellowship of the Faculty of Anaesthetists, RCSI (FFARCSI) taking first place in Part II, and the Fellowship of the Royal College of Anaesthetists (FRCA), both in 1989.

Between 1989 and 1996, George gained further clinical and research experience in the USA, Canada and Western Australia. He held the posts of instructor in anesthesia, clinical research fellow in anesthesia, and assistant professor in anesthesia at the Harvard Medical School, Boston, Massachusetts (MA). At the Beth Israel Hospital, Boston MA he was fellow in cardiac anesthesia, associate anesthetist and was named 'Teacher of the year' in 1995 and 1996. He held the posts of visiting professor in anesthesia at Harvard, Beth Israel and at Saint Louis University, Missouri. In Perth, Western Australia, he was senior registrar at the Department of Anaesthesia, Sir Charles Gairdner Hospital and in Canada, fellow in paediatric anaesthesia at the Hospital for Sick Children, Toronto, Ontario.

George worked closely with Dr Nishan G. Goudsouzian, pediatric anesthesiologist at Massachusetts General Hospital, in assessing the use of the laryngeal mask airway in children.[1] Subsequently he, Goudsouzian and William Denman 'crisscrossed the country, lecturing widely, George Shorten speaking with the mellifluous lilt of his native Cork to presumably bemused American audiences'.[2]

In 1997, he returned to Ireland and was appointed as first professor of anaesthesia and intensive care medicine at University College Cork, with clinical commitments as consultant anaesthetist at Cork University Hospital (CUH) and honorary consultant at the South Infirmary Victoria University Hospital. The immediate challenge facing him was the sustainability of academic departments of anaesthesia which were at risk because universities and governments were prioritising funding for health areas such as cancer and cardiovascular disease. This meant forming strategic alliances and selecting academic projects which could have a lasting impact. Resources were therefore invested in two research themes, acute pain and the science of professional education. The impact of the research outputs improved dramatically as a result and contributed to the establishment of the Masters in Anaesthesia degree (subsequently MSc in Medical Professionalism) at the College of Anaesthetists of Ireland (CAI) and made an important contribution to founding the European Society of Anaesthesiologists' Clinical Trials Network. Extensive work over many years on the science of professional education came to fruition with the publication of a consensus statement on competency-based education and training in anaesthesiology.[3]

George's research interests in human performance in healthcare and innovative training in technical skills were recognised by UCC in 2018 when he received the inaugural President's Lifetime Achievements Award for Teaching and Learning. During his time as dean of the School of Medicine at UCC (2010–13), he established and acted as a foundation director of the Centre for the Application of Science to Simulation in Education, Research and Technology (ASSERT) at University College Cork.[4] He was a coordinating applicant for the Irish Health Research Board infrastructure grant which established UCC's clinical research facility.[5] He has served on many national and international research and education bodies including as chairman of the Education Committee of the European Pain Federation, the Irish Universities and Medical Schools Consortium, the Council of Deans of Medical Schools in Ireland and he was a ministerial appointment to the European Medicines Agency serving as co-chairperson of its Medical Products Committee during Ireland's presidency in 2004.

In 2021, George was conferred with a doctorate in science (DSc) by the National University of Ireland, the first person in the specialty of anaesthesiology to be honoured by NUI with its highest academic award. In May 2021, he became president of the College of Anaesthesiologists of Ireland.

Anaesthetists in Cork have a long and distinguished history of teaching and training and supporting the work of the Faculty of Anaesthetists, RCSI. The anaesthetic department at Cork Regional Hospital played a leading role in establishing the Southern Regional Anaesthetic Training Scheme and the National Senior Registrar Anaesthetic Rotation. A professorship in anaesthesia at UCC was considered long overdue so not surprisingly, when it was finally established, it had widespread enthusiastic support. However, the ultimate success of the new department could not have been achieved without the vision, dynamism and personality of George Shorten.

George won all-Ireland sprint medals with Leevale Athletic Club and Munster Schools Cup medals with PBC in rugby; a sport in which he represented Munster at schools level. In 2003, having climbed four of the 'Seven Summits', George was a member of an Irish team that attempted to reach the summit of Mount Everest. Unfortunately, at 23,000 feet George succumbed to a serious bout of altitude sickness and had to return to base camp.[6] Two members of the team (Mick Murphy and Ger McDonnell) succeeded in reaching the summit on that occasion and in a second attempt a year later, Pat Falvey and Clare O'Leary were successful.[7]

George remains an active mountaineer and completes marathons and ultramarathons regularly at what he describes as a 'leisurely' pace.

In 2004, he married Bronagh McCann. They have two children, Ava and Daniel, and live near the town of Mallow in County Cork.

JC

References

1 King M.R., Mai C.L., Firth P.G., 'Half a century of anesthesia for children: An interview with Dr. Nishan G. "Nick" Goudsouzian', *Pediatric Anesthesia*, 2018, 28, pp. 947–54, https://doi.org/10.1111/pan.13495.

2 Goudsouzian N.G., Denman W., Cleveland R. and Shorten G., 'Radiologic localization of the laryngeal mask airway in children', *Anesthesiology*, 1992, 77, pp. 1085–9.

3 Shorten G.D., De Robertis, E., Goldik, Z., Kietaibl, S., Niemi-Murola, L., Sabelnikovs, O., 'European Section/Board of Anaesthesiology/European Society of Anaesthesiology consensus statement on competency-based education and training in anaesthesiology', *European Journal of Anaesthesiology*, 2020, 37, pp. 421–34.

4 'HRB Clinical Research Facility Cork', available at crfc.ucc.ie (accessed 30 June 2021).

5 'Enabling Safer Better Healthcare', available at https://www.ucc.ie/en/assert/ (accessed 30 June 2021).

6   Tallant N., 'Climbers vow to conquer Everest despite illness of key team member', *Independent*, 6 May 2004, available at https://www.independent.ie/irish-news/climbers-vow-to-conquer-everest-despite-illness-of-key-team-member-25945850.html (accessed 30 June 2021).

7   'First Irish woman reaches summit of Everest', *Irish Times*, 18 May 2004, available at https://www.irishtimes.com/news/first-irish-woman-reaches-summit-of-everest-1.979608 (accessed 30 June 2021).

SECTION 3
Some Other Significant Names in Irish Anaesthesia History

John MacDonnell (1796–1892)

William Brooke O'Shaughnessy (1809–1889)

George Mahood Foy (1843–1934)

Paul Piel (*c.* 1851–1924)

Thomas Percy Claude Kirkpatrick (1869–1954)

Ella Webb (1877–1946)

Ivan Magill (1888–1986)

E. Sheila Kenny (1909–1990)

Edmund Delaney (1925–1979)

Kevin Moore (1936–1997)

Frances Mary Lehane (1944–2013)

Éamon McCoy (1961–)

John MacDonnell (1796–1892)
BA LRCSI MD

John MacDonnell's ancestors arrived in Ireland in 1390 when Ian Vohr MacDonnell, who came from Isla in the Highlands of Scotland, married Marjory Bysset from Glenarm in County Antrim. Ian Vohr's great grandson, Sir Alaster MacDonnell was a major general in the army of the Marquis of Montrose and was successful in six battles in the wars of 1644–5. He was killed at the battle of Nock-na-Noss in Cork. Dr John MacDonnell's father, James, was fourth in descent from Sir Alaster. He was a prominent physician in Belfast and was known as 'the father of Belfast medicine'. He founded the Belfast Dispensary and Fever Hospital, which was the forerunner of the Royal Victoria Hospital. John MacDonnell himself was born at 15 Donegall Place, Belfast on 11 February 1796. He attended school at the Belfast Academy (now the Belfast Royal Academy) and studied afterwards at Trinity College Dublin where he graduated with a BA degree in 1818. He obtained his licence to practise surgery and letters testimonial from the Royal College of Surgeons in Ireland in 1821 and then continued his studies in Edinburgh, London and Paris before receiving his MD from Edinburgh University in 1825. He returned to Ireland where he set up practice in Dublin and was appointed demonstrator in anatomy at the Richmond Medical School, which opened in 1826. This later became the Carmichael School of Medicine in 1865 and eventually part of the RCSI in 1889. Later, he became lecturer in anatomy and physiology through the influence of the surgeon Richard Carmichael. In 1835, a vacancy arose in the Surgical Department at the Richmond and Carmichael tried to persuade the hospital to appoint MacDonnell to the post. When the hospital refused to do so, Carmichael resigned his own position in favour of MacDonnell.[1]

In the same year, 1835, John MacDonnell was elected as the first professor of surgery to the new medical school in Belfast, the Royal Belfast Academical Institution. His father James had been one of the original subscribers to this new Belfast 'Inst' when it was originally incorporated by an act of parliament in 1810 but it had to wait until 1835 before it finally opened. However, in 1836, he eventually received an appointment as visiting surgeon at the Richmond Hospital in Dublin and so he never took up the post as Belfast professor. He was editor of the *Dublin Journal of Medical Science* from 1842–6. This later became the *Dublin Quarterly Journal of Medical Science* under William Wilde.[2]

On 1 January 1847, he was the first doctor in Ireland to perform surgery on an anaesthetised person. Ether was administered (in his report to the *Dublin Medical Press* he wrote, 'we succeeded in establishing complete insensibility' so it is not clear exactly who administered the ether[3]) to a young woman, Mary Kane, for an amputation of the forearm at the elbow and MacDonnell subsequently wrote an account of the procedure for the 6 January edition of the *Dublin Medical Press*.[3]

Later that year, on 23 October, he was appointed professor of descriptive anatomy at the Richmond, a role he held until 1851. He was subsequently appointed as a medical member of the Poor Law Commission, a post he continued in until he was 80 years of age. In his retirement, he found time to write a history of the Irish Rebellion of 1641, which was the start of the Eleven Years War or the Cromwellian War, which he published as *The Ulster Civil War of 1641*. This included an account of the Irish Brigade in Montrose's army as well as the part played in the campaign by his ancestor Sir Alaster MacDonnell.[1]

John MacDonnell was married to Charity, daughter of the Rev. Robert Conway Dobbs of Belfast, and had 11 children, five girls and six boys.[2] His only

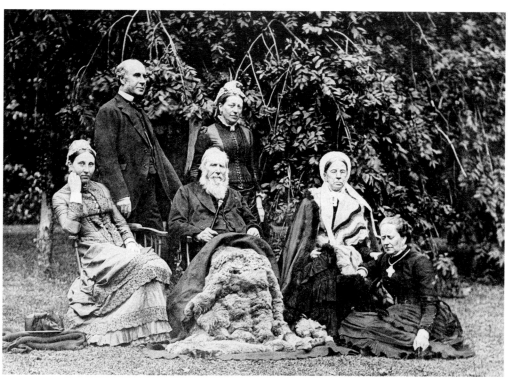

John MacDonnell, seated centre, with his wife Charity on his left, at Kilsharvan in Co. Meath c. 1876. Courtesy of Eoin O'Brien / Anniversary Press.

367

sister married Andrew Armstrong of Kilsharvan, County Meath and their property was left to John's son Robert. He died at his home in Fitzwilliam Square in 1892 aged 96 and was buried in the family plot in Kilsharvan. His son Robert also qualified in surgery, was a visiting surgeon in the Charitable Infirmary, Jervis Street and Dr Steevens' Hospital, Dublin and was president of the Royal College of Surgeons in Ireland 1877–8. He gave the first transfusion of human blood in the country in April 1877.[4]

The MacDonnell coat of arms contains a dolphin in the lower right-hand quadrant and this has been included in the coat of arms of the College of Anaesthetists of Ireland (now the College of Anaesthesiologists of Ireland).

JT

References

1 Froggatt P., 'MacDonnell, Father and Son', *Journal of the Irish Colleges of Physicians and Surgeons*, 1984, 13, pp. 198-206.
2 Breathnach C.S., Moynihan J.B., 'John MacDonnell and insensibility with ether in 1847', *Ulster Medical Journal*, September 2013, 82, pp. 188–91.
3 MacDonnell J., 'Amputation of the Arm, Performed at the Richmond Hospital, without Pain' (letter), *Dublin Medical Press*, 1847, 17, pp. 8–9.
4 Cameron C.A., *History of the Royal College of Surgeons in Ireland and of the Irish Schools of Medicine: Including a Medical Bibliography and a Medical Biography*, Fannin and Co., 1916, pp. 613–16.

William Brooke O'Shaughnessy (1809–1889)
MD FRS

The death occurred in January 1889 of an Irish doctor who may never have practised anaesthesia but whose work in two areas, therapeutic rehydration and the medicinal use of cannabis, still has relevance for present-day anaesthetists. **William Brooke O'Shaughnessy** (1809–1889) was born in Limerick. After spending one year at the medical school of Trinity College Dublin, he moved to the University of Edinburgh, from which he graduated MD in 1829. Shortly afterwards, he relocated to London to pursue his interest in chemistry and toxicology. In late 1831, during a cholera outbreak in Britain, he worked in Newcastle-upon-Tyne studying the blood and excreta of patients with the disease. Referring to the blood he wrote, 'It has lost a large proportion of its water... It has also lost a great proportion of its neutral saline ingredients' and where the excreta were concerned, 'All the salts deficient in the blood, especially the carbonate of soda, are present in the peculiar white dejected matters…'.[1] O'Shaughnessy presented his findings to the Central Board of Health in early 1832 and recommended a revolutionary therapeutic remedy 'the injection into the veins of tepid water holding a solution of the normal salts of the blood'. His report, which laid the foundation for what was to become intravenous fluid and electrolyte replacement therapy, was published later that year.[2] The suggested treatment for cholera was soon put to the test by Dr Thomas Latta of Leith in Scotland who administered salt containing intravenous fluid to 17 cholera patients, eight of whom survived. An editorial in *The Lancet* compared the treatment to 'the workings of a miraculous and

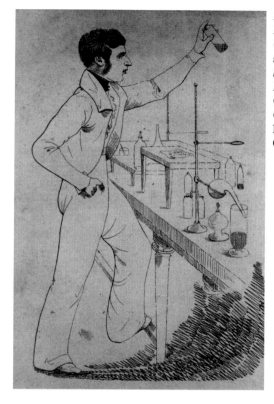

Dr Richard Brooke O'Shaughnessy at work in his laboratory. Drawing by Colesworthey Grant. Courtesy NIH Digital Collections.

supernatural agent'.[3] When the epidemic subsided, interest in the new therapy waned and it was not used again for some decades, not least because Latta died in 1833 and O'Shaughnessy took a position as assistant surgeon with the East India Company.

He continued his chemistry researches in India, becoming professor of chemistry at the Calcutta Medical College. In 1838, he discovered narcotine (noscapine), a previously unknown opium alkaloid, visiting an opium den for himself to see how it was prepared.[4] News of successful ether anaesthesia in Boston, Massachusetts reached the subcontinent during the second week of March 1847 and on 22 March, the first use in India of the agent to relieve the pain of surgery took place under the supervision of O'Shaughnessy, who was the operating surgeon.[5] He explored the potential therapeutic benefits of Indian hemp or cannabis, which at the time was unknown as a drug in Europe, and published his observations.[6] Within a few years, it was being used to treat a wide range of conditions by many of the leading doctors in Britain and Ireland, including

Robert Graves of Dublin.[7] It was not until more specific therapies became available in the early twentieth century that it fell into disrepute. In Ireland, medicinal cannabis can currently be prescribed under the Medical Cannabis Access Programme for a limited number of specific indications.[8] At the time of writing these do not include chronic pain, a condition in which many present-day anaesthetists have a particular interest.

Away from medicine, O'Shaughnessy first published the results of experiments he had carried out with the wire telegraph in 1839.[9] He was appointed Director General of Telegraphs for India in 1852, and his energy in the post is demonstrated by the fact that three years later, the country's telegraph line extended 3,500 miles, connecting Calcutta (now Kolkata) with Agra, Bombay (now Mumbai) and Madras (now Chennai).[7]

Knighted by Queen Victoria in 1856, illness forced this extraordinary Irish doctor to return to England in 1860. He retired during the following year and lived for the remainder of his life in Hampshire.

DW

References

1 O'Shaughnessy W.B., 'Experiments on the blood in cholera', *The Lancet*, 1831–2, 1, p. 490.

2 O'Shaughnessy W.B., *Report on the Chemical Pathology of the Malignant Cholera: Containing analyses of the blood, dejections, &c. of patients labouring under the disease in Newcastle and London, &c*, London: Highley, 1832.

3 'Editorial', *The Lancet*, 1831–2, 2, pp. 284–6.

4 Aldrich M.R., 'The remarkable W.B. O'Shaughnessy', *O'Shaughnessy's: Journal of the Californian Cannabis Research Medical Group*, 2006, Spring, pp. 26–7.

5 Divekar V.M., Naik L.D., 'Evolution of anaesthesia in India', *Journal of Postgraduate Medicine*, 2001, 47, pp. 149–52.

6 O'Shaughnessy W.B., 'On the preparation of the Indian Hemp, or Gunjah (Cannabis Indica), their effects on the animal system in health, and their utility in the treatment of tetanus and other convulsive diseases', *British and Foreign Medical Review*, 1840, 10, pp. 225–8.

7 Coakley D., *Irish Masters of Medicine*, Dublin: Town House, 1992, pp. 149–56.

8 Medical Cannabis Access Programme, available at www.gov.ie/en/publication/90ece9/-medical-cannabis-access-programme/ (accessed 19 January 2021).

9 O'Shaughnessy W.B., 'Memoranda relative to experiments on the communication of telegraphic signals by induced electricity', *Journal of the Asiatic Society of Bengal*, 1839, 8, p. 71.

George Mahood Foy (1843–1934)
LAH FRCSI MD

George Mahood Foy, youngest son of a local merchant, was born in December 1843 in Cootehill, County Cavan. He studied medicine in both Belfast and Dublin, and in 1873, obtained a licence to practice from the Apothecaries Hall of Ireland, becoming both a licentiate and fellow of the Royal College of Surgeons in Ireland during the following year. Foy was appointed surgeon to the Whitworth Hospital, Dublin, in 1876, a position he retained throughout his working life. He was a noted linguist, fluent in seven or eight languages, and also a prodigious reader and writer who, in addition to authoring and translating numerous papers, both

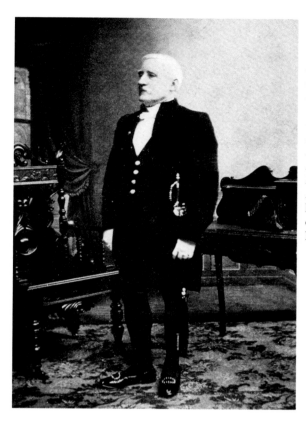

Photograph of George Mahood Foy FRCSI, Dublin surgeon. Reproduced from Taylor FL, Crawford W. Long and the Discovery of Ether Anesthesia, Paul B. Hoeber Inc., 1928. By kind permission of Wolters Kluwer.

scientific and lay, corresponded regularly with medical and popular press publications on both sides of the Atlantic Ocean. He was always interested in history and as early as 1885, his publication titled 'Science and civilisation: their influence on pharmacy' included a brief piece on anaesthetic agents, which contained this sentence: 'Ether, which is so much used as an anæsthetic, was first used for this purpose by Dr Morton, of Boston, during tooth extraction, in 1846'. It can be inferred therefore, that at that time, Foy was unaware of the work of Dr Crawford Williamson Long who had used anaesthetic ether in Jefferson, Georgia from 1842 onwards.

Between October 1888 and June 1889, no fewer than eight lengthy articles by George Foy on 'Anæsthetics' were published in the *Dublin Journal of Medical*

371

Science. Having been revised and improved, this series soon appeared in book form, with the lengthy title and subtitle:

Anæsthetics Ancient and Modern: their Physiological Action, Therapeutic Use, and Mode of Administration; *together with an Historical Resumé of the Introduction of Modern Anæsthetics – Nitrous Oxide, Ether, Chloroform and Cocaine; and also an Account of the more Celebrated Anæsthetics in use from the Earliest Time to the Discovery of Nitrous Oxide.*[1]

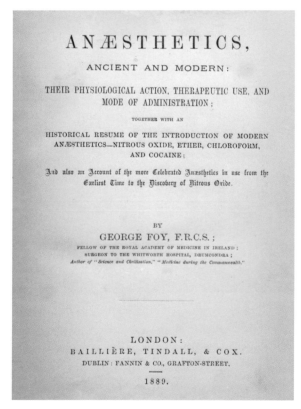

Title page of George Mahood Foy's Anæsthetics, Ancient and Modern, *1889.*

ANÆSTHETICS,

ANCIENT AND MODERN:

THEIR PHYSIOLOGICAL ACTION, THERAPEUTIC USE, AND
MODE OF ADMINISTRATION;

TOGETHER WITH AN

HISTORICAL RESUME OF THE INTRODUCTION OF MODERN
ANÆSTHETICS—NITROUS OXIDE, ETHER, CHLOROFORM,
AND COCAINE;

And also an Account of the more Celebrated Anæsthetics in use from the
Earliest Time to the Discovery of Nitrous Oxide.

BY
GEORGE FOY, F.R.C.S.;
FELLOW OF THE ROYAL ACADEMY OF MEDICINE IN IRELAND;
SURGEON TO THE WHITWORTH HOSPITAL, DRUMCONDRA;
Author of "Science and Civilisation," "Medicine during the Commonwealth."

LONDON:
BAILLIÈRE, TINDALL, & COX.
DUBLIN: FANNIN & CO., GRAFTON-STREET.

1889.

Foy's book was the first on anaesthesia to be written by an Irish doctor who, at the time of publication, was working in Ireland. It commences with an extensive resumé, going back to ancient Greece and Rome, of the evolution of attempts to provide painless surgery. This extends to five chapters and 60 pages and is considered to be the first detailed historical account of anaesthesia's early development. By the time it was published, Foy had become aware of Crawford Long's work and commented, after writing on the latter's March 1842 ether administration to James Venable, 'From deficient inter-State communication in 1842, Dr Long's operation remained unknown until the 1847 controversies of Wells, Morton, and others, caused the past records to be examined'. Later chapters address the advantages and disadvantages of the various anaesthetic agents and techniques, including local anaesthesia, in use at the time of writing. Foy concluded with a list of 'rules' (his word) on the administration of anaesthetics and a series of illustrations, with descriptions, of contemporaneous apparatus.

He dedicated his book to Hunter Holmes M'Guire, a surgeon in Richmond, Virginia, USA, who had previously been medical director of the 'Stonewall' Jackson Corps of the Confederate States Army, and who had visited Dublin in 1878. This visit may have been the catalyst for Foy's enduring interest in the American Civil War, on which he became an expert, writing regularly on the subject for Irish newspapers and journals. An ongoing friendship between the two surgeons ensued, with Foy being hosted by M'Guire when he visited Richmond and the Virginia battlefields in 1892. He later named his only child Charles Hunter M'Guire Foy, after his American colleague.

In 1900, having received assistance from Mrs Frances Long Taylor, a daughter of Crawford Long, Foy published a three-part paper on the life of the Georgian doctor – it was the first detailed account of Long's work and claim to priority, where general anaesthesia for surgery was concerned, to appear in any European publication.[2] It also included considerable detail on his Irish ancestry and early life. The 1910 annual meeting of the British Medical Association (BMA) was held in London. Following discussions with Dr Frederic Hewitt, president of the BMA Anaesthetic Section, George Foy wrote to the Long family inviting members to cross the Atlantic in order to exhibit material relating to Crawford Long. The items were shown at what was termed the 'Medical Museum' held in association with the BMA meeting. They attracted great interest, and were repeatedly discussed with Mrs Long Taylor and her sister by the leading British anaesthetists of the day. Some months later, Foy wrote:

> Today, December 24 1910, I am thankful to say that Dr C.W. Long is acknowledged as the discoverer by every one of our anaesthetists in Great Britain and my arguments in his favour have been translated into all the principal languages in Europe. Of one great fact I am sure, to wit; the principal anaesthetists of London recognise his claim to the discovery of general anaesthesia as well-founded and in their hospital classes they so inform their students.[3]

Foy's final paper on Long appeared in January 1916 – it was written to mark the centenary two months earlier of the Georgian's birth. In her biography of her late father, published in 1928, Frances Long Taylor was fulsome in her praise of the Dublin surgeon. She described his work in advocating on behalf of Long as 'his espousal of such an apparently hopeless cause as my father's appeared to be'.[3] American honours accorded to George Mahood Foy during his lifetime included honorary membership of the Southern Surgical and Gynaecological Association (1895), MD (*honoris causa*) University of Virginia (1897) and honorary membership of the Medical Societies of both Virginia and Georgia.

DW

References

1 Foy G., *Anæsthetics, Ancient and Modern*, London: Baillière, Tindall and Cox, 1889.
2 Foy G., 'Crawford Williamson Long, M.D. The Discoverer of Ether Anaesthesia', *Janus*, 1900, 5, pp. 138–42, 235–8, 285–93.
3 Taylor F.L., *Crawford W. Long & The Discovery of Ether Anesthesia*, New York: Paul B. Hoeber, 1928, pp. 174–5.

Paul Albert Piel (*c*. 1851–1924)
LRCP & SI LM

Paul Albert Piel, the son of a medical doctor, was born in France. It is unclear when he first arrived in Ireland, but it must have been prior to 8 May 1878, the date on which he married Elizabeth de MacMahon, a member of the French aristocracy, in Booterstown Roman Catholic Church, Dublin. He passed the examination in General Education of the Royal College of Surgeons in Ireland in 1879[1] and subsequently graduated LRCSI (1884) and LRCPI (1885). His first wife having died, Piel's second marriage, to Alice Darker, took place in February 1889.

Prior to 1886, anaesthetics required by patients undergoing surgery at the Adelaide Hospital, Dublin were administered, as in many other hospitals, by junior surgeons. This was presumably considered unsatisfactory for, in that year, Piel was appointed as the hospital's first anaesthetist – indeed, he was the first doctor to be appointed to a designated anaesthetic post in any hospital on the island of Ireland. His position was part-time and he also ran a general medical practice from his nearby home in Harcourt Street. He later wrote 'In 1886 I was appointed … at a salary of £50 a year to administer anaesthetics on Tuesdays and Thursdays from 10 a.m. until 12 noon, and to look after the antiseptics of the hospital'. He was paid in part by the hospital's Medical Board, and in part by the Managing Committee.[2]

Piel wrote to the Medical Board in 1899 suggesting that his hours of attendance (and presumably his salary) should be 'redefined' as the amount of

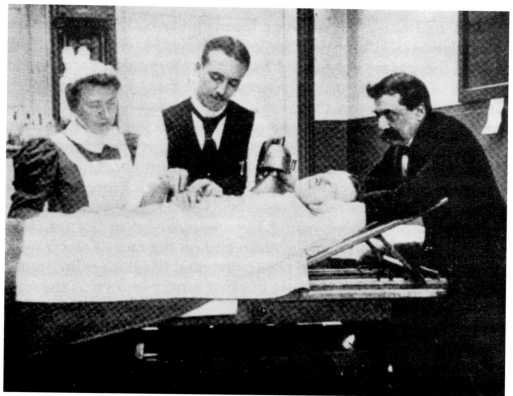

Photograph of an operation in progress at the Adelaide Hospital c.1895 including Dr Paul Piel, anaesthetist. Reproduced from Mitchell D. A 'Peculiar' Place: The Adelaide Hospital, Dublin 1839–1989, Blackwater, 1989.

surgical work had increased greatly over the previous few years and operations were now taking place on most days of the week. He was informed that his duties 'were to be continued as before'. Two years later he wrote again, informing the board of 'the advisability of introducing the use of gas and oxygen by the anaesthetist'. The matter was discussed and it was agreed that the necessary apparatus be obtained. However, it appears that it was never purchased for as late as 1906, Piel felt the need to put pen to paper once more, enclosing estimates for gas and oxygen and gas (alone) appliances for anaesthetic purposes. On this occasion, the board minutes recorded:

> it was determined that the gas alone would meet the requirements of the hospital sufficiently for the present, it being shown that the gas and oxygen apparatus was too complicated for ordinary hospital purposes and also that the expense would be very much greater than for the gas alone.[3]

375

The number of operations taking place in the hospital continued to grow (813 in 1905 compared with 147 in 1885) and Piel's salary was eventually increased in 1909 to £100 per annum. From 1911 onwards, his name appeared on the students' Clinical Card as 'Anaesthetist and Lecturer in Anaesthetics'. However, he was never accorded membership of the hospital's honorary medical staff – he remained a medical officer employed in part by the medical board and in part by the hospital itself. Many years were to pass before anaesthetists were to achieve parity of status with those in the more-established specialties such as medicine and surgery.

Piel's health gradually declined in the final few years of his service to the Adelaide. He retired in 1918, having been awarded a pension of £50 per annum, and was thanked 'for having for over 30 years so ably filled the post of Anaesthetist'. He died at his home in Harcourt Street, Dublin, on 9 January 1924 of cardiac failure and nephritis.

The photograph, taken *c.* 1895, shows Dr Piel, known for his splendid moustache, administering a general anaesthetic. He was using Clover's portable regulating ether inhaler, introduced by Joseph Clover in 1877. The apparatus can be seen 'resting' on the patient's upper thorax, indicating that Piel was employing an intermittent anaesthetic technique. At least one of his hands appears to be supporting the patient's airway.

DW

References

1 'Royal College of Surgeons', *The Freeman's Journal*, 5 August 1879, p. 3.
2 Mitchell D., *A 'Peculiar' Place: The Adelaide Hospital, Dublin 1839–1989*, Dublin: Blackwater Press, 1989, p. 124.
3 Minute book of the Adelaide Hospital Medical Board, Meeting of 2 July 1906. MARLOC 11270/2/3/3/4, Trinity College Dublin.

Thomas Percy Claude Kirkpatrick (1869–1954)
BA MD FRCPI LITT.D (Hon) D.LITT (Hon) FRCP (Hon)

Thomas Percy Claude Kirkpatrick was born in Rutland (now Parnell) Square, Dublin in September 1869, to John Rutherford Kirkpatrick, King's professor of midwifery in Trinity College Dublin, and his wife Catherine (*née* Drury).

He was educated at Foyle College, Londonderry from which he entered Trinity College Dublin, obtaining a first-class honours degree in history before commencing medical studies. Graduating MB BCh BAO in 1895, he proceeded MD in the same year, and was appointed resident surgeon to the County Donegal Infirmary at Lifford. Returning to Dublin in 1897, he waited until his 1899 appointment as anaesthetist to Dr Steevens' Hospital for his first hospital position in the city; thus began an association with the hospital that lasted for the rest of his life. Over the following decades, many aspects of Steevens (as it was known) including its history,

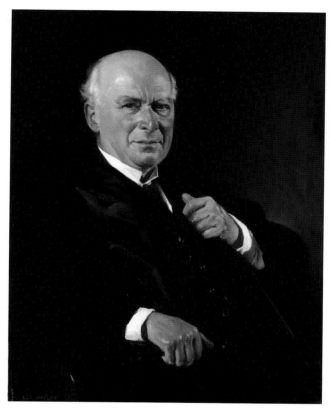

Dr Thomas Percy Claude Kirkpatrick. Oil on canvas by Leo Whelan. Reproduced by kind permission of the Royal College of Physicians of Ireland (1940.2).

fabric and administration concerned him. For 50 years, he gave the hospital's Worth Library his devotion, not only in studying its contents, but in caring for each individual volume in the collection.

The Dr Steevens'Hospital Anaesthetic Register for 1900 reveals that 306 general anaesthetics were administered in the hospital over the course of the year, with Kirkpatrick being the anaesthetist for 268 of these. He used a combination of nitrous oxide and ether in 186 cases, nitrous oxide alone in 45, and chloroform in 27. The same three agents were administered in various other combinations to the remaining 10 patients cared for by him.[1]

At the end of the year 1900, he was promoted to the post of assistant physician, and he became full visiting physician in 1903. His main interest as a practising physician was in venereal disease and to encourage his patients to attend, he held a clinic at a discreet early morning hour to facilitate anonymity.[2] He also continued to practice anaesthesia in Steevens', but more especially in the

Invitation to the inaugural Kirkpatrick Lecture of the Faculty of Anaesthetists, Royal College of Surgeons in Ireland. Reproduced by kind permission of the Royal College of Physicians of Ireland (MS/90).

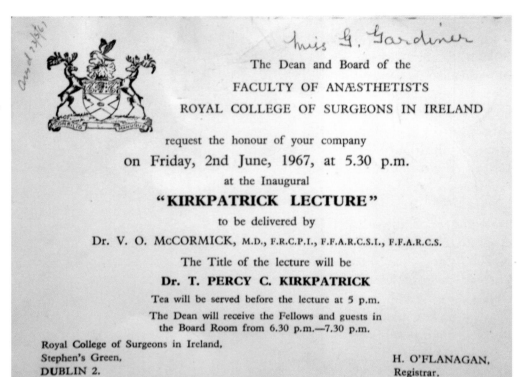

miss G. Gardiner

The Dean and Board of the

FACULTY OF ANÆSTHETISTS

ROYAL COLLEGE OF SURGEONS IN IRELAND

request the honour of your company

on Friday, 2nd June, 1967, at 5.30 p.m.

at the Inaugural

"KIRKPATRICK LECTURE"

to be delivered by

Dr. V. O. McCORMICK, M.D., F.R.C.P.I., F.F.A.R.C.S.I., F.F.A.R.C.S.

The Title of the lecture will be

Dr. T. PERCY C. KIRKPATRICK

Tea will be served before the lecture at 5 p.m.

The Dean will receive the Fellows and guests in
the Board Room from 6.30 p.m.—7.30 p.m.

Royal College of Surgeons in Ireland,
Stephen's Green,
DUBLIN 2.

H. O'FLANAGAN,
Registrar.

Dental Hospital and various smaller Dublin institutions, for the remainder of his medical career.

Kirkpatrick had a particular interest in dental anaesthesia. In 1901, he spoke to dental students on 'The asphyxial factor in nitrous oxide anaesthesia', giving a clear description of the symptoms and dangers of restricting the amount of oxygen delivered to the patient. He wrote of the advantages of administering oxygen along with nitrous oxide as recommended by Frederic Hewitt. He also advocated for separate dentists and anaesthetists where general anaesthesia was used. In subsequent publications, he wrote of his opposition to the use of chloroform in dental practice and discussed the General Anaesthetics Bill of 1908. One of the more interesting of his anaesthetic papers (for he also wrote on many other subjects) was one in which he reported a personal series of over 5,000 anaesthetics given in the Incorporated Dental Hospital of Ireland between 1899 and 1909.[3–6]

He was appointed lecturer in anaesthetics to Trinity College Dublin in 1910, a post he held until 1948. His lectures dealt not only with methods of anaesthesia but also with the history of the emerging specialty.[7] Upon his election in 1946 as the first president of the newly formed Section of Anaesthetics of the Royal Academy of Medicine in Ireland (RAMI), the first all-Ireland body devoted to the specialty, he contributed an address on anaesthesia's early development.

Kirkpatrick became registrar of the Royal College of Physicians of Ireland (RCPI) in 1910, and this role, which continued until his death 44 years later, afforded him the opportunity to indulge his lifelong love of books and medical history, on which he was a prolific author. His major works include his *History of the Medical School in Trinity College, Dublin* (1912), the *Book of the Rotunda Hospital* (1913); and *History of Dr Steevens' Hospital 1720–1920* (1924), which, to this day, is regarded as a classic of its kind. He also wrote numerous pamphlets and articles on Irish hospitals, Irish doctors and other historical topics, and collected and safeguarded much important material which might otherwise have been lost. The Kirkpatrick Archive, consisting of his personal and professional papers and his manuscript collection, forms part of his bequest to RCPI and serves as a unique source of information for researchers of Irish medical history. With the exception of some Irish medical works, also willed to RCPI, his library was auctioned after his death by Sotheby's of London. Of the sale items, 310 dated from the seventeenth century or earlier while 37 were incunabula, i.e. they had been printed before the year 1501. The proceeds amounted to £13,709, equivalent to over £400,000 in 2021.

His book on Trinity College's medical school gained him the Litt. D. (Doctor of Letters) *hon causa* of his own university and in 1933, the National University of Ireland bestowed on him a similar honour. Later, he was elected to honorary fellowship of the Royal College of Physicians, London. He was president of the Irish Historical Society (1948–51), of the Royal Irish Academy (1946–9) and a member and president of both the Friendly Brothers and Strollers Clubs.

The number and quality of Kirkpatrick's anaesthetic papers, his appointment as lecturer in Trinity College (undoubtedly the first such recognition of the specialty by any Irish academic institution) and his presidency of the fledgling Section of Anaesthetics at RAMI reflect the important role played by him in the advancement of Irish anaesthesia during the first half of the twentieth century. His outstanding contribution was recognised by the Faculty of Anaesthetists, RCSI when it established the eponymous Kirkpatrick Lecture, delivered on a number of occasions between 1967 and 1984.[8]

DW

References

1   Dr Steevens' Hospital Register of Anaesthetics, 1900 (TPCK/2/2/3), Royal College of Physicians of Ireland Archive.
2   Kirkpatrick T.P.C., 'The asphyxial factor in nitrous oxide anaesthesia', *Medical Press and Circular*, 1901, 52 NS, pp. 431–4.
3   Kirkpatrick T.P.C., 'The use of chloroform as an anaesthetic for dental operations', *Medical Press and Circular*, 1903, 55 NS, pp. 129–32.
4   Kirkpatrick T.P.C., 'The General Anaesthetics Bill, 1908', *Dublin Journal of Medical Science*, 1909, 127, pp. 411–7.
5   Kirkpatrick T.P.C., 'Ten years' anaesthetic practice at the Incorporated Dental Hospital', *Medical Press and Circular*, 1910, 89 NS, pp. 463–6.
6   Lyons J.B., 'Kirkpatrick, Thomas Percy Claude' in *Dictionary of Irish Biography*, vol. 5, Kane–McGuinness, Cambridge: Royal Irish Academy and Cambridge University Press, 2009, pp. 230–1.
7   T.G., 'In Memoriam. T.P.C. Kirkpatrick MD, FRCP, MRIA', *Irish Journal of Medical Science*, 1954, 29, pp. 364–70.
8   McCormick V.O., 'Dr. T. Percy C. Kirkpatrick'. Inaugural Kirkpatrick Lecture of the Royal College of Surgeons in Ireland, 2 June 1967.

Ella Webb (1877–1946)
MBE BSc MA MD

Isabella (later shortened to Ella) Ovenden, was born in Dublin in 1877 and schooled in Dublin, London and Göttingen, Germany. An 1899 science graduate of the Royal University of Ireland, she enrolled in the Catholic University School of Medicine in Cecilia Street and qualified MB BCh BAO in 1904, obtaining first place and winning a travelling scholarship. She was awarded a doctorate in medicine (MD) in 1906.

Writing the following year, Ovenden outlined the qualities required of female doctors. She discussed the cost of training and remuneration, remarking that the profession was not one which gave 'quick returns', to women in particular. She stated that prospects were improving, but that a woman's position would only be secure if she showed that she had taken up medicine as a serious scientific or philanthropic undertaking.[1] In December 1907, she married George Webb, philosopher and mathematician.

Ella Webb became active in the Women's National Health Association which focused on finding ways to eradicate tuberculosis by coordinating pasteurised milk distribution, opening healthcare centres and addressing conditions surrounding the high infant mortality rates in Ireland at the time. She taught anatomy in Trinity College Dublin and physiology in Cecilia Street while also working on a voluntary basis in two Dublin 'Babies Clubs'. The clubs had free doctors' clinics for infants and assisted mothers by holding classes on cookery, home hygiene and sewing. Webb was an advocate of breastfeeding and in 1913, published an analysis of why 200 of her patients commenced the practice but then abandoned it, outlining measures that could be taken to improve matters.

As Lady District Superintendent in the St John Ambulance Brigade during the 1916 Easter Rising, she took command of and transformed the St John headquarters at

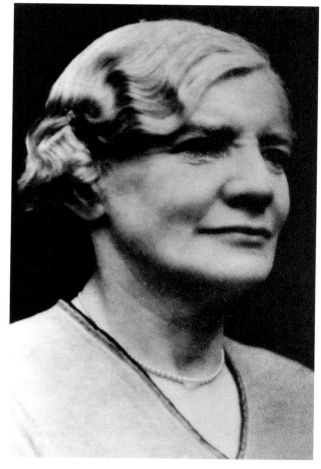

Photograph of Dr Ella Webb. Reproduced by kind permission of the Royal College of Physicians of Ireland (SU/8/3/8).

Merrion Square, Dublin into an emergency hospital, cycling through the firing lines to attend there and at other St John locations. Webb was later made a Member of the Most Excellent Order of the British Empire (MBE) in recognition of her efforts. She continued to write and authored an important 1917 paper on maternal and child welfare in Dublin.[2]

In 1918, Dr Paul Piel retired as anaesthetist to Dublin's Adelaide Hospital. He was succeeded by the first female to become a member of the Adelaide medical staff, Ella Webb.[3] Although Dr Sara McElderry in the Mater Infirmorum Hospital, Belfast and Drs Ina Clarke and Nina McCarthy in the Richmond Hospital, Dublin had provided some anaesthetic services in earlier years, their roles appear to have been relatively informal and Webb is considered to have been the first 'official' female appointee to such a post in an Irish hospital. In addition to her anaesthetic duties, she ran a children's dispensary in which she laid emphasis on the child's social circumstances and sought help in addressing this aspect of her patients' care. Winifred Alcock, who had been training as an almoner in London responded to her plea for assistance and began what was a novel arrangement of making home visits to those in need, thereby originating medical social work in Ireland.

St Ultan's Hospital for Infants, Charlemont Street, Dublin was founded in 1919 by female doctors and activists who were concerned at the level of infant mortality in the city. Initially, it worked primarily to combat ill-health experienced because of poverty but later assumed a major role in the fight against tuberculosis and was the first hospital in Britain or Ireland in which the BCG vaccine was administered. Ella Webb worked there from its foundation and for most of the remainder of her life.

In her work at the Adelaide and St Ultan's Hospitals, she treated many cases of childhood rickets and was aware that poor diet and living conditions were significant factors in the causation of the disease. By the early 1920s, sunlight was being promoted for prevention and healing. Following the discovery in 1923 that ultraviolet (UV) light could provide the same protection as sunlight, Webb began to use the treatment. However, many of her patients lived in slums and she knew that they could not be permanently cured without adequate food and care after hospital discharge. She and her friend Letitia Overend searched for somewhere to look after them during convalescence. In 1924, a site became available in Stillorgan, County Dublin and following fundraising, a bungalow-type house with two wards was built; the Children's Sunshine Home opened in March 1925.[4]

Webb was now committed to the Sunshine Home, was working in St Ultan's, was anaesthetist to the Adelaide and running a children's dispensary. She was attending at least one Babies Club, and volunteering with St John Ambulance. In late 1925, she resigned from St Ultan's citing pressure of work elsewhere, but offered care for babies needing artificial sunlight treatment at her home until the hospital possessed its own lamp. One year later, she stepped down as Adelaide Hospital anaesthetist but retained her dispensary until 1929. She returned to St Ultan's that same year and became involved in postgraduate paediatric education. In 1935, Webb wrote of the first decade of the Sunshine Home, describing the management of rickets there.[5] Children were nursed outside on verandas when possible, often for 24 hours a day in summertime. The cure rate in 477 patients admitted over 10 years was 56 per cent, with most others showing improvement.

By the mid-1940s, her health was failing; she continued to work until shortly before her death in 1946. In her limited spare time, she had been an enthusiastic gardener and took great delight in listening to sacred music. She is remembered by the Webb Ward in Tallaght Hospital and the Dr Ella Webb Room in LauraLynn House, Ireland's first children's hospice.

While Webb's anaesthetic career of nine years was relatively short, her 1918 appointment to the Adelaide Hospital helped 'open the door' for others, and a number of female doctors obtained anaesthetic posts throughout Ireland in the following decade.

DW

References

1   Ovenden E.G.A., 'Medicine', in M. Bradshaw (ed.), *Open Doors for Irishwomen*, Dublin: Irish Central Bureau for the Employment of Women, 1907, pp. 35–6.
2   Webb E.G.A., 'Report on Maternity and Child Welfare in Dublin County Borough', *Dublin Journal of Medical Science*, 1917, 144, pp. 86–97.
3   Minute book of the Adelaide Hospital Medical Board, Meeting of 15 January 1918. MARLOC 11270/ 2/3/3/4, Trinity College Dublin.
4   Kelly L., 'Rickets and Irish Children: Dr Ella Webb and the Early Work of the Children's Sunshine Home', in A. MacLennan and A. Mauger (eds), *Growing Pains: Childhood Illness in Ireland, 1750–1950*, Dublin: Irish Academic Press, 2013, pp. 141–58.
5   Webb E., 'Ten Years' Work at the Children's Sunshine Home', *Irish Journal of Medical Science*, 1935, 10, pp. 225–9.

Ivan Whiteside Magill (1888–1986)
KCVO MB BCh BAO DA DSc (Hon) FFARCS FRCS (Hon) FFARCSI (Hon)

Every anaesthetist in the world has been influenced by the work of Sir Ivan Whiteside Magill and benefited from his foresight.[1]

Ivan Whiteside Magill, arguably the greatest anaesthetist of the twentieth century, was born in July 1888 in Larne, County Antrim to Samuel Magill, a draper, and his wife Sara. He proceeded from Larne Grammar School to Queen's University Belfast from which he graduated MB BCh BAO in 1913. A certificate from the Royal Victoria Hospital stating that he had administered an anaesthetic had been signed by the honorary secretary of the medical staff and the surgical registrar; no anaesthetist was involved, evidence of the standing of anaesthesia at the time.[2] Three years later, he married Edith Robinson, also a doctor.

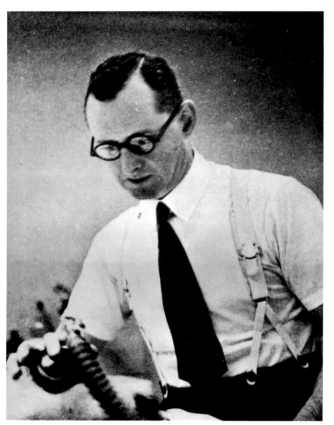

Photograph of Sir Ivan Whiteside Magill. Courtesy of the Anaesthesia Heritage Centre.

After qualifying, Magill spent a short period in general practice. He became house surgeon and then resident medical officer (RMO) at the Stanley Hospital in Liverpool, and was RMO at the Walton Hospital in the city when World War One broke out in 1914. He took a temporary commission in the Royal Army Medical Corps (RAMC) and served, with the rank of captain, for the remainder of the War. In autumn 1915, he was medical officer to the Irish Guards throughout the Battle of Loos, at the time the largest British offensive of the conflict.[2] When hostilities ceased, he was posted to Barnet War Hospital where he occasionally administered anaesthetics. Responding to a questionnaire pertaining to possible demobilisation, he described himself as an anaesthetist and was soon posted to Queen Mary's Hospital for Facial and Jaw Injuries, in Sidcup, Kent. Coincidentally, Stanley Rowbotham, also to become an eminent anaesthetist, was appointed to Queen Mary's at approximately the same time. Most anaesthetists there were non-resident civilians, but the newly posted officers were resident and immediately plunged into administering some of the most challenging anaesthetics that one could meet, as much of the surgery was for facial reconstruction in soldiers following severe injuries sustained during the war. Magill set about the twin tasks of improving his own skills and of perfecting and improving the methods then in use. Rowbotham later wrote that these challenges not only intrigued his colleague, but perhaps as a result of his Northern Ireland descent, stimulated in him an obstinate tenacity![3]

The problem of maintaining an airway was always present, and severely hampered the surgeon in his work. Oral airways and intratracheal insufflation via fine catheters were frequently used with anaesthesia maintained by ether and air. For operations on the mouth, nasal catheters were passed, viewed in the pharynx and inserted into the larynx with a forceps. Magill devised a special forceps, still used today, for this purpose – it later found many roles besides that originally intended by its inventor.[4]

He next introduced the passing into the trachea of wide-bore rubber tubes through which the patient could breathe to and fro, inhaling and exhaling from a constant flow apparatus with a reservoir bag and exhaust valve which later became known as the Magill or Mapleson A anaesthetic circuit. The technique had great advantages – the airway was secure, the anaesthetist was at a distance from the operative field and a pure mixture of gas, e.g. nitrous oxide and oxygen or air, could be used for long operations. Concentrating on nasal rather than oral intubation, he persuaded manufacturers to produce a series of tubes in graduated sizes; as a result of his efforts, blind nasal intubation became firmly established.[2,3] His surgical colleague at Sidcup, Howard Gillies, later commented 'Plastic surgery was founded on Magill and his tube; it would not have been possible without it'.[5]

He invented and perfected many other instruments and pieces of apparatus for use in anaesthesia. After his appointment to the Brompton Hospital for Diseases of the Chest, London, in 1923, he introduced methods that revolutionised thoracic surgery. Chest diseases, in particular tuberculosis, for which there was little in the way of drug therapy, were rife. Magill described his modification of Chevalier Jackson's laryngoscope in 1926.[6] Some years later, he devised a suction catheter with an inflatable cuff as a bronchial blocker, so that secretions could be aspirated from the lung being operated on, and his ingenious endobronchial tubes with bronchoscopic introducers for one lung anaesthesia.[7,8] Appointed to the Westminster Hospital, London in 1924, he adopted the use of dry flowmeters for the measurement of gases four years later. He was an early advocate of using rotameters for the same purpose although it was not until 1935 that he was able to obtain them made to his own specification. In addition to developing new equipment, Ivan Magill also actively promoted advances in anaesthetic drugs and other agents. He described cyclopropane as 'a godsend in surgery of the chest'[8] but considered that trichloroethylene, when introduced, had little advantage over other anaesthetics available at the time. In 1930, he returned from the United States with pentobarbital and was responsible for its introduction into anaesthetic practice in the United Kingdom.[9]

Towards the end of his long life, Magill said that he was most proud of the part he had played in the establishment of anaesthesia as a specialty. In 1931, he had proposed to the Council of the Anaesthetic Section of the Royal Society of Medicine that a diploma be instituted. The society, under its charter, could not undertake this task. However, members of the section met during 1932 and it was decided to form an independent Association of Anaesthetists having as a prime objective the introduction of a postgraduate qualification in the specialty. The first examination for the Diploma in Anaesthetics of the Conjoint Examining Board of the Royal College of Physicians of London and the Royal College of Surgeons of England, the world's first such in anaesthesia, was held in 1935. Magill had been involved in defining the entry requirements and was a member of the first board of examiners. The Irish equivalent followed in 1942. The establishment of the two diplomas subsequently led to the foundation of the Faculties of Anaesthetists of the Royal Colleges of Surgeons in England and Ireland. In December 1946, he delivered the opening address at the inauguration of the Section of Anaesthetics of the Royal Academy of Medicine in Ireland.

Magill's work was recognised by many honours, too numerous to list in full. In 1937, he was elected president of the Section of Anaesthetics of the Royal Society of Medicine. The section presented him with the Henry Hill Hickman Medal during the following year – this was the highest award his fellow anaesthetists could make at the time. In 1945, Queen's University Belfast conferred him as a Doctor of Science *honoris causa*, having many years earlier rejected his MD thesis based on his most famous achievement, blind nasal intubation, in the mistaken belief that it would not prove to be of use! His services to members of the British Royal Family were recognised in 1946 when he was invested as a Commander of the Royal Victorian Order; he was knighted by Queen Elizabeth II in 1960. Magill was elected to Fellowship of the Faculty of Anaesthetists of the Royal College of Surgeons of England in 1948, and was later conferred with honorary fellowships of the Royal College of Surgeons of England (1951), the Royal Society of Medicine (1956), and the Faculty of Anaesthetists, RCSI (1961). As a token of his appreciation of the latter honour, Magill presented to the Irish faculty a silver medal and chain of office to be worn by the dean on formal occasions. In 1966, he became the first recipient of the prestigious Ralph Waters Award of the Illinois State Society of Anesthesiologists.

After retirement from his National Health Service posts in 1955, he continued working in the independent sector and gave his last anaesthetic at 84 years of age. He had been a useful rugby player and boxer in his youth. Later fishing, at which he excelled, occupied much of his spare time; he caught a trout weighing five pounds on his 97th birthday. He was kindly, loyal to his friends and specialty, and loved good company. He continued to attend the Royal Society of Medicine until shortly before his death, in his 99th year, in November 1986.[1,5,9]

Perhaps the best account of the excellence of Magill's care for his patients was provided by fellow anaesthetist Anthony Edridge:

> He never taught save by example and it was obvious that, no matter how effortless or even casual his work might seem, every anaesthetic was the best he could give, having made sure by meticulous preparation that he would never be let down by his apparatus. Magill was a superb anaesthetist … Nothing, one felt, could surprise him and nothing could go wrong. His hand never left the bag and years of the keenest observation had endowed him with almost an uncanny feel for the condition of the patient.[9]

An Irish-language saying comes to mind: 'Ní fheicimid a leithéid arís' ('We will not see his like again').

DW

References
1 A.W.E., 'Obituary. Ivan Whiteside Magill', *The Lancet*, 1987, 1, p. 55.
2 McLachlan G., 'Sir Ivan Magill KCVO, DSc, MB, BCh, BAO, FRCS, FFARCS (Hon), FFARCSI (Hon), DA, (1888–1986)', *Ulster Medical Journal*, 2008, 77, pp. 146–52.
3 Rowbotham S., 'Ivan Magill', *British Journal of Anaesthesia*, 1951, 23, pp. 49–55.
4 Magill I.W., 'Forceps for intratracheal anaesthesia', *British Medical Journal*, 1920, 2, p. 670.
5 W.K.P., 'Obituary. Sir Ivan Magill', *British Medical Journal*, 1987, 294, pp. 62–3.
6 Magill I.W., 'An improved laryngoscope for anaesthetists', *The Lancet*, 1926, 1, p. 500.
7 Magill I.W., 'Modern views on anaesthesia', *Newcastle Medical Journal*, 1934, 14, pp. 67–78.
8 Magill I.W., 'Anaesthesia in thoracic surgery, with special reference to lobectomy', *Proceedings of the Royal Society of Medicine*, 1936, 29, pp. 643–53.
9 Edridge A.W., 'Editorial. Sir Ivan Whiteside Magill', *Anaesthesia*, 1987, 42, pp. 231–3.

Ethel Sheila Kenny (1909–1990)
BA MB BCh BAO FFARCS FFARCSI

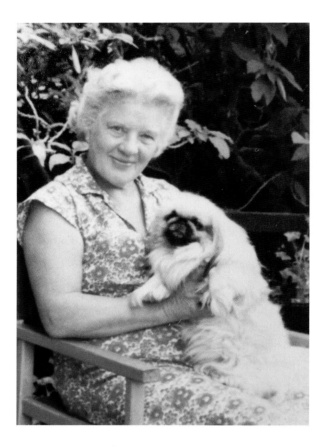

Sheila Kenny was born in Boltown, Kilskyre, County Meath on 24 August 1909, daughter of William James Wilson, a landowner, originally from County Tyrone, and his wife Ethel, who was from County Cavan. She was the eldest of five children, four girls and one boy. She was probably home-schooled initially and then went as a boarder to the Hall School in Belgrave Square, Monkstown, County Dublin in 1921. This prestigious establishment for young ladies merged with a number of others in 1973 to become Rathdown School. While at school, she had private tuition in Latin, Trigonometry and Mechanics which were not taught at the Hall but were necessary for the Senior Cambridge Examination. She passed the Cambridge exam (which was the same as the General Certificate of Education) and entered Trinity to study medicine in 1928. She received her BA in 1931 and qualified MB BCh BAO in 1933.

In her personal diaries, she wrote of having a 'wonderful dinner' with Mr Seton Pringle, a surgeon in the Adelaide Hospital, Dublin at this time. This was evidently her job interview as she was appointed as an anaesthetist to the Adelaide in the following year. At the time, anaesthetic posts in hospitals were honorary so that anaesthetists had to earn their income from either private or general practice. In 1934, Sheila Wilson married Hamilton Kenny, an official in the Bank of Ireland and this, as suggested by Fitzpatrick,[1] may have provided her with enough financial independence to develop her career. She had two daughters, Ann-Elizabeth and Hilary, one of whom now lives in the UK[2] and the other in Australia.

Sheila had a very strong forceful character, worked well with men and seems to have had total control over her surgical colleagues.[2] She worked not only in the Adelaide but also at the National Children's Hospital on Harcourt Street (which was within walking distance), the Royal Victoria Eye and Ear Hospital on Adelaide Road and the Rotunda Hospital. She had a very busy private practice at the Portobello, the Burlington and Herbert nursing homes as well as in Mount Carmel Hospital (which opened in 1958).

The first examination for the Conjoint Diploma in Anaesthetics of the Royal College of Physicians of Ireland and the Royal College of Surgeons in Ireland was held in December 1942. There were eight candidates in total of whom four passed. Ethel Sheila Kenny was one of the four; she was the only female candidate and thus was the first woman in Ireland to be conferred with the diploma.

Seventeen years later, on 15 December 1959, the first meeting of the board of the new Faculty of Anaesthetists, RCSI took place in the college's council room. The board was formally inaugurated by the president of RCSI in July 1960. Sheila Kenny was the only female member. In 1964, when Dr Joseph Woodcock became dean of the faculty, Kenny was appointed vice dean. She was never elected dean and no woman ever held that position in the 28 years of the faculty (it would take until 2009 before the first woman, Dr Jeanne Moriarty, would become president of the College of Anaesthetists of Ireland). She was a member of the Council of AAGBI from 1967–70.

She was an innovator and was involved in the development in 1958 of the 'Adelaide respirator'.[3] In 1965, along with the surgeon Mr Nigel Kinnear and financed by 'the Shilling Fund', she established a four-bedded intensive care unit across the corridor from the operating theatre in what had formerly been the children's ward. It was one of the first intensive care units in Ireland. She also set up a blood gas laboratory in an adjoining office; it was a significant innovation at the time.[4] In 1967, Sheila Kenny had a seminal paper published in the *British Journal of Anaesthesia* (her third in that journal) titled 'The Adelaide Ventilation guide'[5] (the guide was more commonly known as 'the Adelaide nomogram'; it correlated the volume of ventilation of the lungs required to the body weight of the patient).

At the Adelaide Hospital on Peter Street, there was a parcel of waste ground lying idle between a couple of buildings. Kenny, along with the Countess of Iveagh and others, reclaimed this ground and developed it into 'The Adelaide

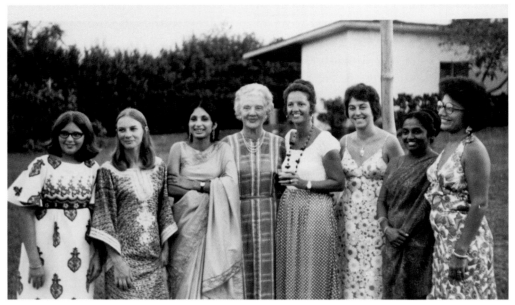

Garden' which was formally opened by Dr G.O. Simms, the Church of Ireland Primate of All Ireland in June 1971. A garden party was held there every summer.

She was a member of council and also served as president (1960) of the Section of Anaesthetics, Royal Academy of Medicine in Ireland. Her presidential address titled 'In Somno Securitas' was a tour-de-force on ventilation and blood gas analysis as well as other aspects of safety in anaesthesia.[6] She retired in 1974 and then went to Nigeria to help establish a medical school there along with Dr Gerry Jessop, who had been dean of the medical school in Trinity. She spent three years in Africa before returning to Ireland where she continued to be active in the Association of Old Adelaide Students and also maintained her involvement with the hospital garden. She was involved in a motor accident in 1987 and suffered severe injuries. She was treated at Our Lady of Lourdes Hospital in Drogheda by an anaesthetist who had studied under her, Dr Carlos McDowell. Although she recovered from her injuries, her health deteriorated and she died on 24 May 1990.[2]

In 2012, the Sheila Kenny Room was opened in the operating theatre suite at Tallaght University Hospital, County Dublin; the hospital incorporates the Adelaide Hospital which closed in 1998. The room was funded by the Association of Old Adelaide Students.

References

1 Paper read by Mr David Fitzpatrick, surgeon at the Adelaide and Tallaght Hospitals, on the occasion of the opening of the Sheila Kenny Room in the theatre suite at Tallaght University Hospital , October 2012.
2 Personal insights into Dr Kenny's life were provided by Dr Carlos McDowell.
3 Kenny S. and Lewis W., 'The Adelaide respirator', *British Journal of Anaesthesia*, 1960, 32, pp. 444–6.
4 Docrat K. and Kenny S., 'The accuracy of capillary sampling for acid-base estimations', *British Journal of Anaesthesia*, 1965, 37, pp. 840–4.
5 Kenny S., 'The Adelaide ventilation guide', *British Journal of Anaesthesia*, 1967, 39, pp. 21–3.
6 Kenny S., 'In somno securitas', *Irish Journal of Medical Science*, 1960, 415, pp. 292–309.

JT

Edmund J. Delaney (1925–1979)
MB BCh BAO DA FFARCS FFARCSI

Edmund James Delaney was born in Dublin in 1925. He was the second youngest of four children of James and Christina Delaney (*née* Lally).

James Delaney was a publican with a business address at St James's Street, Dublin while the family home was on the North Circular Road and in later years in Malahide, County Dublin. Edmund was educated at Belvedere and Clongowes Wood Colleges. He studied medicine at University College Dublin graduating MB BCh BAO in 1949. Having completed his intern year at the Mater Misericordiae Hospital, Dublin he began training in anaesthesia, firstly

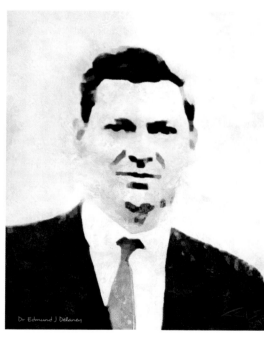

Dr Edmund J Delaney. Portrait by his son Richard P Delaney. With kind permission of Richard P Delaney

at Blackburn in Lancashire, and later as a registrar at the Norfolk & Norwich Royal Infirmary in East Anglia. Despite his commitment to work and study, he proved no less susceptible to romance than any other young man and while working in East Anglia, he met and fell in love with Catherina Hubertina Isabella

Schweitzer, a young Dutch lady who was a staff nurse at the National Hospital for Neurological Diseases in Queen Square, London. Edmund and Catherina (known affectionately thereafter as Kitty) were married in September 1953. Edmund's training continued and after he had obtained the Fellowship of the Faculty of Anaesthetists of the Royal College of Surgeons of England, he and Kitty and their first child, James, who had arrived in July 1954, moved to Dundee where Edmund became senior registrar and tutor in clinical anaesthetics at the University of St Andrews.[1] Dundee proved to be a particularly happy and successful location not just for Edmund's anaesthetic career but also for the Delaney family with the birth of their second child, Richard, in 1956.

In 1958, the family relocated to Dublin where Edmund was appointed consultant anaesthetist at Dr Steevens' Hospital which was Dublin's second oldest, having first opened its doors in 1733 with capacity for 40 patients. By the early 1960s it had over 200 beds and was well established as a teaching centre for undergraduate and postgraduate medical students and for nursing. It was also gaining recognition for its specialist expertise in orthopaedic, maxillofacial and plastic surgery, including the management of congenital defects of the lip and palate. The National Burns Unit was later based at the hospital. The task of providing anaesthesia to support these areas fell to the newly appointed Dr Delaney and his senior colleague, Arthur 'Alfie' Jessop. Delaney's appointment proved to be a huge fillip to the hospital and its anaesthetic department, not least because it ended the near intolerable demands of the 'single consultant service' – single-handed anaesthetic units were not uncommon in the 1960s. His interest in introducing new techniques, for example the provision of neuraxial anaesthesia for major orthopaedic and gynaecological surgery,[2, 3] his skills as a paediatric anaesthetist and his undoubted gifts as a teacher and educator quickly established Dr Steevens' as one of the most sought-after postings for trainee anaesthetists. The early 1960s also saw the development of the Faculty of Anaesthetists, RCSI and Edmund Delaney played a major role in this, serving as a board member (1965–9 & 1974–8) and as vice dean (1971–3). He was lecturer in anaesthetics at Trinity College Dublin, and a frequent speaker at faculty scientific meetings. He was a regular contributor on the Primary and Final fellowship courses and had a particular interest in anatomy, recognising its importance for anaesthetists, something that not all of his colleagues had always appreciated!

Quite apart from his clinical and academic skills, Edmund Delaney was blessed with great charm, wit kindness and generosity which endeared him to all who met him. He inspired confidence and calm in the operating theatre but could equally be the source of uproarious laughter on social occasions with his storytelling and gift for mimicry. He realised the importance of the social and recreational aspects of lecturing and speaking at scientific meetings and the famed Dublin Anaesthetists Travelling Club became the vehicle for many of these undertakings.

Edmund Delaney died in October 1979. He was just 54 years of age. In recognition of his contribution to the hospital and to the specialty of anaesthesia, his colleagues at Dr Steevens' erected a memorial plaque in his memory. When the hospital closed in 1987, the plaque was recovered by a number of former nursing and medical colleagues including Dr Patrick Mullin, and was given to his widow, Kitty, who donated it to the Faculty of Anaesthetists, RCSI. It currently 'resides' in the lecture theatre at the College of Anaesthesiologists of Ireland in Merrion Square North, Dublin.

In 1980, the Faculty of Anaesthetists, RCSI had a medal struck, the Delaney Medal, in his honour, which was awarded to Dr Frank Jennings, a senior registrar who had been working closely with Edmund Delaney in the area of chronic pain management prior to his death. The following year, the Delaney Medal competition for

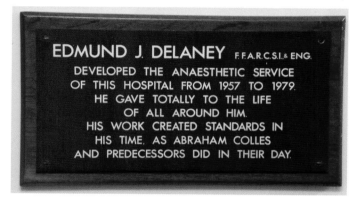

Commemorative plaque erected at Dr Steevens' Hospital by colleagues of Dr Edmund Delaney.

EDMUND J. DELANEY F.F.A.R.C.S.I.& ENG.
DEVELOPED THE ANAESTHETIC SERVICE
OF THIS HOSPITAL FROM 1957 TO 1979.
HE GAVE TOTALLY TO THE LIFE
OF ALL AROUND HIM.
HIS WORK CREATED STANDARDS IN
HIS TIME. AS ABRAHAM COLLES
AND PREDECESSORS DID IN THEIR DAY.

registrars was established. It is open to trainee anaesthetists for work carried out in Ireland on a subject related to anaesthetic practice. The winner of the first competition held in 1981 was Dr Charles O'Hagan with a presentation entitled 'A prototype blade to measure the force generated during laryngoscopy'.

JC

References

1   Delaney E.J., 'Cardiac irregularities during induction with halothane', *British Journal of Anaesthesia*, 1958, 30, pp. 188–91.
2   Delaney E.J., 'Pelvic floor repair under lumbar epidural analgesia and promazine (sparine)', *Irish Journal of Medical Science*, 1960, 35, pp. 187–92.
3   Hill P., Wharton L. and Delaney E.J., 'Extradural block in major surgery of the hip', *British Journal of Anaesthesia*, 1962, 34, pp. 107–14.

Kevin P. Moore (1936–1997)
MB BCh BAO FFARCSI

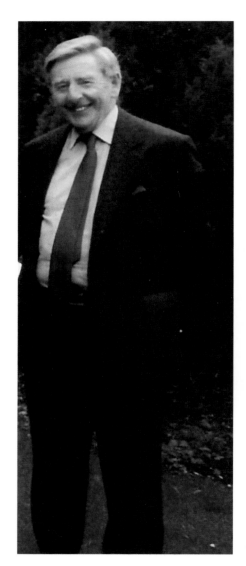

Kevin Patrick Moore was born in Glasgow in 1936. He was an only child. His father Frank was a publican whose parents had emigrated from County Kilkenny to Scotland where Frank was born. Kevin's mother, Kathleen (*née* Diggin) was from Kerry but had moved to the UK to train as a teacher. In 1950, the family moved to Dublin, primarily to escape the notorious smog which at the time plagued all major cities in the UK including Glasgow – Kevin's mother had a long history of respiratory problems. The first Clean Air Act was only introduced in England and Scotland in 1956. Kevin was 14 years of age when the family relocated to Dublin and he continued his education with the Jesuits at Belvedere College having previously attended St Aloysius' College in Glasgow, also a Jesuit school.

He went on to study medicine at University College Dublin (UCD) graduating MB BCh BAO in 1961. He completed his internship at the Mater Misericordiae Hospital and immediately began training in anaesthesia at the Leeds General Infirmary and St James' Hospital, Leeds, West Yorkshire.

Having obtained the Fellowship of the Faculty of Anaesthetists, RCSI in December 1964, he returned to Dublin two years later to continue his training and was the first registrar in anaesthesia to be appointed to Our Lady's Hospital for Sick Children (later renamed Our Lady's Children's Hospital) in Crumlin. In 1968, he returned to the UK to complete his training at the Queen Elizabeth Hospital, Birmingham.

In 1964, Kevin married his childhood sweetheart, Helen Hilliard. They had met and dated while still at school and had three children, all boys. The eldest was born in Leeds and his two younger brothers in Dublin.

Kevin and Helen and their 5-year-old son returned to Dublin in 1970 when Kevin was appointed as a consultant anaesthetist in Our Lady's Hospital for Sick Children.

Although the hospital had been opened in1956, Kevin Moore was just the second full-time consultant anaesthetist there. The development of paediatric anaesthesia in Crumlin, as the hospital was known, and of training in anaesthesia in general, were closely linked over the following decades and Kevin Moore was at the heart of both. The Eastern Regional Anaesthetic Training Scheme was established in 1972 and the National Senior Registrar Training Scheme followed shortly afterwards in 1976. Both were administered and run by the Medical Advisory Committee of the Faculty of Anaesthetists, RCSI which was chaired by Kevin Moore for many years. Dr Moore also served as an elected member of the Board of the Faculty of Anaesthetists, RCSI (1982–92) and as vice dean (1991–2). A gifted clinician and paediatric anaesthetist, Kevin Moore was also revered as a teacher, an administrator, for his wit, his kindness and his indomitable spirit. Our Lady's Hospital for Sick Children was the largest of the three specialist paediatric hospitals in the state and offered unique opportunities for trainee anaesthetists to gain experience in the specialty and Kevin Moore was always available to encourage and advise trainees on how best to take full advantage of their time there and advance their careers.[1-4]

For most of his consultant career, Kevin Moore had to contend with chronic ill health necessitating renal dialysis on a regular basis. That a burden of such magnitude was never allowed to curtail his clinical duties, not to mention his work with the Faculty of Anaesthetists, RCSI, is testament not only to an extraordinary dedication and commitment on his part but also to the unwavering support and affection of his wife Helen and their three sons, Colm, Eoin and Kevin Brian.

During a career spanning more than 25 years at 'Crumlin'– he never retired – Kevin Moore inspired numerous anaesthetic trainees and helped to equip them with a knowledge and appreciation of paediatric anaesthesia which has remained a cornerstone of their own careers as consultants in Ireland and abroad.

In 2012, the College of Anaesthetists of Ireland established the KP Moore Medal competition to acknowledge his outstanding contribution to the specialty and pay tribute to a revered colleague. The competition is organised by the Committee of Anaesthesia Trainees (CAT) and is open to trainees in the first years of training for work based on clinical cases in anaesthesia, intensive care medicine and pain medicine.

JC

References

1   MacDonald N.J., Fitzpatrick G.J., Moore K.P., Wren W.S. and Keenan M., 'Anaesthesia for congenital hypertrophic pyloric stenosis. A review of 350 patients', *British Journal of Anaesthesia*, 1987, 59, pp. 672–7.
2   Cahill J., Moore K.P. and Wren W.S., 'Nasopharyngeal Continuous Positive Airway Pressure in the Managements of Bronchiolitis', *Irish Medical Journal*, 1983, 76, pp. 191–3.
3   Lyons B., Casey W., Doherty P., McHugh M. and Moore K.P., 'Pain relief with low dose Clonidine in a child with severe burns', *Intensive Care Medicine*, 1996, 22, pp. 249–51.
4   Chambers F.A., Casey W., Dowling F. and Moore K.P., 'Malignant hyperthermia during isoflurane anaesthesia', *Canadian Journal of Anaesthesia*, 1994, 41, pp. 355–6.

Frances Mary Lehane (1944–2013)
MB BCh BAO FFARCSI

Mary (Frances Mary) Lehane was born in 1944 in Wallasey, Cheshire. She was educated at Maris Stella Convent, New Brighton and Holt Hill Convent, Birkenhead. Mary was the second eldest of eight children of Dermot Lehane and his wife Joan (*née* McGinty).

Mary's father, Dermot Lehane, graduated in medicine at University College Cork in 1937. He spent his career in the UK and was awarded the CBE in 1977 for his outstanding work as director of the Regional Transfusion Centre in Liverpool.

Mary's brother John also qualified in medicine, in Liverpool in 1974, and chose a career in anaesthesia. In 1984, he and a colleague, R.S. Cormack, published the seminal paper describing four distinct views seen at laryngoscopy, two of which (grade III and IV) are associated with difficult intubation, and setting out a safety drill to anticipate and manage such emergencies.[1]

Mary was determined to follow in her father's footsteps and study medicine. Her strength of character and obvious academic ability convinced her school to make special provisions to enable her to study A-level physics and chemistry, not normally part of the school curriculum, which were required to enter medical school. Having completed her A levels in Birkenhead, Mary enrolled in the school of medicine at University College Cork (UCC), and graduated MB BCh BAO in 1970. On completing her house jobs, she began training in anaesthesia at St Finbarr's Hospital, Cork. She obtained the Fellowship of the Faculty of Anaesthetists, RCSI in 1973 and was appointed to a senior registrar post at the Birmingham Group of Hospitals in 1975. She returned to Cork three years later and became a consultant anaesthetist at St Finbarr's and associated

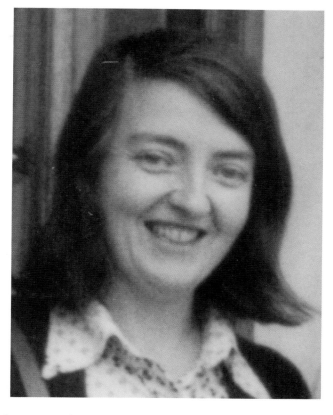

hospitals. When the new Cork Regional Hospital opened at Wilton (later Cork University Hospital) in 1979, Mary played a pivotal role in setting up the new intensive care unit.

Despite a busy clinical commitment Mary became involved in a research and diagnostic project at UCC which was to bring international renown and make a major contribution to patient safety. In a collaborative effort with Profs James Heffron and Thomas McCarthy of the Department of Biochemistry, Mary took on the role of clinical lead of the team investigating the recently described condition Malignant Hyperthermia (MH). MH is an inherited condition which lies dormant unless triggered by certain commonly used anaesthetic agents. Once triggered, MH causes a profound hypermetabolic upset with a significant mortality rate if not immediately recognised and appropriately treated. Diagnosing susceptibility to the condition (MHS) required laboratory testing (halothane/caffeine muscle contracture test carried out at UCC) of a tissue sample from patients suspected of having the condition but obtaining such samples necessitated a general anaesthetic. Mary took on the task of providing a specifically designed anaesthetic service for these patients and the anaesthetic department at CUH became the national referral centre for patients requiring muscle biopsies as part of their MHS investigations. Over the years, a wealth of crucial clinical and laboratory information was accumulated and Mary's calm authoritative voice reassured many patients and clinicians who sought her advice.

The European Malignant Hyperthermia Group (EMHG) was established in 1983 and Mary was one of the founding members. Her quiet unassuming persona and her clinical and research excellence were recognised at the many EMHG meetings she attended throughout Europe.[2] Diagnosing and advising on the management of patients who were susceptible to MH (MHS) was only part of the research project. Mapping the genetic profile of the condition took many years but in 1990, Mary and her colleagues published a paper in *Nature* showing a linkage between MHS and deoxyribonucleic acid (DNA) markers from the glucose phosphorolate isomerise (GPI) region of human chromosome 19.[3] These results indicated that human (and porcine) MH was most probably due to mutations in homologous genes, and also provided a potentially accurate and noninvasive method of diagnosis for MHS. Somewhat ironically, the results of the group's laboratory work meant that the dedicated anaesthetic service at CUH which Mary had built up over the years would soon become redundant.

Mary was an outstanding teacher – she was a lecturer in the Department of Pharmacology at UCC, and an examiner in the Primary fellowship examination of the Faculty of Anaesthetists, RCSI and later the College of Anaesthetists of Ireland. She was also a linkman for the Association of Anaesthetists of Great Britain & Ireland (AAGBI).

Outside her clinical duties, Mary's two passions were gardening and rugby. Her love of Munster rugby as well as her encyclopaedic knowledge of gardens were given memorable expression on two notable occasions at CUH. In 2007, Mary and her colleague Dr Ken Walsh converted two small courtyards in the grounds of the hospital into gardens that would be accessible to patients and staff and, in 2008, members of the victorious Munster rugby team, champions of Europe, complete with Heineken Cup, visited the hospital. Mary was a huge supporter of the therapeutic garden project at CUH, and more such gardens have now been installed in many other locations in the hospital grounds.[4,5]

In 2007, Mary Lehane was awarded the President's Medal of the College of Anaesthetists of Ireland for her major contribution to anaesthesia and patient safety both nationally and internationally and for her role in anaesthetic research and education.

In 2015, the College of Anaesthetists of Ireland instituted the Mary Lehane Medal competition. The winner of the inaugural competition was Dr Paudie Delaney. The title of his presentation was 'Patient frailty as a prognostic indicator in cardiothoracic surgery – a pilot study'.

JC

Mary Lehane holds the Heineken Cup aloft during a visit of the victorious Munster team to Cork University Hospital. Munster were crowned European Rugby Champions following their 16 -13 victory in the final against Toulouse at the Principality stadium in Cardiff in May 2008. With kind permission of Finbarr Buckley.

References

1   Cormack R.S. and Lehane J., 'Difficult intubation in obstetrics', *Anaesthesia*, 1984, 39, pp. 1105–11.
2   'Mary Lehane', available at https://www.emhg.org/in-memoriam/2018/6/26/mary-lehane (accessed 30 June 2021).
3   McCarthy T.V., Healy J.M., Heffron J.J., Lehane M., Lehmann-Horn T., Farrall M. and Johnson K., 'Localization of the malignant hyperthermia susceptibility locus to human chromosome 19ql2–13.2', *Nature*, 1990, 343, pp. 562–64, https://doi.org/10.1038/343562a0
4   St Leger A., *Cork University Hospital. Celebrating forty years 1978–2018*. Cork: Health Service Executive – Cork University Hospital, 2018, pp. 163–5.
5   Images of gardens at CUH, available at https://www.cuhcharity.ie/wp-content/uploads/2015/07/PV-Garden-12.jpg (accessed 30 June 2021).

Éamon Paul McCoy (1961–)
MB BCh BAO FFARCSI MD

Éamon McCoy was born on 23 November 1961 in Kisumu, Kenya where his father, Dr Derek McCoy was a missionary doctor and his mother Breda a teacher. The family returned to Ireland in 1963 and settled in Bantry, County Cork when his father was appointed as a consultant physician at St Joseph's County Hospital. He attended secondary school in Cistercian College, Roscrea, County Tipperary before studying medicine in University College Cork (UCC). He graduated MB BCh BAO in 1986. On completing his intern year in Cork University Hospital,

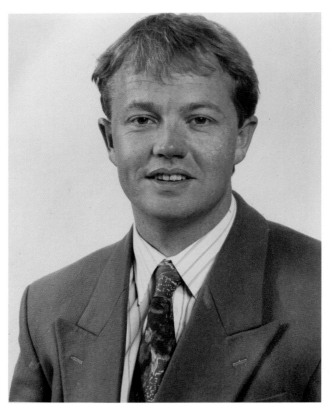

he then went to the Royal Victoria Hospital (RVH), Belfast for anaesthetic training.[1] This programme included rotations to the Ulster Hospital (Belfast), Daisy Hill Hospital (Newry), Altnagelvin Hospital (Derry) and finally the Royal Victoria Hospital and Mater Infirmorum Hospital in Belfast. He became a Fellow of the Faculty of Anaesthetists of the Royal College of Surgeons in Ireland in 1990. In 1992, he was appointed to the Academic Anaesthetic Department at Queen's University Belfast (QUB), where he was mentored by Rajinder Mirakhur (see Biographies). He has published widely with over 60 scientific papers mainly on pharmacokinetics and was awarded an MD by QUB in July 1995 for his research on the pharmacology of neuromuscular blocking agents. In August of that year, he moved to the Royal Adelaide Hospital in South Australia as an overseas fellow with Prof. John Russell, where he gained experience in clinical anaesthesia and in air retrieval of the critically ill. He returned to Belfast in 1996 as a consultant anaesthetist at the Royal Victoria Hospital.

In recognition of his clinical research, particularly in difficult airway management, he was awarded the Dr A. Harvey Granat Memorial Prize by the Neuroanaesthetists Society of Great Britain and Ireland in 1993 and the President's Medal of the Association of Anaesthetists of Great Britain and Ireland in the same year. He received the Registrars' Prize from the Society for Computing and Technology in Anaesthesia in 1994 and was awarded the Cutler's Surgical Prize by the Royal College of Surgeons of England in the following year. Éamon was named the United Kingdom Doctor of the Year in May 1995 and in 1999

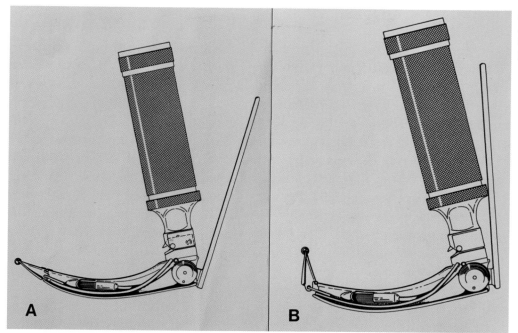

McCoy Laryngoscope. Courtesy of Eamon McCoy.

he was awarded the Alumnus Achievement Award by UCC.[1]

He has been involved in providing medical care in war zones throughout his career. He co-founded (with Mr John Beavis, an English orthopaedic surgeon), the medical aid charity International Disaster and Emergency Aid with Long Term Support (IDEALS.org.uk) while they were working in the State Hospital, Sarajevo when that city was under siege during the Bosnian civil war (1993–5). He continued his links with Sarajevo and Mostar after the war had ended (1995–2003). Since then he and other members of IDEALS have provided medical care and training as well as material aid to the Federally Administered Tribal Areas in Pakistan (2003–7) and to Tengalle, Sri Lanka after the Asian tsunami (2005–8). Since 2009, he has continued his medical aid interest by working in Al Shifa Hospital, Gaza city, in the Gaza strip.

His areas of clinical interest are emergency and trauma anaesthesia, difficult airways management, error analysis, clinical research and audit. He is an examiner in the Membership examination of the College of Anaesthesiologists of Ireland and is a reviewer for the *European Journal of Anaesthesiology*.

The McCoy Laryngoscope

As a registrar in Belfast during his training years, McCoy invented the 'McCoy Laryngoscope'.[2] He designed it to help in the management of both normal as well as difficult airways and it overcame some of the problems associated with endotracheal intubation. The development and research into the design was carried out over three years before it was marketed by the equipment manufacturers Penlon in 1993. At the time, it was a huge success both commercially and medically and resulted in a large number of reports on its use in difficult airways. The first paper on the McCoy laryngoscope[2] was described by the editor of the journal *Anaesthesia* as one of the ten most significant anaesthetic papers published in the previous 19 years.[3] It was widely recommended by various specialist difficult airway societies throughout the world. Even though it may have been superseded in more recent years by fibreoptic intubation devices, the McCoy is easy to use even for inexperienced operators and is relatively inexpensive. It was chosen in 2000 as a Millennium Product in the UK at a time when over 100,000 McCoy laryngoscopes had been sold in over 60 countries worldwide.[1]

Éamon is married to Angela, a practitioner, and they have three children, Claire, a midwife in the Royal Victoria Hospital, Mark, a chemical engineer, and Ciara, a geographer. His other interests include boating, cycling, travel and photography.

JT

References

1 Curriculum vitae and description of the McCoy laryngoscope provided by Dr McCoy.
2 McCoy É.P. and Mirakhur R.K., 'The Levering Laryngoscope', *Anaesthesia*, 1993, 48, pp. 516–19.
3 Morgan M., 'Retrospective Soliloque', *Anaesthesia*, 1998, 53, pp. 935–6.

Appendices

Appendix 1
Foundation Fellows of the Faculty of Anaesthetists, RCSI 1960.
S.N. Basu (South Africa)
Kathleen Bayne
William Bingham (Lurgan)
James Daniel Bourke (Cork, in absentia)
John Boyd (Belfast)
George J.C. Brittan (Wigan)
Arthur Barclay Bull (South Africa, in absentia)
Francis Mc Dermott Byrn (in absentia)
Daniel Gerard Coleman (Cork)
W. Davis (Omagh)
Raymond Davys (Dublin, Board member)
Patrick Drury-Byrne (Dublin, Board member)
John W. Dundee (Belfast, Board member)
Thomas J. Gilmartin (Dublin, Board member)
Kevin B. Glynn
Thomas Francis Heavey (Bath)
John C. Hewitt (Coleraine)
Anthony Halton Kasasian (South Africa, in absentia)
Sheila Kenny (Dublin, Board member)
Ordino Victor Steyn Kok (South Africa, in absentia)
Zoltan Lett (in absentia)
Harold Love (Belfast, Board member)
M.M. Vida Lemon (Belfast)
Brendan Vincent Lyne (New Zealand, in absentia)
Paul Ronald Mesham (South Africa, in abstentia)
Maureen Murphy (Dublin, in absentia)
Paul F. Murray (Dublin, Board member)

John Alan MacAuley (Belfast)
Victor O. McCormick (Dublin, Board member)
Patrick Joseph Nagle (Dublin, Board member)
Mary J. Ahern O'Connor
Silver Deane Oliver (Dublin)
Lady F. Edna Read
David Lindsay Scott (Sweden, in absentia)
Richard H. Shaw (Dublin)
David Lindsay Scott (Sweden, in absentia)
Joseph A. Woodcock (Dublin, Board member)
W.A.Woods (Ards)

Appendix 2
Fellowship by Election (without examination) 1961
Henry Edmund Bell
Gerry W. Black
J.K. Black
Alexander Blayney
John Patrick Conroy
Cecil Francis Cunniffe
Brendan Joseph Daly
Ian Walton Davidson
Edmund J. Delaney
Deirdre Donovan
Patrick Anthony Foster
J. Des Gaffney
W.R. Gilmore
Arthur John Lawrence Haley
Samuel Hoffman
Nasi Jafrey
W.R. Lambey
P.V. Long
Joseph George Lomaz
J.M. Lynham
Leo McArdle
Joseph McAuley
Patrick Fenton McGarry
Ian Donald Michie
William J.K. Morrow

Cecil Moss
Stephen Paul Murphy
Austin P. O'Connor
Kevin P. O'Sullivan
D. Power
A. Owen Flood
Joseph Ozinsky
F.W. Parke
Subramaniam Ponnambalam
Yee Kit Poon
Mukteshwar Prosad
John Rothwell Radcliffe
Hugh Raftery
Oscar Schmahmann
Doris Euphemia Verlet
R.D. Walsh
K. Hilde Wayburne
Frank De Burgh Whyte
Douglas Spencer Wilson

Fellowship by Election (without examination) 1962
M.W. Abrams (Johannesburg)
Fiona Mary Acheson (Dublin)
John Pentland Alexander (Belfast)
Charles Arthur Gibbons Armstrong (Magherafelt)
Miriam Brereton Barlow (Johannesburg)
Hyman Bentel (Johannesburg)
Mary Maud Bergin (Crowthorne)
James Thomas Bolger (Galway)
Thomas Albert Brown (Belfast)
Una B. Byrne (Enniskillen)
Peter Anthony Caswell (Johannesburg)
Anthony Joseph Crehan (Limerick)
Jay Fleming (Dublin)
John G. Goodbody (Dublin)
Robert C. Gray (Belfast)
J. Greenan (Wyhtenshawe)
William M. Jones (Glasgow)
W.P. Lee (Tralee)

Leslie Cecil Luck (British Guiana)
S.G. de Clive-Lowe (Blackheath)
John R. McCarthy (Dublin)
John R. McCormack (Limerick)
James Valentine McDermott (Limerick)
Michael Francis McGrath (Dublin)
James Alexander McNeilly (Belmont)
Dermot Leo McQuillan (Cottingham)
Nathaniel James Michlen (Salisbury)
Margaret N. Mills (Dublin)
Edward Morrison (Hendon)
Michael Nash (Dublin)
James North (Shalford)
Sister M. Bridget O'Leary (Drogheda)
Eugene Francis O'Riordan (Massachusetts)
J.S. Ruddel (Alberta)
John Tait S. Russell (Port Elizabeth)
J. Declan Ryan (Wigan)
W.H. Scriven (Farnham)
Mary Solan (Cork)
Peter Kenneth Storah (Northern Rhodesia)
George Tay (Singapore)
Richard Thomas (North Merthyr Tydfi)
James Tyrrell (Wakefield)
Charles Herbert Wilson (Dublin)

Appendix 3
Honorary Fellowship, Faculty of Anaesthetists, RCSI
1960 Dr John Gillies, Dr Geoffrey Organe
1961 Sir Ivan Magill
1962 Dr Ritzema Van Eck, Prof. William Woolf Mushin, Prof. Cecil Gray
1964 Prof. Robert Reynolds Macintosh, Prof. Henry Beecher
1968 Dr Robert Patrick Webb Shackleton, Prof. Eric Neilsen
1970 Dr Robert Dunning Dripps, Dr Ronald Jarman, Maj. General Keith
        Stephens OBE
1971 Dr William Derek Wylie
1972 Dr Harry Seldon, Dr Kevin McCaul
1973 Dr J. Alfred Lee, Dr Bjorn Ibsen
1974 Prof. Alexander Forrester, Prof. Jacques Boureau

1975 Dr John Joseph Downes, Prof. Emanuel M. Papper
1977 Dr Cyril Frederick Scurr, Prof. Jean Lassner
1978 Prof. Marion Thomas Jenkins
1979 Dr Francis F. Foldes
1980 Prof. Gordon Robson, Dr Thomas Joseph Walsh
1982 Prof. Tess Rita O'Rourke Brophy (*née* Cramond)
1984 Prof. Guy Vourc'h, Dr Gordon Jackson Rees
1985 Dr John Francis Nunn
1987 Dr Edmond 'Ted' I. Eger
1988 Dr Ephraim S. Siker
1989 Dr Richard J. Kitz
1990 Prof. Michael Rosen
1991 Dr Alan Sessler
1993 Dr Ronald Miller
1995 Prof. David Morrell
1996 Prof. John William Hall
1997 Prof. Cedric Prys-Roberts, Dr William MacRae
1998 Dr Mary McAleese, first Fellow of the College of Anaesthetists of Ireland

Appendix 4
Gilmartin Lecturers
1985 Prof, John Wharry Dundee, 'From small beginnings'
1986 Sir Gordon Robson
1987 Dr Edmond Eger II, 'What is the inhaled anaesthetic of the future?'
1988 Dr Ephraim S. Siker, 'A measure of vigilance'
1989 Prof. Richard Kitz, 'Muscle relaxants and anti-cholinesterase agents'
1990 Prof Anthony Clare, 'Medical aspects of alcoholism'
1991 Peter D. Sutherland S.C., 'Europe 1992'
1992 Dr Maurice Hayes, 'Subsidiarity breeds consent'
1993 Mr John Gilmartin, 'Works of art of medical interest'
1994 Dr John Nunn, 'Egyptian medicine'
1995 Prof. Seamus Heaney, 'The operation of poetry'
1996 Prof. Mary McAleese, 'Learning to unlearn'
1997 Dr Art Cosgrove, 'The Universities Bill 1996'
1998 Ms Pauline Marrinan Quinn, 'What is an ombudsman?'

Select Bibliography

Boulton T.B. *The Association of Anaesthetists of Great Britain & Ireland 1932–1992 and the Development of the Specialty of Anaesthesia*, London: Association of Anaesthetists of Great Britain and Ireland, 1999.

Buxton D.W. *Anæsthetics: Their Uses and Administration*, London: Lewis, 1888.

Cameron C.A. *History of the Royal College of Surgeons in Ireland*, 2nd Edition, Dublin: Fannin, 1916.

Casey C. *The Eighteenth-Century Dublin Town House*, Dublin: Four Courts Press, 2010.

Casey P.J., Cullen K.T. and Duignan J.P. *Irish Doctors in the First World War*, Dublin: Merrion Press, 2015.

Clarke R.S.J. *A Directory of Ulster Doctors (who qualified before 1901)*, Belfast: Ulster Historical Foundation, 2013.

Clarke R.S.J. *The Royal Victoria Hospital Belfast: A History 1797–1997*, Belfast: Blackstaff, 1997.

Duncum B.M. *The Development of Inhalation Anaesthesia*, London: Oxford University Press, 1947.

Foy G. *Anæsthetics, Ancient and Modern*, London: Baillière, Tindall and Cox, 1889.

Hewitt F.W. *Anæsthetics and Their Administration*, London: Charles Griffin, 1893.

Kelly L. *Irish Women in Medicine, c. 1880s–1920s*, Manchester and New York: Manchester University Press, 2012.

Love H. *The Royal Belfast Hospital for Sick Children – A History, 1948–1998*, Belfast: Blackstaff, 1998.

Lyman H.M. *Artificial Anæsthesia and Anæsthetics*, New York: Wood, 1881.

Mitchell D. *A 'Peculiar' Place: The Adelaide Hospital, Dublin 1839–1989*, Dublin: Blackwater Press, 1989.

Nolan E. *Caring for the Nation: A History of the Mater Misericordiae University Hospital*, Dublin: Gill and MacMillan, 2013.

O'Donnell B. *Irish Surgery and Surgeons in the Twentieth Century*, Dublin: Gill & MacMillan, 2008.

Snow J. *On Chloroform and Other Anæsthetics: Their Action and Administration*, London: Churchill, 1858.

Stratmann L. *Chloroform, the Quest for Oblivion*, Stroud: Sutton, 2003.

Wren M.-A. *Unhealthy State: Anatomy of a Sick Society*, Dublin: New Island, 2003.

Index

Note: References in captions or illustrations are indicated by page numbers in bold.

411